PARADIGMS OF PERSONALITY ASSESSMENT

PARADIGMS OF PERSONALITY ASSESSMENT

JERRY S. WIGGINS

In collaboration with

Rebecca S. Behrends, Yossef S. Ben-Porath, Sidney J. Blatt,
Paul T. Costa, Jr., Michael B. Gurtman, Dan P. McAdams,
Ralph L. Piedmont, Aaron L. Pincus,

and

Krista K. Trobst

THE GUILFORD PRESS
New York   London

© 2003 The Guilford Press
A Division of Guilford Publications, Inc.
72 Spring Street, New York, NY 10012
www.guilford.com

Printed in the United States of America

This book is printed on acid-free paper.

Last digit is print number: 9 8 7 6 5 4 3 2 1

Library of Congress Cataloging-in-Publication Data

Wiggins, Jerry S.
  Paradigms of personality assessment / by Jerry S. Wiggins.
    p. cm.
Includes bibliographical references and index.
  ISBN 1-57230-913-X
  1. Personality assessment. I. Title.
  BF698.4.W525 2003
  155.2′8—dc21

                                        2003005958

About the Author

Jerry S. Wiggins, PhD, has been contributing to the scientific literature in personality assessment for over 45 years; his approximately 100 publications include six books. He has held faculty positions at Rochester University (1956–1957), Stanford University (1957–1962), the University of Illinois (1962–1973), and the University of British Columbia (1973–1996), where he is Emeritus Professor. Since 1999, he has been an adjunct professor at York University.

While at the University of Illinois, Dr. Wiggins completed the undergraduate textbook *The Psychology of Personality* (1971), and its sequel *Principles of Personality* (1976), with three of his colleagues. In 1973 he published the now-classic volume *Personality and Prediction: Principles of Personality Assessment*, which was characterized by Goldberg (1974) in his seminal overview for the *Annual Review of Psychology* as "the most important single volume written about assessment." Despite the 30 years that have passed since its original publication, this characterization still remains apt.

Dr. Wiggins is also well known for his construction of the original content scales for the MMPI and for his contributions to the development and validation of interpersonal circumplex models of personality. He is the author of the Interpersonal Adjective Scales (including the revised, Big Five version), coauthor of the Inventory for Interpersonal Problems—Circumplex, and editor of the widely regarded volume *The Five-Factor Model of Personality: Theoretical Perspectives* (1996). In addition, he has been a prolific reviewer of empirical articles, serving as a member of the editorial board for nine psychology journals and as an ad hoc reviewer for over 30 psychology journals. In 2002, Jerry S. Wiggins was honored by the Society for Personality Assessment with the Bruno Klopfer Award, which is given each year to someone who has made an outstanding, long-term contribution to the field of personality assessment.

Contributing Authors

Rebecca S. Behrends, PhD, is Assistant Clinical Professor of Psychology in the Department of Psychiatry at Yale University.

Yossef S. Ben-Porath, PhD, is Professor of Psychology at Kent State University. He has published extensively on the MMPI-2 in particular and personality assessment more generally and is a frequent presenter on using the MMPI-2 in continuing education workshops. Dr. Ben-Porath also serves as a consultant to the University of Minnesota Press. He is a codeveloper of many of the MMPI-2's more recently developed scales and a coauthor of the test's manual.

Sidney J. Blatt, PhD, is Professor of Psychiatry and Psychology at Yale University and Chief of the Psychology Section in the Department of Psychiatry at the Yale University School of Medicine. He is also coauthor of the volume *The Interpretation of Psychological Tests* (with Joel Allison and Carl Zimet; 1988).

Paul T. Costa, Jr., PhD, is Chief of the Laboratory of Personality and Cognition, Intramural Research Program, at the National Institute on Aging in Baltimore. With long-term collaborator Robert R. McCrae, he is the coauthor of the NEO Personality Inventory— Revised (NEO PI-R) and a book, *Personality in Adulthood* (2nd ed., 2002; Guilford Press).

Michael B. Gurtman, PhD, is Professor of Psychology at the University of Wisconsin–Parkside. His recent research has focused on applications and development of the interpersonal circumplex model of personality. Dr. Gurtman is also a founding member of the Society for Interpersonal Theory and Research.

Dan P. McAdams, PhD, is Professor of Human Development and Social Policy and Professor of Psychology at Northwestern University. He is also the Director of Northwestern's Foley Center for the Study of Lives, a research center dedicated to the study of personality and social development in the adult years. Dr. McAdams has championed the use of narrative methods and concepts in the study of adult personality development. His research and writing have focused on the topics of life stories and narrative identity in adulthood, generativity, and intimacy motivation. He the author of *The Person: An Integrated Introduction to Personality Psychology* (2000).

Ralph L. Piedmont, PhD, is Associate Professor in the Department of Pastoral Counseling at Loyola College in Columbia, Maryland. He is also the Director of the Institute for Religious and Psychological Research. Dr. Piedmont is author of *The Revised NEO Personality Inventory: Clinical and Research Applications* (1998).

Aaron L. Pincus, PhD, is Associate Professor of Psychology at The Pennsylvania State University. His work focuses on interpersonal theory and assessment, conceptualization and assessment of personality disorders, and the interface of personality and clinical psychology. Dr. Pincus is also a licensed psychologist and regularly supervises a clinical training practicum on contemporary psychotherapy for personality disorders. He is a founding member and past president of the Society for Interpersonal Theory and Research.

Krista K. Trobst, PhD, is Assistant Professor of Psychology at York University in Toronto. She received her doctorate in Clinical Psychology from the University of British Columbia in 1997 after completing an internship at the Yale University School of Medicine. She completed 2 years of postdoctoral training in Paul T. Costa, Jr.'s, Laboratory of Personality and Cognition at the National Institute on Aging, National Institutes of Health, from 1997 to 1999. Dr. Trobst's research focuses primarily on the application of the interpersonal circumplex model and five-factor model in clinical and social psychology, including the development and application of an interpersonal circumplex measure of social support transactions. She is a founding member and president-elect of the Society for Interpersonal Theory and Research.

Acknowledgments

This book was written with more than a "little help from my friends." The individuals listed as "Contributing Authors" were directly involved in the case study (Part II) as representatives of their respective paradigms. Many of them also reviewed earlier drafts of my chapters in Part I that cover their particular paradigms. For critical reviews of material related to their own paradigms, I am also grateful to Lewis R. Goldberg, John A. Johnson, Robert R. McCrae, David S. Nichols, and William McKinley Runyan. When Thomas A. Widiger heard of this project, he kindly volunteered to provide critical feedback and suggestions on drafts of the entire book! Although I would never have dared ask him to take on such a time-consuming task, he is the person I would have selected to do this, if given a free choice. I would also like to thank Dan Ozer and Howard Tennen for their critical comments on the manuscript.

Krista K. Trobst is my principal collaborator, wife, and best friend. To say that this book could not have been written without her help would seriously understate her contribution. Among many other things, she took on the unenviable task of teaching an aging dog the most recent tricks of word processing. She also provided help, support, and advice at every stage of this project.

Contents

PART II. A Collaborative Case Study

No matter how helpful a clinical tool it may be, a psychological test cannot do its own thinking. What it accomplishes depends upon the thinking that guides its application. This guiding thought is psychological theory, whether explicit and systematized or implicit and unsystematized.

—SCHAFER (1954, p. xi)

Introduction

PERSONALITY, MEASUREMENT, AND ASSESSMENT

This book is concerned with the history and development of five major traditions in personality assessment, which, for reasons that will become clear, may be regarded as "paradigms" within that field. Each of these paradigms has provided different answers to the fundamental questions of "What is personality?," "How should we measure it?," and "What should we measure?" In Table Int.1, developments over time are read within rows (and across columns), and alternative interpretations (not necessarily during the same time period) are read within the columns (and down the rows). The five great theorists who interpreted the concept of "personality" in different ways were Sigmund Freud, Harry Stack Sullivan, Henry A. Murray, Sir Francis Galton, and Emil Kraepelin.

Freud believed that human transactions are not as they appear on the surface, and that the wellsprings of human behavior are to be found in socially unacceptable unconscious drives; these drives express themselves in disguised form in such phenomena as slips of the tongue, dream symbols, and psychiatric symptoms. Sullivan could not conceive of personality as apart or separate from interpersonal relationships, and he defined personality in terms of recurrent patterns within such relationships. Murray maintained that the history of the personality *is* the personality. Galton believed that character has a corporeal basis, which can be inferred from an individual's actions, in much the same way that we infer intelligence from intelligent actions. And Kraepelin believed that disturbances in personality have an organic basis, and that they are best understood with reference to clusters of symptoms (as is done with physical symptoms in medicine).

1

Conceptions of personality are of little scientific value unless they can be operationalized and translated into concrete measurement procedures. The methodologists listed within the "Measurement" column of Table Int.1 were pioneers of personality measurement who developed psychological testing procedures to operationalize the concepts of their intellectual forebears. David Rapaport used projective and cognitive tests to measure the psychodynamic concepts of Freud. Timothy Leary devised concrete measurement procedures to operationalize Sullivan's concepts. David C. McClelland developed a variety of procedures to measure the personological concepts of Murray in the study of lives. Raymond B. Cattell, following Galton and others, applied the statistical methods of intelligence testing to the personality sphere and operationalized both phenotypic (language) and genotypic (traits) aspects of personality. And Starke R. Hathaway operationalized his measures of psychopathology by contrasting responses of psychiatric patients in different Kraepelinian categories with the responses of normal individuals.

Personality assessment involves the gathering and evaluation of various sources of information about individuals (e.g., psychological tests, interviews, biographical material) to serve various purposes (e.g., selection, placement, diagnosis, case formulation). In the present context, "assessment" may be thought of as the application of measurement procedures (that were developed to operationalize personality concepts) to newer and broader domains. The persons listed in the final column of Table Int.1 are contemporary personality assessment psychologists who have extended the lines of inquiry of their respective paradigms. The work of these individuals, and many others, is the subject matter of this book. For that reason, many of the following comments may not be meaningful to some readers and should be regarded as a preview rather than as an exposition.

Sidney J. Blatt has extended and refined the Freud–Rapaport psychodynamic paradigm to include more recent concepts of development, attachment, and object relations. Donald J. Kiesler has consolidated work within the Sullivan–Leary paradigm by demonstrating the heuristic potential of the interpersonal paradigm for integrating highly diverse conceptual and applied areas of research. Dan P. McAdams has reformulated the personological traditions of Murray and McClelland to include the formulations of Erik Erikson and to place the personological paradigm at the center of the recently revived interest in narrative life history. Following the language path of Cattell's contributions, Lewis R. Goldberg has developed a rigorous taxonomy of trait-descriptive terms that provides a psycholinguistic foundation for contemporary studies of personality dimensions. Paul T. Costa, Jr., and Robert R. McCrae have consolidated the 65-year-old tradition of dimensional measurement begun by Cattell into a program of research that has revitalized work within this paradigm. And Paul E. Meehl expanded

TABLE Int.1. Personality, Measurement, and Assessment Components of the Five Paradigms

Paradigm	Personality (What is it?)	Measurement (How should we measure it?)	Assessment (What should we measure?)
Psychodynamic	*Sigmund Freud* Unconscious sexual and aggressive drives express themselves in disguised form in psychiatric symptoms.	*David Rapaport* Used a battery of cognitive and projective tests to measure the psychodynamic concepts of Freud.	*Sidney J. Blatt* Expanded and refined the paradigm to include more recent concepts of development, attachment, and object relations.
Interpersonal	*Harry Stack Sullivan* Personality is a person's recurrent patterns of interpersonal relationships.	*Timothy Leary* Developed a battery of interpersonal personality tests to operationalize the concepts of Sullivan.	*Donald J. Kiesler* Demonstrated potential of the paradigm for integrating diverse conceptual and applied areas of research.
Personological	*Henry A. Murray* The history of the personality *is* the personality.	*David C. McClelland* Developed a variety of procedures to measure the personological concepts of Murray in the study of lives.	*Dan P. McAdams* Reformulated the paradigm to include formulations of Erikson and to place it at the center of recently revived interest in narrative life history.
Multivariate	*Sir Francis Galton* Like intelligence, character has a corporeal basis that can be inferred from actions.	*Raymond B. Cattell* Applied the statistical methods of intelligence testing to the measurement of personality in both its (1) phenotypic (language) and (2) genotypic (traits) aspects	*Lewis R. Goldberg* Developed a rigorous taxonomy of personality *language.* *Paul T. Costa, Jr., and Robert R. McCrae* Developed an inventory of personality *traits* that revitalized the paradigm.
Empirical	*Emil Kraepelin* As in medicine, personality disturbance has an organic basis inferred from clusters of symptoms.	*Starke R. Hathaway* Contrasted the item responses of patients in different Kraepelinian categories with responses of a normal control group to develop an empirical measure of psychopathology.	*Paul E. Meehl* Expanded the scope and rationale of Hathaway's measurement procedures, and thereby influenced the theory and practice of clinical psychology.

Note. Movement within rows (across columns) indicates temporal sequence, showing evolution over time. Movement within columns (across rows) indicates alternative interpretations made.

the scope and rationale of Hathaway's measurement procedures in ways that have profoundly influenced the theory and practice of contemporary clinical psychology.

PARADIGMS IN THE NATURAL AND SOCIAL SCIENCES

> How does one elect and how is one elected to membership in a particular community, scientific or not? What is the process and what are the stages of socialization to the group? What does the group collectively see as its goals; what deviations, individual or collective, will it tolerate; and how does it control the impermissible aberration?
> —KUHN (1996, p. 209)

By "paradigm," I mean the background of a set of generally accepted beliefs or orienting attitudes within and against which personality tests are constructed, administered, and interpreted. I also wish to make it clear from the outset that there are major differences between paradigms in the social and behavioral sciences and paradigms in the natural sciences, which Kuhn (1996) has described in his classic book *The Structure of Scientific Revolutions* and in subsequent essays (Kuhn, 2000). In fact, the differences between the social and natural sciences that Kuhn (1996) observed during his tenure at the Center for Advanced Studies in the Behavioral Sciences were what first led him to recognize the unique role that paradigms play in the natural sciences (pp. ix–x). Nevertheless, I believe that some of Kuhn's ideas about scientific *communities* may be applied fruitfully to paradigms of personality assessment.

The history of natural science was once viewed as an unbroken accretion of knowledge, in which finished scientific achievements built cumulatively upon one another and eventuated in the scientific achievements of today. In contrast to this view, Kuhn characterized the historical development of science as involving extended periods of "normal science," during which concerted efforts are made to force nature into the prevailing conceptual orientation ("paradigm") by investigating "puzzles" created by the paradigm according to the methods and standards for evaluating solutions provided by the paradigm. When this puzzle solving ceases to be successful or when it yields results that are inconsistent with the paradigm, a "scientific revolution" may occur. The distinction between the new and old paradigms may represent "incommensurable ways of seeing the world and of practicing science in it" (Kuhn, 1996, p. 4). Once a revolutionary "paradigm shift" has occurred, there is no going back to the older, incommensurable world view; the notion of "progress" as a cumulative series of advancements leading toward eventual enlightenment no longer makes sense.

SCIENCE AND PERSONALITY ASSESSMENT: LIMITATIONS OF THE ANALOGY

> It remains an open question what parts of social science have yet acquired such paradigms at all. History suggests that the road to a firm research consensus is extraordinarily arduous.
> —KUHN (1996, p. 15)

It must be recognized at the outset that descriptions of the paradigms of personality assessment must differ in several major, if not crucial, ways from the descriptions of the paradigms of physical science provided by Kuhn: (1) the reasons for membership within communities of like-minded practitioners within the two fields, (2) the degree of fit between theory and data that obtains within the two fields, and (3) the decided lack of consensus among assessment psychologists on the nature of "normal science."

With respect to the first of these aspects, Kuhn (1996) observed that in the natural sciences, "it is sometimes just its reception of a paradigm that transforms a group previously interested merely in the study of nature into a profession or, at least, a discipline" (p. 19). In this context, Kuhn specifically excluded medicine, technology, and law from that generalization because for those fields, "the principal *raison d'être* is an external social need" (p. 19). By similar reasoning, many paradigms of personality assessment might also be excluded from this generalization. For example, from his historical survey of objective assessment instruments, Goldberg (1971) concluded that "new personality scales and inventories are at least as likely to be focused upon constructs arising out of *societal pressures* as upon theories of personality" (p. 335; emphasis added).

Although a paradigm "forces scientists to investigate [a very small] part of nature in a detail and depth that would otherwise be unimaginable" (Kuhn, 1996, p. 24), it also "leads to a detail of information and to a precision of the observation–theory match that could be achieved in no other way" (p. 65). In fact, the fit between observation and theory in contemporary natural sciences may often be so close, and so routine, that departures may go unnoticed. But when noticed, such departures may lay the grounds for an eventual paradigm shift. In contrast, within personality assessment the road to consensus on a common paradigm is made even more arduous by the comparative lack of precise fit between theory and data. In my view, it is highly unlikely that there will ever be a common paradigm for personality assessment that is acceptable to members of the five paradigms I have distinguished. What may happen—and in fact has already happened to some extent—is a greater agreement on the *kinds* of constructs to be measured (e.g., "attachment"), as well as a recognition of the value of *multimethod assessment*, which is provided by the application of more than one paradigm to a given assessment problem.

THE DEVELOPMENT OF PERSONALITY
ASSESSMENT COMMUNITIES

Scientific knowledge, like language, is intrinsically the common property
of a group or else nothing at all. To understand it we shall need to
know the special characteristics of the group that create and use it.
—KUHN (1996, p. 210)

Quite independently of the ideas of revolution and scientific progress, the
notion of "paradigm"—or as Kuhn (1996) later preferred, "interdisciplinary matrix"—would seem to capture some of the group dynamics within
the various subdisciplines of personality assessment in useful ways. Kuhn
placed heavy emphasis on the need for a common set of received beliefs
about the nature of the world and the practice of science within it among
members of a given scientific community. Such unanimity of belief is ensured by the "educational initiation that prepares and licenses the student
for professional practice" (p. 5). The student is indoctrinated into a paradigm with reference to the earlier scientific accomplishments that have occurred within that paradigm, and is informed of the range of phenomena
that may be investigated within the purview of that paradigm. This intense
level of specialization, in turn, creates a community of scientists whose
journal articles are largely unintelligible to those who are not members of
their professional group.

Education in Personality Assessment

Psychology is currently among the most popular majors for students in col-
leges of arts, and many future professionals receive their first exposure to
the field through introductory textbooks in personality, clinical, and abnormal psychology. Such textbooks share, to a limited extent, characteristics of
science textbooks as described by Kuhn (1996, Ch. 11). That is, they are
"systematically misleading" with respect to the chaotic history of the field
and its major shifts of emphasis and false starts. Instead, textbooks often
present an orderly sequence of contributions extending from past to present, suggesting a long-standing tradition "often compared to the addition
of bricks to a building" (p. 140).

In general, a psychology student's orientation toward research and
practice will be influenced by the graduate school he or she attends and by
the particular advisor and/or clinical supervisor with whom he or she
works most closely. Thus, for example, one can identify combinations of
institution–advisor–orientation that have historically predisposed students
toward a particular paradigm:

1. Yale–Blatt–psychodynamic
2. Virginia Commonwealth–Kiesler–interpersonal

3. Harvard–Murray–personological
4. Illinois–Cattell–multivariate
5. Minnesota–Meehl–empirical

However, the foregoing generalizations are perhaps more accurately characterized as prototypes at best, or stereotypes at worst, because they are likely to apply to a relatively small proportion of the professional work force. A more substantial proportion of practitioners identify themselves as "eclectic"—reflecting the fact that most institutions, including those just mentioned, have faculty members who represent several orientations within personality assessment. From my reading of Kuhn, this combination of "eclecticism" in education and professional practice is almost inconceivable in contemporary physical science.

In approaching the task of individual assessment, a practitioner is typically committed to a set of received beliefs concerning human nature and its assessment that were acquired in the course of the practitioner's graduate education. These prior conceptual and methodological commitments determine the assessment procedures that the practitioner will employ, the conceptual significance assigned to them, the conclusions drawn from them, and the professional recommendations that the practitioner will make. A graduate student is prepared for membership in the particular assessment community in which he or she will later practice through the study of a particular paradigm of personality assessment. Such a paradigm may be thought of as a set of shared beliefs concerning human nature and its assessment held by a particular community of assessment psychologists and acquired through the attendance of specialized courses, practica, internships, and workshops, as well as through the reading of specialized textbooks, journals, and newsletters.

The Nature of Assessment Communities

The field of personality assessment may thus be thought of as consisting of several different communities of psychologists. In comparison with contemporary communities of natural scientists, these communities are in a "preparadigm" period of development in which there are many competing schools of thought, each of which questions the theories, methods, and standards of other schools. In the absence of a collective consensus on these matters, there does not appear to be anything comparable to the practice of the "normal science" that has characterized the daily activities of scientific communities during most periods of their historical development. Thus, despite evidence of advances within schools of personality assessment, there has been little that would be considered "progress" in the specific sense of an addition to the *collective* achievement of all communities (Kuhn, 1996). However, although the nature of assessment communities clearly differs from that of scientific communities, it should not be axiomatically assumed that it does so with reference to ultimate external standards of truth, progress, or maturity.

Accomplishments and Paradigms

Current practice and research within a paradigm of personality assessment are based on the accomplishments of an earlier worker or group of workers in the field. These accomplishments are acknowledged by a particular assessment community as providing the foundation for its current and future practice. The accomplishments are emphasized in the training of practitioners by reviewing the previously successful applications of the paradigm and by providing examples of the applicability of the paradigm to current concerns. As a consequence, practitioners whose work is based on a shared paradigm are committed to a common set of rules and standards for assessment practice. It is at this point, however, that our extension of Kuhn's formulations of paradigms in natural science to paradigms in personality assessment begins to break down.

As Kuhn (1996) observed, "Though many scientists talk easily and well about the particular individual hypotheses that underlie a concrete piece of research, they are little better than laymen at characterizing the established bases of their field, its legitimate problems and methods" (p. 47). It would appear that competent scientists are so well and, to an extent, so narrowly trained that they can go about their business in an extraordinarily effective manner without reflecting upon its "paradigmatic" or other abstract qualities. Kuhn also called attention to Polanyi's (1966) notion of "tacit knowledge," whereby successful scientists have mastered the essential, but not explicitly verbalized, tricks of their respective trades: "That scientists do not usually ask or debate what makes a particular problem or solution legitimate tempts us to suppose that, at least intuitively, they know the answer" (Kuhn, 1996, p. 46).

Perhaps because of the subject matter involved, practitioners of personality assessment appear to be more self-conscious about their activities than practicing physical scientists are. This may also reflect the fact that this youthful discipline has not yet developed a canonical paradigm comparable to what Kuhn has called "normal science." As a consequence, the task of describing the major shifts of emphasis within personality assessment is lightened by the availability of a number of soul-searching books and articles on the assumptions, achievements, and shortcomings of different paradigms within that field. Within the natural sciences, soul searching is notably absent, except during those infrequent historical periods when normal science goes awry, setting the stage for a scientific revolution.

PARADIGMS OF ASSESSMENT IN CLINICAL PRACTICE
Assessment Procedures

Clinical psychologists often employ a range of assessment instruments (singly or in combination) to address the range of diagnostic issues posed by their clients. These assessment techniques are generally well validated, at a level comparable to and at times even exceeding medical tests for physical disease and lesions (Meyer et al., 2001). When thought disorder is suspected, psychologists may administer a Rorschach. Some may routinely administer the Interpersonal Adjective Scales (IAS) to assess the character and quality of a client's interpersonal relationships. From most clients they will obtain a case history, and their clients may be asked to fill out the Revised NEO Personality Inventory (NEO PI-R) to clarify dimensions of normal personality functioning, or the Minnesota Multiphasic Personality Inventory—2 (MMPI-2) to assess psychological abnormality.

The majority of clinicians describe their theoretical orientation as "eclectic," and indeed that appears to be true. But they also may be operating, perhaps unknowingly, within larger historical contexts of assumptions and beliefs that may include traditions of thought as diverse as psychoanalysis, symbolic interactionism, psychobiography, psychometrics, and empirical realism (respectively, for the tests just mentioned). These contexts are referred to as "assessment paradigms," by which I mean the background of a set of unquestioned beliefs or orienting attitudes within and against which personality tests are administered and interpreted.

The paradigms to be considered in this book are referred to as "psychodynamic," "interpersonal," "personological," "multivariate," and "empirical." Such paradigms are related, but *not* equivalent, to certain theories of personality (Hall & Lindzey, 1978) or theories of psychopathology (Millon, 1969). Similarly, these paradigms are related, but *not* equivalent, to certain kinds of personality tests. Thus the MMPI and MMPI-2 have been associated with a distinctive philosophy of science (empirical realism), rather than with a particular theory of psychopathology. The Rorschach test and the Wechsler scales have figured prominently within the ego-psychological perspective of the psychodynamic paradigm, although both tests were originally constructed for quite different purposes.

Ranges and Foci of Convenience of Assessment Paradigms

Although some instruments have been described as omnibus measures of personality, this is at best an unwarranted generalization. Different assessment contexts require the assessment of different aspects of personality, often from quite different conceptual perspectives. In this sense, the five paradigms of personality assessment are not competing, but instead represent what Kelly (1955) has called different "ranges of convenience" and "foci of convenience." The "focus of convenience" of a paradigm is typically that aspect of personality with which the founders of the paradigm were initially most concerned. Thus Freud was most concerned with the vicissitudes of instinct, Sullivan with interpersonal relations, Murray with the complete life course, Cattell with the structure of traits, and Hathaway with psychiatric diagnosis. In general, although there are exceptions, assessment paradigms work best within their original foci of convenience. The foci of convenience of the five paradigms are summarized in Table Int.2.

The "range of convenience" of a paradigm describes the breadth or scope of personality attributes that may be usefully assessed within that paradigm. For example, as will become evident later, the psychodynamic paradigm appears to have a smaller range of application than originally claimed, and the empirical paradigm appears to have utility beyond the limited range of psychiatric diagnosis.

I believe that these paradigms reflect different and potentially useful ways of viewing the entire psychodiagnostic enterprise. I also believe that these paradigms have contributed to the building of more or less invisible barriers to communication among clinicians who work, knowingly or not, within them. This state of affairs is unfortunate, because "membership" in a paradigm is mainly determined by where one went to graduate school, with whom one studied, and the particular clinical setting in which one finds oneself operating. Furthermore, I am convinced that some remarkably similar ideas are presently being advocated about the nature of personality and its assessment among those working within several different para-

TABLE Int.2. Foci of Convenience of the Five Assessment Paradigms

Paradigm	Focus of convenience
Psychodynamic	The manner in which the individual deals with the competing demands of relatively unconscious sexual and aggressive drives and the prohibitions of society against their direct expression.
Interpersonal	The patterned regularities in the individual's relations with other persons (who may be real, personified, or imagined).
Personological	The psychological life history of the individual.
Multivariate	The individual's relative standing on dimensions of individual differences in personality traits that are moderately heritable, and that are relatively stable over the adult life span.
Empirical	The established empirical correlates of the individual's classification with respect to the traditional categories of psychiatric impairment.

digms, and that recognition of these commonalities might advance the field as a whole.

I would venture to suggest that most readers will be familiar with a few of these paradigms, but not with some of the others. For example, those intimately familiar with the psychodynamic paradigm are unlikely to be familiar with the multivariate and empirical paradigms, and vice versa. And even those who are fond of obtaining life history data from semi-structured interviews may not be fully aware of the rich history of the personological paradigm, or of the exciting recent developments that have occurred within that paradigm. And many may not be aware that the interpersonal paradigm has fostered a strong "underground movement" within clinical psychology for many decades.

PLAN OF THE BOOK
Personality Theory and Personality Assessment

An earlier volume of mine consistently advocated theory-based personality assessment, but was mainly concerned with the details of the assessment process itself (Wiggins, 1973b). The present text emphasizes both theory and assessment by placing assessment procedures within the different conceptual paradigms from which they arose. The order in which the paradigms are presented reflects both historical and conceptual trends in the relation between theory and assessment. The different paradigms have been ordered in terms of the years in which they were first articulated. They are also ordered in terms of the extent to which they are theory-driven, from the elaborate theoretical edifice of psychoanalysis to the ultraempiricism of the empirical paradigm.

Referring to the fifth paradigm as "empirical" is not meant to imply that the other paradigms lack adequate interest in empiricism or lack adequate empirical support. As will become apparent in the following chapters, the psychoanalytic, interpersonal, personological, and multivariate paradigms have a rich and compelling empirical foundation. The term "empirical," however, is often attached to the Kraepelinian paradigm because of its particular emphasis on the construction and validation of scales through empirically contrasted groups (see Chapter 5).

Overview of the Field of Personality Assessment

Table Int.3 is meant to provide an overview of the historical development of the five major personality assessment paradigms and to also provide a suggestion as to the structure of subsequent chapters in this book. The rows of the table are divided into decades. The columns list contributions within decades—giving the author or authors, the date, and either the title or the subject matter of each publication. For example, the first entry in Table Int.3 is Freud's 1908 paper on "Character and Anal Erotism," which is discussed in Chapter 1 on the psychodynamic paradigm. (All references cited may be found in the References list at the end of the book.)

This table represents my attempt to list the individuals who were among the most influential in consolidating a particular paradigm at a given period of time. It would be presumptuous to claim that these citations represent a "top three" list for each decade, and no such claim is made. Chapters 1–5 present the five paradigms listed in the columns of Table Int.3 and are contained within Part I of the book. The historical development of each paradigm is considered separately, and each chapter treats the conceptual framework, assessment instruments, interpretive principles, and the applications and current status of each paradigm.

Chapter 6 also appears within Part I and is concerned with recent conceptual and empirical convergences among the five paradigms that have occurred with reference to the "metaconcepts" of agency and communion. Part II of the book consists of Chapters 7–12 and presents the results of a collaborative case study that was conducted specifically for the present book; the same individual was assessed from the perspectives of five different paradigms by leading exponents of each paradigm.

The references cited in Table Int.3 are meant to be representative rather than definitive, although considerable thought has gone into their selection. The reader who is already familiar with a particular paradigm might constructively question the specific selections for a given decade and propose alternatives that capture this decade with greater fidelity. The novice for whom these selections are intended may find the selections helpful in "concretizing" what seem, to me at least, to be rather complicated sociocultural/historical developments over the decades.

E. G. Boring (1950a, 1950b), perhaps our foremost historian of psychology, was much concerned with the issue of whether "great men" (columns of Table Int.3) or the *Zeitgeist* (rows of Table Int.3) determined the history of experimental psychology. My emphasis in this book on the columns of Table Int.3 is pedagogical rather than "historical" in any deep sense. I am aware that study of the rows in Table Int.3 would facilitate the kind of historical perspective taking advocated by Kenneth Craik (1986), in whose classes at the University of California different graduate students were assigned the literature of different decades of personality research and then asked to share their impressions with one another. Although Table Int.3 was not constructed with this type of historical comparison in mind, I have personally found this procedure to be useful in arriving at a "big picture" of the various decades of personality assessment. But regardless of whether the reader attends to rows or columns, frequent reference to Table Int.3 while reading the chapters that follow may serve as a useful road map to what is admittedly a rather long and arduous journey.

TABLE Int.3. Milestones in the Historical Development of the Major Assessment Paradigms

Decades	Psychodynamic	Interpersonal	Personological	Multivariate	Empirical
Origins	Freud (1908) "Character and Anal Erotism" Abraham (1921) Oral and genital characters Rorschach (1921) Inkblot test	Breuer and Freud (1893–1895) "Studies on Hysteria" Meyer (1907) Schizophrenia White (1922) Outline of Psychiatry	Freud (1910) "Leonardo da Vinci . . ." Jones (1910) Hamlet and Oedipus Abraham (1911) "Giovanni Segantini"	Galton (1888) Measurement of "co-relations" Pearson (1896) Correlation coefficient Spearman (1904) Factor analysis of abilities	Woodworth (1917) First inventory: Personal Data Sheet Pressey (1921) "Cross-out" measure of emotional adjustment Strong (1927) Vocational Interest Blank (contrasted groups)
1930s	Reich (1933) Character Analysis Erikson (1937) Children's play Hartmann (1939) Ego psychology	Cooley (1930) Looking-glass self Mead (1934) Symbolic interactionism Sapir (1935) Importance of language	Dollard (1935) Criteria for the Life History Allport (1937) Personality Murray (1938) Explorations in Personality	Cattell (1933) Factor analysis of temperament Thurstone (1934) Factor analysis of trait ratings Guilford and Guilford (1936) Early "Big Four"	Landis and Katz (1934) Validity of neuroticism questionnaires Humm and Wadsworth (1935) Humm–Wadsworth Temperament Scale (contrasted groups) Landis et al. (1935) Empirical validity of adjustment inventories
1940s	Rapaport (1942) First manual of diagnostic testing Rapaport et al. (1946) The Menninger assessment Schafer (1948) The Clinical Application of Psychological Tests	Sullivan (1940) "Conceptions of Modern Psychiatry" Sullivan (1948a) Meaning of anxiety Sullivan (1949) Multidisciplinary approach	Allport et al. (1941) Lives within Nazi Germany Allport (1942) The Use of Personal Documents . . . OSS Assessment Staff (1948) Selection of intelligence agents	MacKinnon (1944) Classic literature review Eysenck (1947) Extraversion and Neuroticism Fiske (1949) Five factors in different rating sources	Hathaway and McKinley (1940) Construction of the MMPI Hathaway and McKinley (1943) MMPI manual Meehl (1945) "The Dynamics of 'Structured' Personality Tests" (continued)

TABLE Int.3. (*continued*)

Decades	Psychodynamic	Interpersonal	Personological	Multivariate	Empirical
1950s	Rapaport (1951) Psychoanalytic conceptual model Fairbairn (1952) Object relations theory Jacobson (1954) *The Self and the Object World*	Freedman et al. (1951) Interpersonal model Sullivan (1953b) *The Interpersonal Theory of Psychiatry* Leary (1957) *Interpersonal Diagnosis of Personality*	McClelland (1951) *Personality* Stern et al. (1956) *Methods in Personality Assessment* Erikson (1958) *Young Man Luther*	Eysenck (1953) Multivariate position statement Cattell (1957) Multivariate position statement Guilford (1959) *Personality*	Meehl (1954) *Clinical versus Statistical Prediction* Cronbach and Meehl (1955) "Construct Validity in Psychological Tests" Welsh and Dahlstrom (1956) *Basic Readings on the MMPI . . .*
1960s	Holt (1966) Aggression and the Rorschach Mayman (1967) Rorschach object representations Allison, Blatt, and Zimet (1968) Test interpretation	Schaefer (1961) Maternal and child behavior Lorr and McNair (1963) "An Interpersonal Behavior Circle" Carson (1969a) *Interaction Concepts of Personality*	Allport (1965) *Letters from Jenny* Murray (1967a) "The Case of Murr" Erikson (1969) *Gandhi's Truth*	Tupes and Christal (1961) Five-factor model (FFM) strongly replicates Norman (1963) "Toward an Adequate Taxonomy . . ." Borgatta (1964) Replication with different items	Dahlstrom and Welsh (1960) *An MMPI Handbook* Marks and Seeman (1963) *The Abnormal Actuarial Description of Personality* Wiggins (1966) Content scales for the MMPI
1970s	Bowlby (1973) *Attachment and Loss: Vol. 2. Separation* Blatt (1974) Object representation in depression Blatt et al. (1976) Concept of object on Rorschach	Benjamin (1974) "Structural Analysis of Social Behavior" Kiesler (1979) Relationship in psychotherapy Wiggins (1979) Interpersonal taxonomy	Block (1971) *Lives through Time* Levinson (1978) *The Seasons of a Man's Life* Tomkins (1979) "Script Theory"	Wiggins (1973b) First discussion of FFM in textbook Goldberg (1977) "Language and Personality" Digman (1979) "The Five Major Domains . . ."	Butcher (1972) *Objective Personality Assessment* Hathaway (1972) "Where Have We Gone Wrong?" Dahlstrom et al. (1972, 1975) *An MMPI Handbook* (rev. ed., 2 vols.)

1980s	Blatt and Lerner (1983a) Object representation Greenberg and Mitchell (1983) *Object Relations in Psychoanalytic Theory* Main et al. (1985) Security and representation	Anchin and Kiesler (1982) *Handbook of Interpersonal Psychotherapy* Kiesler 1983) "The 1982 Interpersonal Circle" Horowitz et al. (1988) Inventory of Interpersonal Problems	Runyan (1982) *Life Histories and Psychobiography* Runyan (1988a) *Psychology and Historical Interpretation* McAdams and Ochberg (1988) *Psychobiography and Life Narratives*	Goldberg (1981) "Language and Individual Differences" Costa and McCrae (1985) NEO Personality Inventory Hogan (1986) Hogan Personality Inventory	Dahlstrom and Dahlstrom (1980) *New Basic Readings on the MMPI* Morey et al. (1985) MMPI personality disorder scales Butcher et al. (1989) MMPI-2 manual
1990s	Westen (1991) Object relations and TAT Blatt and Zuroff (1992) Prototypes for depression Blatt and Blass (1996) "Relatedness and Self-Definition"	Wiggins (1995) Interpersonal Adjective Scales Kiesler 1996) Interpersonal textbook Plutchik and Conte (1997) *Circumplex Models . . .*	Alexander (1990) *Personology* McAdams (1993) *The Stories We Live By* Elms (1994) *Uncovering Lives*	McCrae and Costa (1990) *Personality in Adulthood* Costa and Widiger (1994) Personality disorders and the FFM Wiggins (1996a) Theoretical perspectives on the FFM	Butcher et al. (1990) MMPI-2 content scales Ben-Porath et al. (1991) MMPI-2 content scales in diagnosis Butcher et al. (1992) MMPI-A manual

WHAT THIS BOOK IS *NOT* ABOUT

The principal reason for writing this book was to introduce the reader to
the notion of paradigms of personality assessment, which in my view provides a useful way of viewing the several (often conflicting) programs of
personality assessment that have been proposed over the last 50 years. It is
my hope that those already committed to a paradigm may come to understand their own paradigm better when contrasting it with alternative paradigms. I also hope that those who may be "shopping" for a paradigm may
gain a clearer idea of the market.

This book is *not* meant to be a compendium of personality tests; excellent compendia are available elsewhere (e.g., Aiken, 1997). Instead, I have
tried to illustrate each paradigm with one or two "paradigmatic" tests for
that paradigm. The absence of detailed treatment of a particular test is *not*
meant as a negative judgment on the merits of that test. This book is also
not meant to be a survey of the art and science of personality assessment;
many materials are available for this purpose, ranging from out-of-date
"classics" (e.g., Wiggins, 1973b) to up-to-date gems (e.g., Lanyon &
Goodstein, 1997).

PERSONAL RECOLLECTIONS OF PARADIGMS

Disclaimer

As Part I will make clear, I have been influenced in different ways by each
of the five major paradigms of personality assessment and by prominent
members within those paradigms. Because I am more than a little self-conscious about writing an autobiographical section, I would like to make it
clear that at least part of my reason for doing so was a suggestion from my
good friend and frequent advisor William McKinley Runyan, one of the
leading exponents of the personological paradigm. Runyan has convinced
me that potential readers, particularly graduate students, may have some
interest in my particular life story as it relates to the subject matter of this
book. Partial confirmation of Runyan's position was obtained earlier when
I presented some of this material to graduate students at the 1997 Summer
School for Personality Assessment held in Vienna; many of the students
there were kind enough to say that they found this material interesting. But
then, what else could they have said?

Assessment in General

I have had an enduring interest in the so-called "milestone assessment studies" for many years, since Lew Goldberg introduced me to the Kelly and
Fiske (1951) study on the selection of graduate students in clinical psychol-

ogy. In my book *Personality and Prediction* (Wiggins, 1973b), I featured these studies and gave heavy emphasis to the conceptualizations of Stern, Stein, and Bloom (1956), who unfortunately are still underappreciated. Again, with a little help from Goldberg, I was appointed as a selection officer for the Peace Corps in its early and exciting days, and was able to obtain invaluable hands-on experience on that project, some of which is also described in *Personality and Prediction*. And I, like so many other assessment psychologists, eventually had the honor of participating as an assessor in one of the projects conducted by the Institute of Personality Assessment and Research (IPAR) at the University of California–Berkeley, when IPAR was still housed in its historic fraternity house. I greatly enjoyed this and other "applied" work, and consider myself fortunate to have had these experiences.

Psychodynamic Paradigm

I read Freud in high school, probably because of his emphasis on sex. This particular reading habit was actively discouraged by my father, who provided me with a copy of Overstreet's (1949) *The Mature Mind*—a highly puritanical treatment of matters sexual (as an antidote to my salacious reading preferences). Under the influence of my older sister, my parents recanted when I became a student at American University in Washington, D.C.; they gave me the five-volume *Collected Papers* of Freud as a birthday gift, which was greatly appreciated and is still in use.

I had somewhat of a "peak experience" in a course in English literature during my freshman year when I elected to write a term paper on "Hamlet and Oedipus," which I now know is part of the personological paradigm. The peak experience occurred during a Christmas break when I was able to spend many wonderfully long days at the fabulous Library of Congress researching this topic. Despite my relative youth and inexperience, I felt I belonged there, and the librarians made me feel that way. My English professor was also extremely kind and encouraging about the term paper itself. A few years later, when Lawrence Olivier's film version of *Hamlet* appeared, I was able to impress the young lady who accompanied me to the film by my in-depth knowledge of its "Oedipal implications." By that time I had adopted the affectation of smoking a pipe, often referred to James Agee's articles on film (which were then appearing in *Partisan Review*), and generally behaved as an obnoxious teenage "intellectual."

My interest in Freud and in psychoanalysis continued even during my graduate training, which was conducted in a rigorously behavioristic setting. It was, and to some extent still is, a "hobby" of mine. As a young faculty member in clinical psychology at Stanford, I realized that quite distinguished personages, such as Robert Sears, Ernest Hilgard, and Lee Winder, took the psychodynamic point of view seriously. In fact, Lee was able to secure training funds (from the National Institute of Mental Health) for providing analytic consultation to both faculty and graduate students in the clinical program from a number of distinguished analysts in the Bay Area. Undergoing personal analysis was also an option, and because of this, I was able to undergo a brief psychoanalysis with a highly competent ego psychologist.

In the course of team-teaching the introductory personality course at the University of Illinois with three of my young colleagues there, we decided to write a textbook (Wiggins, Renner, Clore, & Rose, 1971). I took this opportunity to present David Rapaport's (1959b) distinction among the five metapsychological "points of view" of psychoanalytic theory in a chapter that I thought would be of great interest to undergraduates. When this textbook was reviewed in *Contemporary Psychology*, the reviewer directed a comment to me: " . . . you must be kidding if you think undergraduates will be able to follow a meta-theoretical account of psychoanalytic theory" (Mosher, 1972, p. 523). The textbook was eventually adopted at such places as Berkeley and Oxford—but, perhaps unsurprisingly, not many other places.

I continued to present this material in undergraduate lectures, using what I considered to be a very useful mnemonic device: The *D*ynamic point of view relates to instinctual forces and the directionality they impart to behavior; the *E*conomic point of view relates to instinctual energies and the manner in which they are discharged, distributed, and transformed; the *G*enetic point of view relates to the history and development of mental life and the manner in which past experiences influence current structures and functions; the *A*daptive point of view relates to the manner in which the organism effects adaptive coordinations between instinctual drives and the demands of external reality; and the *S*tructural point of view relates to psychological processes characterized by a relatively slow rate of change and by a permanence of organization and function.

I told my undergraduate students that if they could remember the name of the famous French Impressionist painter Edgar *DEGAS*, they would have a very good start in answering final-exam essay questions on the metapsychological viewpoints of psychoanalytic theory. During one of these examinations, one of the students stayed longer than the other students and appeared to be having considerable difficulty. I looked over the student's shoulder at the paper and found only the barest beginnings of an answer: *M*, motivation; *O*, Oedipus; *N*, narcissism; *E*, energy; and *T*, transference. So much for my mnemonic device!

Roy Schafer's (1948) book on psychodynamic test interpretation had a profound, but quite unexpected, positive influence on my career in psychology. I acquired a copy of the book for practically nothing from a "born-again behaviorist," one Neal Kent, who was a fellow graduate student and good friend at Indiana University. Neal had been trained at another institution before he saw the behaviorist light and was eager to unload his psychodynamic textbooks on anyone who was interested. I read the book with great interest as part of my continuing "hobby."

In Arnold Binder's graduate course in assessment at Indiana, the final exam consisted of a Rorschach, Thematic Apperception Test (TAT), and Wechsler protocol that we were supposed to interpret more or less "blindly." He had selected the protocol of a person with a narcissistic character disorder from Schafer's (1948) book, on the very plausible assumption that graduate students in this Mecca of behaviorism would not have encountered it before. I almost fainted when I recognized it, but was able to pull myself together and employ a bit of gamesmanship that I had learned from Stephen Potter's (1950) book—another "hobby" of mine. In my answer, I first identified the protocol and its source, and then outlined the general nature of the interpretations given by Schafer. I then, with all due respect (and arrogance), proposed some alternative interpretations. Once I had established myself as somewhat of a "genius" in Binder's mind, it was inevitable that he should subsequently recommend me so strongly to his alma mater (Stanford) when I was later very much in need of a faculty position.

Interpersonal Paradigm

While I was still an undergraduate at American University, I had the opportunity to meet people who were either directly or indirectly associated with the Washington School of Psychiatry. For example, a fellow student in a French language course was a woman whose husband was a psychiatrist in training at the Washington School. She recommended to me her husband's assigned text for a course he was taking: Mullahy's (1948) *Oedipus Myth and Complex*, which pretty much changed my life. The book focused on the theories of both Freud and the neo-Freudians, especially Harry Stack Sullivan, whose major works had not yet been published. I was intrigued by this book, although it would be many years before I appreciated the full significance of Sullivan's work.

Victor Lovell is among the most colorful and memorable persons I have ever met, and I consider myself fortunate to have known him as a graduate student and friend (at Stanford). He was associated with many members of the "counterculture" that existed in and around San Francisco in the late 1950s and early 1960s, and he had a hand in the introduction of LSD to this counterculture (see Wolfe, 1969, pp. 39–54). Vic and I shared an interest in the interpersonal paradigm, and because he took courses at both Stanford and Berkeley (an unprecedented state of affairs), he was able to report to me on the doings of the then relatively obscure and somewhat mysterious Timothy Leary. In any event, some 30 years later, Vic appeared at an invited address I was giving at an American Psychological Association meeting in San Francisco and surprised me with a copy of a monograph in which Sullivan (1949) reported what might be considered the first interpersonal circumplex, to which Vic had added the inscription: "Harry did it first." Vic never stopped being an invaluable colleague and good friend.

Personological Paradigm

My acquaintance with Dan McAdams began when I adopted his wonderful introductory personality text (McAdams, 1990) and used it in reorganizing my undergraduate personality course at the University of British Columbia to conform to his personological orientation. My students loved the book, as well as their assignment to write a psychobiography of someone who interested them. McAdams and I have had a number of occasions to interact since that time in connection with our mutual interests. I was especially pleased when he asked me to contribute to a special issue of the *Journal of Personality* he was editing, in which, for the first time, I carried out a psychobiographical analysis of a colorful individual from the perspective of the interpersonal paradigm (Wiggins, 1997). I consider McAdams to be among the finest minds in contemporary personality psychology.

I have been acquainted with William McKinley Runyan (known to his friends as "Mac") for a longer period of time. We have always had a common interest in personality assessment; more recently, he has been unstinting in his efforts to educate me about life histories and psychobiography. Mac is the most deeply scholarly person I know (a *real* intellectual) and also one of the most caring. As mentioned earlier, he is responsible for my writing the present section of this introductory chapter.

Multivariate Paradigm

By the time I left Stanford in 1962 for a position at the University of Illinois, I was on my way to becoming a full-fledged member of the multivariate paradigm. This was to be somewhat of a baptism under fire, however. One of my first graduate teaching assignments at Illinois was to present a lecture in the Measurement Section of the Departmental Graduate Proseminar in Psychology. My fellow contributors to this section included such superstars as Raymond Cattell, Lee Cronbach, Lloyd Humphreys, Henry Kaiser, and Ledyard Tucker. As a consequence, I developed a deeply personal appreciation of the "imposter syndrome," which some of my colleagues generously interpret to this day as "modesty" on my part.

All of these men have influenced me in different ways, but my memories of Cattell are perhaps the most vivid. In preparing my *Annual Review of Psychology* contribution on "Personality Structure" (Wiggins, 1968), I took on the impossible self-appointed task of summarizing Cattell's work; fortunately, I received some help on this project from both Cattell and members of his lab. One of the infamous obstacles to achieving a deep appreciation of the significance of Cattell's work is his use of neologisms in naming his many factors. Being a rigorous empiricist, Cattell eschewed the use of popular labels for his factors, preferring to use a neologistic shorthand label describing what had been empirically established about the factors. Thus, for example, "comention" is the name of a factor that is to be read as "conformity or cultural amenability through good parent self-identification." When I asked a member of Cattell's lab how they kept track of all of these neologisms, he replied, "We don't. Not even Dr. Cattell has memorized these labels; he has to look them up." Being a great fan of Cattell's, I must also point out that some of his other neologisms, such as "ipsative," "itemmetric," and "surgency," now appear in the supplement to the *Oxford English Dictionary*. But what I remember most are the great kindness, warmth, and sensitivity of this brilliant scholar and the many ways in which he enriched both my personal and professional life.

My fondest recollection of another warm and wise scholar, Donald Fiske, is of the year he visited the University of British Columbia and we cotaught a graduate course in personality assessment—he using his excellent book *Measuring the Concepts of Personality* (Fiske, 1971) and I using *Personality and Prediction* (the title of which was suggested by Don in his helpful prepublication comments). Don's tough-minded approach to the measurement of personality has kept our field on course at many points in our stormy history.

My 45-year association with Lewis R. Goldberg has provided me with a constant set of high standards and a most enduring friendship. For many years the Oregon Research Institute was my "home away from home," and the professional and social atmosphere that Lew created there had a highly significant impact on my career, as well as on the careers of literally dozens of other investigators (including the late Warren Norman, whom I first met there).

Over the course of our extensive professional interactions, Paul Costa and I have become friends. Paul was the best man at my wedding; my wife, Krista Trobst, and I were then visitors at his lab for 2 years, during which time we discussed further integration of the five-factor and circumplex structural models of personality. I consider Paul to be *the* most influential figure in the evolution of the multivariate paradigm during the past decade.

Empirical Paradigm

As a graduate student, I was fortunate enough to receive classroom instruction in the MMPI paradigm from Alexander Buchwald and, on internship, clinical tutorials from Bernard Aaronson. All of this was supplemented by what I have described elsewhere as "a total and joyful immersion in Meehl's early and classic writings (1945–1956)" (Wiggins, 1991, p. 109) and an attempt to keep up with the burgeoning empirical literature of the MMPI during that period. Instruction in the MMPI paradigm and in clinical applications during those days relied heavily on direct contact with Minnesotans (for a fortunate few) and on the circulated (mimeographed) lecture notes and presentations of such luminaries as Paul Meehl and Harrison Gough (for the rest of us). Consequently, when I assumed a teaching position in the clinical program at the University of Rochester in 1956, a just-published canonical volume of readings (Welsh & Dahstrom, 1956) served well as a required textbook for my frighteningly bright and eager graduate students at that institution.

In my subsequent position at Stanford, I had the opportunity of presenting a series of lectures on the MMPI at the Menlo Park Veterans Administration Hospital to an extraordinary group of trainees from both Berkeley and Stanford. In addition to such notables as Victor Lovell and Rudolph Moos, I was fortunate to have in the audience a trainee from Berkeley named Kenneth Craik, who still likes to tease me by insisting that he is one of my "students" (although the converse would be a more accurate characterization).

Final Thoughts

In the course of editing a book on the five-factor model (Wiggins, 1996a), it became most evident to me that my own life story is intricately related to the development and interrelations among the major paradigms of personality assessment. That some of the contributors to the book—David Buss, Paul Costa, Lew Goldberg, Bob Hogan, and the late Jack Digman—happened to be friends of mine is not entirely accidental. Nor is the fact that they each represent quite distinctive views on the nature and interpretation of the five-factor model. Bringing together this distinguished group of scholars warmed my Kellyian–constructivist heart. And I think my own achievement was in carrying it off, since the members of this particular group did not always see eye to eye on many matters psychological.

However, the foregoing account of my acquaintance with members of each of the five paradigms of personality assessment is not meant to demonstrate that I have "paid my dues." Rather, it is intended to emphasize how very fortunate I have been to have had the opportunity to associate with so many kind and generous colleagues.

PART I

THE FIVE PARADIGMS
AND THEIR CONVERGENCES

The Psychodynamic Paradigm

> Properly speaking, the unconscious is the real psychic; its inner nature is just as unknown to us as the reality of the external world, and it is just as imperfectly reported to us through the data of consciousness as is the external world through the indications of our sensory organs.
>
> —FREUD (1900, p. 486)

THE TWO DISCIPLINES OF PSYCHOANALYSIS

As may be seen from Table Int.3 of the Introduction, the writings of Sigmund Freud provided the initial conceptual bases for three of the five paradigms of personality assessment considered in this book, and a case could be made for his having had some influence on the remaining two paradigms as well. However, the nature of Freud's influence on different paradigms varied in ways that will become evident in this chapter and in the chapters to follow, which emphasize differences among paradigms. In Chapter 6, I consider the differences and similarities between the psychodynamic paradigm and each of the other paradigms. Underlying these differences and similarities is a fundamental conceptual distinction between the drive/structure and relations/structure models of psychoanalytic theory—a distinction that was first emphasized by Greenberg and Mitchell (1983).

Drive/Structure Model

Freud's original psychoanalytic model was stated in the language of the biological and physical sciences of the 19th century, in terms of energy, force, and structure; "structure" was defined as psychological processes characterized by a relatively slow rate of change (Rapaport, 1959b). The principal energy sources of human behavior were held to be innate and largely unconscious sexual and aggressive drives that are directed toward "objects" (persons) in the environment, and that are opposed by both external and internalized societal prohibitions. In this model, "cathexes"[1] of external objects serve mainly as vehicles through which instinctual energies are discharged.

Relations/Structure Model

In a radical departure from Freud's drive/structure model, Harry Stack Sullivan (1953b) maintained that human behavior is comprehensible only within the context of interpersonal relations, the "relatively enduring patterns of recurrent interpersonal situations which characterize a human life" (p. 111). As Greenberg and Mitchell (1983) noted, "Every major feature of Sullivan's theory reflects his shift from Freud's drive/structure theory to relational/structural premises" (p. 100). Whereas Freud's model is primarily "biological," Sullivan's is primarily sociological and cultural.

> The models, to use Kuhn's term, are "incommensurable"; they rest on fundamentally different a priori premises. Any dialogue between their adherents, although useful in forcing a fuller articulation of the two models, ultimately falls short of a meaningful resolution. (Greenberg & Mitchell, 1983, p. 404)

Relational Psychoanalysis

During the years since Greenberg and Mitchell (1983) declared the drive/structure and relations/structure models to be "incommensurable," there appears to have been a shift in the received view on this matter. Greenberg (1998) has qualified the original Greenberg–Mitchell position by emphasizing changes that had occurred in the use of the term "relational" since their earlier book. In their original usage, Greenberg and Mitchell meant to distinguish orthodox "drive/structure" theorists (such as Freud, Hartmann, and Rapaport) from "relational" theorists (such as Sullivan, Thompson, and Fromm).

Freud's earliest versions of the drive/structure perspective focused on inherent biological drives that presumably "provide the energy for, and the goals of, all mental activity" (Greenberg & Mitchell, 1983, p. 3). In order to incorporate "object relations" into this theory, it was necessary to view relationships as "vicissitudes" of drives that facilitate or inhibit drive discharge. Thus "all facets of personality and psychopathology are understood essentially as a function, a derivative, of drives and their transformations" (Greenberg & Mitchell, 1983, p. 3).

---

[1] Investment of feelings or emotions in others.

In contrast to the drive/structure perspective, the "relational" theorists assume that we humans are "genetically predisposed to relate to others— relating to others is not a byproduct of something else (i.e., drive discharge or gratification)" (Eagle, 2000, p. 674). This school of thought includes such theorists as Sullivan (1953b), Thompson (1964), and Fromm (1947), as well as "object relations" theorists such as Fairbairn (1952), Guntrip (1961), and Winnicott (1965).

More recently, there has occurred what one reviewer described as a "miniparadigm shift" in classical psychoanalysis (Eagle, 2000) with respect to what is now called "relational psychoanalysis" (Mitchell & Aron, 1999). Although the two models may not be "incommensurable," they are sufficiently different to be treated separately, as I have done in this chapter and the next. Subsequent developments within the drive/structure theoretical framework, such as object relations theory, were attempts to incorporate interpersonal relations within the drive/structure model, and these developments are discussed in the present chapter. Further complicating matters, an even greater crossover has recently occurred within object relations theory; this is known as "attachment theory." Although attachment theory has historical roots in the drive/structure model, it is clearly based on a relations/structure model, and for that reason is mentioned in this chapter. Finally, in Chapter 6 I argue that on a higher level of abstraction, the drive/structure and relations/structure models are not necessarily "incommensurable."

CONCEPTUAL BACKGROUND
OF THE PSYCHODYNAMIC PARADIGM

Of the five paradigms of personality assessment to be considered in this book, the psychodynamic paradigm is by far the most conceptually rich, stemming as it does from the elaborate theoretical edifice of Sigmund Freud's psychoanalytic theory of personality. The psychodynamic paradigm is distinguished not so much by the assessment instruments employed within it, but by the conceptual framework that guides the interpretation of results obtained from these instruments. Thus, although the Rorschach inkblot test was originally the principal assessment instrument employed within the psychodynamic paradigm, the test itself is now frequently employed without reference to any theory at all (e.g., Exner, 1993).

Because Freud aspired to nothing less than a complete theoretical account of the workings of the human mind, his work has been frequently evaluated from philosophical as well as psychological perspectives (e.g., Bouveresse, 1995; Grunbaum, 1993). Therefore, it is not surprising that within the psychodynamic paradigm itself, conceptual issues have been as numerous as empirical issues. This is particularly true of psychoanalytic "metapsychology"—Freud's (1917) term for the study of the assumptions upon which the system of psychoanalytic theory is based.

The Assumptions and Points of View of Psychoanalytic Metapsychology

In response to a request from the American Psychological Association to summarize the scientific status of psychoanalytic theory, David Rapaport (1959b) produced what can only be described as a masterpiece of formal systematization: He integrated the historical background and metapsychological assumptions of the theory in modern terms, while retaining and extending Freud's original concepts expressed in the natural science terminology of "structures," "forces," and "energies."

In his papers on metapsychology, Freud (1915–1917) discussed the basic conceptual assumptions underlying his evolving theory of the mind. In their totality, these papers provide a chronicle of the occasionally contradictory revisions and elaborations of his basic concepts over time. Rapaport's (1959b) incomparable achievement was to organize and formalize the minimal set of assumptions underlying psychoanalytic theory that he considered both necessary to and sufficient for a complete explanation of human behavior. A basic premise of psychoanalytic theory is that behavior is *multiply determined*. The different sources of determination may be thought of as different conceptual "points of view" on the same behavior sequence (Rapaport & Gill, 1959). These viewpoints, and the metapsychological concepts on which they are focused, appear in Table 1.1.

Freud's earliest writings emphasized the motivating forces of largely unconscious sexual and aggressive drives (dynamic) and their vicissitudes in a prohibitive society (economic). His original topographic conception of the mind (unconscious, preconscious, conscious) was never explicitly replaced by a structural viewpoint (Rapaport & Gill, 1959), the latter being one of Rapaport's more enduring clarifications. Similarly, although psychoanalytic theory is clearly a genetic psychology, Freud did not formulate this explicitly.[2] The adaptive point of view was clarified in the ego psychology of Hartmann, Erikson, and Rapaport, all of whom argued that this point of view had always been implied in Freud's work.

The Language of Psychoanalysis

[Psychoanalysts] have attempted to formulate explanations of action in the mode . . . of natural science explanation. . . . In line with this strategy, reasons become *forces*, emphases become *energies*, activity becomes *function*, thoughts become

---

[2] The term "genetic" in psychoanalytic theory concerns developmental experiences, as indicated in Table 1.1, not biogenetic heritability.

representations, affects become *discharges* or signals, deeds become *resultants*, and particular ways of struggling with the inevitable diversity of intentions, feelings and situations become *structures*, *mechanisms*, and *adaptations*.
—SCHAFER (1976, p. 103; emphasis added)

Although Freud's metapsychology was initially meant to clarify the precise nature of his constructs, his use of the language of 19th-century natural science to describe the relations among his constructs eventually generated more heat than light, as it were. For example, his mechanistic, anthropomorphic personifications of metapsychological constructs "interacting" with each other (e.g., instinctual energy vs. countercathectic forces) generally lacked any reference to what actual persons might be doing or in what situations they might be doing it. These ambiguities posed serious problems for both analytic practitioners and theorists. Some practitioners found it difficult to "translate" back and forth between metapsychological constructs and the lives and problems of their patients. By the 1960s, a considerable number of theorists had become highly critical of this metapsychological "language problem" (e.g., Grossman & Simon, 1969; Guntrip, 1967; Holt, 1965; Home, 1966; Klein, 1967; Rycroft, 1966). It was in this context that Roy Schafer (1976) boldly published a book proposing *A New Language for Psychoanalysis*.

Using the writings of prominent linguistic philosophers as a guide (e.g., Austin, 1970; Hampshire, 1959; Ryle, 1949; Wittgenstein, 1958), Schafer devised an "action language" for psychoanalysis, with the fundamental rule that

> we shall not use nouns or adjectives to refer to psychological processes, events, etc. In this, we should avoid substantive designations of actions as well as adjectival or traitlike designations of modes of action. Thus, we

TABLE 1.1. Metapsychological Points of View in Psychoanalytic Theory

Viewpoint	Focus
Dynamic	Instinctual forces and the directionality they impart to behavior
Economic	Instinctual energies and the manner in which they are discharged, distributed, and transformed
Structural	Psychological processes characterized by a relatively slow rate of change and by a permanence of organization and function
Genetic	History and development of mental life, and the manner in which past experiences influence current structures and functions
Adaptive	Manner in which the organism affects adaptive coordinations between instinctual drives and the demands of external reality

Note. Data from Rapaport (1959b).

should not use such phrases as "a strong ego," "the dynamic unconscious," "the inner world," "libidinal energy," "rigid defense," "an intense emotion," "autonomous ego function," and "instinctual drive." (Schafer, 1976, p. 9)

The bulk of Schafer's revolutionary book is devoted to reworking the language describing the fundamental concepts of psychoanalytic metapsychology into an unambiguous language of action and modes of action. Schafer's perspective, although much more detailed and rigorous, was not entirely "new" to classical psychoanalytic thought. Psychoanalysts have always been aware of their analysands' tendencies to deny or to be unaware of their *own* contributions "to such puzzling or seemingly absurd phenomena as dreams, symptoms, errors, repetitive self-injurious behavior, and emotionality that is inappropriate in kind or object or intensity" (Schafer, 1976, p. 61). And in the classical analytic intervention strategy, "The patient's attention is drawn to his own *activity*; *he himself* has been bringing about that which up to now he has thought he was experiencing passively" (Fenichel, 1941, p. 52; emphasis in original). By emphasizing the problematic actions of the analysand, Schafer's reworking of the formal language of psychoanalytic metapsychology reconciled the theory and practice of psychoanalysis, and thus must be counted among the more salutary and original contributions to the psychodynamic paradigm.

With reference to the quotation from Schafer given at the beginning of this section, it might be said that Schafer, and the considerable number of contemporary psychodynamic theorists who share his sentiments, have "reversed" Freud's original translations. "Force" has become reason, "energies" have become emphases, "function" has become activity, and so on. Within psychoanalytic metapsychology, the formal replacement of natural science metaphors with psychological constructs is similar to what Kuhn (1996) has called a "paradigm shift."

Evolving Psychoanalytic Perspectives on Personality

Psychoanalytic Characterology

The notion of "character" forms the earliest link between psychoanalytic theory and personality assessment. In Allport's (1937) classic distinction, "*Character is personality evaluated, and personality is character devaluated*" (p. 52; emphasis in original). Because "character" implies a moral evaluation of an individual's comportment, Allport suggested that the term not be used in the objective study of personality. However, within early psychoanalytic medical practice, the term "character" was used to denote what was "wrong" with a person, and that usage persists. In later psychiatric nosology, the phrase "character disorders" was employed to describe persons who behaved in unacceptable (antisocial) ways, and the current term "personality disorders" (American Psychiatric Association, 1994) retains a similar evaluative component. Indeed, such expressions as "personality *assessment*," "personality *evaluation*," and "personality *appraisal*" are still with us today.

The conceptual history of psychoanalytic characterology has been a checkered one. Within classical psychoanalysis, the focus was on the vicissitudes of infantile instinctual development that are prolonged or sublimated in adult character traits. Freud (1908) was the first to note the relation between anal eroticism (or, as the *Standard Edition* spelled it, "erotism") in children and the characterological triad of orderliness, parsimony, and obstinacy in the adult "anal character." Abraham (1921) expanded this conception with clinical data, and later gave extended accounts of "oral character" and "genital character" as well. Freud (1931) returned to the concept of character with a tripartite classification based on his structural theory of "id" (erotic type), "ego" (narcissistic type), and "superego" (obsessional type). Reich's (1933) later concept of "character armor" stressed the adaptive limitations on character flexibility imposed by ego defenses against repressed instincts, and he did so with a considerably broader range of character types (e.g., passive–feminine, paranoid–aggressive, masochistic).

The paradox of psychoanalytic characterology became evident in the contrast between the intuitive appeal of certain clusters of adult personality traits (such as the anal triad of orderliness–parsimony–obstinacy) on the one hand, and the lack of empirical evidence from prospective studies establishing linkages with early experiences (e.g., toilet training) on the other. Such paradoxes highlighted the need for an ego psychology that would extend the scope of classical psychoanalytic theory by emphasizing such aspects of the ego as cognitions, attitudes, and modes of experiencing affect. More than 30 years passed before Shapiro (1965, 1981) attempted to resolve this paradox by offering an ego-psychological formulation of neurotic styles. Such styles are "ways of thinking and perceiving, ways of experiencing emotion, modes of subjective experience in general, and modes of activity that are associated with various pathologies" (Shapiro, 1965, p. 1). Shapiro's (1965) formulations of obsessive–compulsive, paranoid, hysterical, and impulsive "styles" are classics of the ego-psychological perspective.

Ego Psychology

In Freud's tripartite division of personality structure into id, ego, and superego, the ego was assigned a rather impotent and ambiguous role in the development of the individual and in the individual's adjustment to changing social environments. The ego was seen as "the helpless rider of the id horse" (Rapaport, 1959a, p. 9). Psychoanalytic ego psychology was (and is) an attempt to extend classical psychoanalysis by revising Freudian concepts related to the ego, while retaining much of the original theoretical framework.

Freud's original notion of ego made reference to the "person" or "conscious self." Memories that are incompatible with the conscious self (particularly sexual seduction by an adult) were thought to be dissociated from consciousness. When Freud discovered that reports of infantile seduction were based on fantasies rather than on actual occurrences, he temporarily put aside the role of reality experience in psychosexual development and returned to his original emphasis on instinctual drives and their derivatives. His later concepts of the reality principle and of secondary process extended the role of the ego somewhat, but without granting the ego an energy source that was independent of instinctual drives. Later, in "The Ego and the Id," Freud (1923) described the ego as a coherent organization of mental processes, but he still did not provide the ego with independent (from drive) energy of its own. Over time, the ego concept assumed a less subservient role in Freud's theory; eventually, in "Analysis Terminable and Interminable," Freud (1937) implied that the ego might have independent energy sources of its own (see Rapaport, 1959a, p. 11).

Heinz Hartmann (1939) provided a systematic account of an ego that has independent (from drive) energy sources from birth and that operates in a conflict-free ego sphere:

> I refer to the development *outside of conflict* of perception, intention, object comprehension, thinking, language, recall phenomena, productivity, to the well-known phases of motor development, grasping, crawling, walking, and to the maturation and learning processes implicit in all of these and many others. (p. 8; emphasis in original)

It should be clear from this quotation alone that ego psychology aspires to be a general psychology (Loewenstein, Newman, Schur, & Solnit, 1966) of contemporary rather than of historical significance, and that it is much more compatible with mainstream psychological research and theory.

Object Relations Theory

> . . . recent developments within psychoanalytic theory are an integral part of an attempt to extend the "experience-distant" metapsychology, which uses concepts of structures, forces, and energies to describe the functioning of the mind—concepts based primarily on a model related to the natural sciences, to a more "experience-near" clinical theory . . . primarily concerned with concepts of self and others in a representational world.
> —BLATT and LERNER (1983b, p. 88)

The generally increased emphasis upon ego functions in postclassical psychoanalysis was also reflected in the currently important psychodynamic alternative of object relations theory. Proponents of this view challenged the classical idea that cathexes of external "objects" (persons) serve mainly as vehicles through which instinctual energies are discharged. Instead, it was postulated that early interactions with significant others ("objects") lead to internalized representations of both others (Jacobson, 1954; Sandler & Rosenblatt, 1962) and self (Kohut, 1971) that serve as "internal working models" (Bowlby, 1973) for later interpersonal relationships. From this perspective, the person is, from birth (Main, Kaplan, & Cassidy, 1985), an object seeker (Fairbairn, 1952; Winnicott, 1965) who establishes a "gratifying involvement" with other persons (Behrends & Blatt, 1985).

As will become evident in this chapter, the shift in emphasis within psychoanalytic theory from the early characterology based on drives, to the ego-psychological perspective, and finally to the internalized representations of object relations theory is to some extent paralleled in the corresponding shifts in rationales for personality assessment from the ego-psychological approach to character assessment (e.g., Prelinger & Zimet, 1964), to the more general ego-psychological approach (e.g., Allison, Blatt, & Zimet, 1988), and more recently to the object relations perspective (e.g., Blatt & Lerner, 1983a).

CONCEPTUAL BACKGROUND OF PROJECTIVE METHODS

> Coming directly to the topic of projective methods for personality study, we may say that the dynamic conception of personality as a process of organizing experience and structuralizing life space in a field, leads to the problem of how we can reveal the way an individual personality organizes experience, in order to disclose or at least gain insight into that individual's private world of meanings, significances, patterns, and feelings.
> —FRANK (1939, p. 402)

As will become apparent in both the present chapter and the one to follow, advances in physics in general and the formulations of physical field theory in particular had a decided influence on the conceptual foundations of both the psychodynamic and interpersonal paradigms of personality assessment. With respect to the psychodynamic paradigm, Lawrence K. Frank's (1939) article "Projective Methods for the Study of Personality" became an instant classic within the psychodynamic paradigm, and it is still widely cited today. Using Kurt Lewin's (1935) notion of "structuralizing" one's life space according to one's private world, Frank argued that this principle of organizing experience "leads to the problem of how we can reveal the way an individual personality organizes experience, in order to disclose or at least gain insight into that individual's private world of meanings, significances, patterns, and feelings" (p. 402).

THE PSYCHODYNAMIC TRADITION
IN CLINICAL PERSONALITY ASSESSMENT

David Rapaport was not only a major systematizer of psychoanalytic theory; he was the originator of a now standard psychodiagnostic test battery and a highly influential mentor of the principal architects of the psychodynamic tradition in personality assessment. After receiving his PhD from the Royal Hungarian University, he emigrated to the United States in 1938 and shortly thereafter joined the staff of the Menninger Clinic in Topeka, Kansas, where he eventually became chief psychologist and head of the Research Department. During and shortly after World War II, the results of an extensive program of collaborative research were summarized in a two-volume *Manual of Diagnostic Psychological Testing* (Rapaport, 1944–1946), which eventually "revolutionized clinical psychology and influenced clinical psychologists the world over" (Gill & Klein, 1967, p.18). While at Menninger, Rapaport developed an internship program for graduate students in psychology that emphasized psychodiagnostic assessment with a standard test battery (Rapaport & Schafer, 1946). This program (Challman, 1947) consolidated the psychodynamic paradigm by training many of its future contributors.

In 1948, Rapaport moved to the Austin Riggs Center in Stockbridge, Massachusetts and continued his extensive collaborations with colleagues at such institutions as the Menninger Foundation, the Yale University Department of Psychiatry, and the Research Center for Mental Health at New York University. Speaking collectively for workers at these and other institutions, Roy Schafer (1967) observed that "All of us are working within the psychoanalytic psychodiagnostic tradition crystallized by David Rapaport" (p. 2). The Rapaport disciples whose work is considered in the present chapter are listed in Table 1.2.

At the Menninger Clinic, Rapaport was assisted by Merton Gill, a psychiatrist; Martin Mayman, a psychology intern; and the precocious Roy Schafer, who had a bachelor's degree at the time. All three of these clinicians would later have distinguished careers in their own right. Rapaport and several other members of the Menninger staff moved to the Austin Riggs Center and were later joined there by Erik Erikson and by Roy Schafer (who had, in the interim, completed his doctorate at Clark University). Under the tutelage of this distinguished group, David Shapiro produced his classic *Neurotic Styles* (1965). Schafer eventually left Austin Riggs to accept a position as chief of the Psychology Section in the Department of Psychiatry at Yale University. While at Yale, Schafer recruited Carl

TABLE 1.2. Genealogy of the Psychodynamic Paradigm

Menninger Foundation	Austin Riggs Center	Yale University
David Rapaport	David Rapaport	
Merton Gill	Erik Erikson	
Roy Schafer	Roy Schafer	Roy Schafer
Martin Mayman	David Shapiro	Carl Zimet
		Sidney Blatt

Zimet for a staff position in the Department of Psychiatry. The circuitous route whereby Sidney Blatt arrived at the Yale University Department of Psychiatry is a story in itself (see Auerbach, 1999). But the collaboration of Blatt, Zimet, and Allison (who had interned with Schafer) resulted in a textbook (Allison, Blatt, & Zimet,[3] 1988) that contributed to the continuing survival of the Rapaport tradition in psychodiagnostic testing.

THE MENNINGER ASSESSMENT BATTERY

Rationale

Prior to Rapaport's writings in the 1940s, assessment psychologists were primarily technicians who administered IQ tests. Since that time, they have become clinicians who administer batteries of both structured and projective tests of personality and cognition. At Menninger, a multitest battery was advocated in view of the apparent complexity of personality and cognition and their interrelated functions, as well as for the purpose of gathering normative data that would shed light on those complexities (Rapaport, Gill, & Schafer, 1946). The composition of the battery reflected judgments regarding the potential of each instrument to yield measures that might be interpreted within the ego psychological framework of Rapaport and his associates.

Composition

The projective component of the original Menninger battery included the Rorschach test (Rorschach, 1921), the Thematic Apperception Test (TAT; Morgan & Murray, 1935), and a locally constructed Word Association Test. The nonprojective component included the Bellevue Scale (Wechsler, 1941), the Babcock Test of mental efficiency (Babcock, 1933), the Sorting Test of concept formation (Goldstein & Scheerer, 1941), and Hanfmann

---

[3] "The authors are listed in alphabetical order and each of us came to this task better equipped because of contact with Roy Schafer as colleague or teacher" (p. x).

and Kasanin's (1937) test of concept formation. Experience with this battery led to the deletion of Hanfmann–Kasanin and Babcock instruments, as well as a revision of the Word Association Test items (Schafer, 1948). As this revised test battery evolved over a 20-year period, the Rorschach, the TAT, and the Wechsler Adult Intelligence Scale (WAIS; Wechsler, 1958) became the more or less standard core of the psychodynamic test battery (e.g., Allison et al., 1988) to which a variety of supplemental tests might be added (e.g., Sentence Completion, Draw-a-Person, and Bender Gestalt; see Piotrowski & Zalewski, 1993).

Interpretive Principles

Only a few tests have been constructed specifically for use within a classical psychoanalytic framework (e.g., Blum, 1968). The major assessment instruments employed in the Menninger battery were all originally developed in quite different theoretical contexts. Rorschach may never have intended his test to be interpreted in terms of psychoanalytic theory (Exner, 1974, p. 222); Murray developed his elaborate taxonomy of needs and the TAT in reaction to the paucity of drive variables postulated by psychoanalytic theory (Anderson, 1988); and, perhaps most obviously, the mental testing tradition within which the WAIS was constructed bears little resemblance to the psychodynamic tradition. The vast literature on psychodynamic interpretive principles associated with the instruments employed in the Menninger battery defies easy summarization. The following statements are meant to convey only some of the flavor of three, among many, interpretive principles.

Projective Hypothesis

The projective hypothesis states that "All behavior manifestations of the human being, including the least and the most significant, are revealing and expressive of his personality, by which we mean that individual principle of which he is the carrier" (Rapaport, 1942, p. 92). Thus an individual's possessions—clothes, automobile, furniture—are expressive of his or her personality and reflect single acts of choice; in their totality, they reflect the organization of such choices (Frank, 1939). Responses to the ambiguous stimuli of projective tests may also be thought of in terms of "choice," although such choices are much less conscious or volitional in nature. Thus responses to a Rorschach inkblot may be thought of as reflecting "choices" between forms, colors, shadings, and so forth, to which a subject imparts meaning through organization. Responses to a TAT card also involve both choice (e.g., with which figure to identify) and organization (e.g., sequence of events) (Rapaport, 1942, pp. 92–94). Responses to intelligence and concept formation tests involving choice and organizational processes may be used as "nonprojective tests of personality," given an adequate theory of "functions underlying the reactions and achievements on these tests" (Rapaport, 1946, p. 228).

Levels of Functioning

The psychoanalytic model of primary (pleasure principle) and secondary (reality principle) modes of thought is meant to account both for a developmental sequence and for characteristics of the mature adult (Rapaport, 1951). Consequently, there is a *continuum* of adult psychological functioning that may be assessed with an appropriate battery of tests.

> This continuum ranges from functioning in situations which put a premium on highly logical, reality-oriented secondary modes of thought (WAIS) to those which allow for more personal, less conventionally constrained thinking (TAT) and finally those which allow for considerably novel, personalized, and regressive modes of thinking (Rorschach). (Allison et al., 1988, p. vii)

Assessment of level of functioning has been greatly facilitated by Holt's innovative procedures for assessing primary and secondary process in the Rorschach (Holt & Havel, 1960).

Psychological Adjustment

The Rorschach, TAT, and WAIS may be employed both to assess adaptive capacities and impairments in psychological functioning and to identify the functions impaired in different psychiatric diagnostic groups. Adjustment and maladjustment may be assessed with reference to the following postulated sequence:

> . . . certain patterns of defense mechanisms are adopted and these determine specific strengths and weaknesses in psychological functioning which then become characteristic of the adjustment of the personality; with the onset of maladjustment, an exaggeration or breakdown in these strengths and weaknesses characteristic for that maladjustment occurs which can be measured; this leads to a diagnostic differentiation. (Rapaport, Menninger, & Schafer, 1947, p. 249)

THE RORSCHACH INKBLOT TEST
Origins and Development of the Test

The origins and development of the Rorschach are best understood by considering the contributions since the 1920s of the many, often colorful, individuals who have, at different times, proposed quite differing rationales and scoring procedures for quantifying and interpreting responses to the test. The 10 standard inkblots that make up the test are indeed ambiguous and inviting of "projection"; different theorists have seen a remarkable variety of potentialities for psychodiagnosis in the same inkblots. Table 1.3 provides a rough chronology of these developments.

Hermann Rorschach

The following pages describe the technic of and the results thus far achieved in a psychological experiment which, despite its simplicity, has proved to be of value in research and in general testing. At the outset it must be pointed out that all of the results are predominantly empirical. . . . The conclusions drawn, therefore, are to be regarded more as observations than as theoretical deductions. The theoretical foundation for the experiment is, for the most part, still quite incomplete.
—RORSCHACH (1921, p. 13)

Although several psychologists had previously considered the use of inkblots as test material for eliciting imaginative productions (e.g., Binet & Henri, 1895–1896; Whipple, 1910), it was the Swiss psychiatrist Hermann Rorschach (1884–1922) who launched a 10-year systematic investigation of the usefulness of such stimuli in the experimental study of concept formation. From among thousands of trial blots, Rorschach eventually selected a standard set of 10 blots that constituted what he called the "form interpretation test" and that now make up the Rorschach test. Rorschach's (1921) monograph Psychodiagnostik (translated into English later as Psychodiagnostics) was a "preliminary report" of an experiment conducted on a variety of normal and psychiatric patients using the standard inkblots.

In discussing the results of his experiment, Rorschach (1921) indicated the part of the inkblot used in a response as whole (W), common detail (D), or small detail (Dd). He distinguished among responses that were mainly determined by the form of the blot (F), by the chromatic color of the blot (C), by both (FC, CF), and by the attribution of human movement to the blot (M). Rorschach invoked the notion of "kinesthesia" with reference to the capacity to produce human movement responses (M) to the blots, and contrasted such responses with color responses (C), which he thought reflected extraversion and affectivity. The ratio of M to total C was called the Erlebnistyp ("experience balance"), and it corresponded roughly to Jung's introversion–extraversion distinction. He also classified the content of the response (e.g., A = animal figure) and noted original percepts (Orig.). In comparing contemporary scoring categories with those suggested by Rorschach over 80 years ago, one is struck by the extent to which this system appeared to spring almost "full-blown" from a single highly creative person.

TABLE 1.3. A Selected Chronology of Rorschach Scoring and Interpretive Systems

1920s–1930s: Rorschach (1921); Klopfer and Sender (1936); Beck (1937)

1940s: Klopfer and Kelley (1942); Beck (1944, 1945, 1949); Rapaport et al. (1946); Schafer (1948)

1950s: Beck (1952); Phillips and Smith (1953); Klopfer et al. (1954, 1956); Schafer (1954); Piotrowski (1957)

1960s: Beck (1960); Rickers-Ovsiankina (1960); Klopfer and Davidson (1962); Allison et al. (1968); Exner (1969)

1970s: Klopfer et al. (1970); Exner (1974, 1978)

1980s: Exner and Weiner (1982); Exner (1986)

1990s: Exner (1990, 1991, 1993)

Rorschach's untimely death in 1922 at the age of 37 left many unanswered questions concerning such matters as the directions in which his work might have proceeded and the conceptual orientation within which his work might eventually have been organized. Shortly after Rorschach's death, his closest coworker, the psychoanalyst Emil Oberholzer, published a manuscript of Rorschach's titled "The Application of the Interpretation of Form to Psychoanalysis" with Oberholzer's own extensive annotations (Rorschach & Oberholzer, 1924). Although this paper suggested to some later workers that Rorschach would have continued within the psychoanalytic tradition along Freudian lines (e.g., Klopfer & Kelley, 1942), Rorschach's original monograph appears to reflect mainly the influence of associationist psychology, Bleuler, and the early Freud and Jung (Schafer, 1954). Rorschach's definitive biographer has suggested that his orientation was moving in the direction of phenomenology (Ellenberger, 1954), and others have suggested that Rorschach was developing his own theory of personality based on his test (e.g., Acklin & Oliveira-Berry, 1996). Regardless of the direction in which Rorschach might have been moving, his test soon found fertile soil within the psychodynamic community in the United States.

Bruno Klopfer

Bruno Klopfer came upon the American scene in 1934 and kindled a flame which has since illuminated the paths of thousands of students and colleagues. . . . More than any other teacher in the field, Klopfer demonstrated how clinical judgments and "intuitive feel" can be developed and communicated and how subjective evaluations can be made public with proper teaching, training and experience.

—HERTZ (1970, pp. ix–xii)

Bruno Klopfer (1900–1971) was born in Augsburg, Bavaria, and attended the University of Munich, where he received a PhD at the age of 22. He developed an early interest in Jungian theory and served as a staff member at the Berlin Institute for Child Guidance. When Hitler came to power in 1933, Klopfer moved his family to Zurich, Switzerland, with the help of Carl Jung. While serving as a technician at the Psychotechnic Institute there, he learned how to administer the Rorschach for purposes of employee selection. In 1934 he accepted a position as research associate for Franz Boas in the Department of Anthropology at Columbia University. As Handler (1994) observed,

> Americans were starved for information about the Rorschach in 1934, for there were few people available who could offer training in administration and interpretation. When several graduate students at Columbia University discovered that Klopfer knew the Rorschach, word went through the department like wildfire. (p. 569)

Klopfer's charismatic personality and his insightful analyses of Rorschach protocols created a demand for instruction that was barely met by the many workshops he gave at Columbia; at the University of California–Los Angeles; at Crafts, New York, for armed services personnel; and elsewhere. In contrast to Rorschach's more narrow scientific approach, Klopfer's interpretive style was subjective, intuitive, and broadly eclectic. His contributions to Rorschach scoring and interpretation were prodigious (e.g., Klopfer, Ainsworth, Klopfer, & Holt, 1954; Klopfer & Davidson, 1962; Klopfer et al., 1956; Klopfer & Kelley, 1942; Klopfer, Meyer, Brawer, & Klopfer, 1970).

From a historical standpoint, Klopfer's lasting contributions to the psychodynamic paradigm were as much organizational and administrative as substantive. In 1936 he organized and edited a mimeographed newsletter called the *Rorschach Research Exchange* (Klopfer, 1936), which became the *Rorschach Research Exchange and Journal of Projective Techniques* (Murphy, Stone, Hutt, Deri, & Frank, 1947), which in 1950 became the *Journal of Projective Techniques*, and which in 1971 became the present-day *Journal of Personality Assessment*. In 1939 Klopfer organized and formed the Rorschach Institute to ensure the availability of training in the Rorschach method, and that institute eventually became the Society for Personality Assessment.

Samuel J. Beck

My general orientation remains as stated in 1944. In limiting itself to the individual associations, the book stops short of interpretation. It does not concern itself with whole personality structures. The sole purpose here is to provide students with a steady frame of reference. The hope is that, given such a manual of constant usage, it will be possible to work with the test as a stable instrument. . . . To the extent that this is achieved, Rorschach test scoring would become an *operationalist* technic.

—BECK (1949, p. xi; emphasis in original)

In contrast to Klopfer's more intuitive interpretive style, Beck was the prototype of the *empirical* Rorschach scientist. For example, whereas Klopfer emphasized clinical judgment in determining whether the form of a response to a given location of an inkblot was of "good" (F+) or "poor" (F–) quality, Beck insisted on making such judgments with reference to empirical normative data. Nevertheless, Beck's (1960) skill in making "blind" interpretations of Rorschach protocols (given only the age and sex of the respondent) became as legendary as Klopfer's performances (Viglione, 1993).

Upon completing his doctoral dissertation on the Rorschach at the strongly scientific Psychology Department of Columbia University in 1932, Beck studied the Rorschach with Oberholzer in Zurich and, for the most part, remained within the Rorschach–Oberholzer orientation (Beck, 1959, p. 273). Nevertheless, Beck (1936) felt that the Zurich scoring procedures were more artistic than scientific, and he insisted on fixed standards in scoring and interpretation (Beck, 1937). As Exner (1974) noted, "It was almost inevitable that Beck and Klopfer were to disagree on many basic Rorschach issues" (p. 9). Yet these two scoring systems eventually became canonical, and the net effect was that clinical graduate students in the early 1950s (including myself) had to master *both*.

David Rapaport

How can man know of, and act in accordance with, his environment when his thoughts and actions are determined by the laws of his own nature?

—RAPAPORT (1959b, p. 57)

In summarizing the contributions of David Rapaport (1911–1960) to psychoanalysis and psychology, Gill and Klein (1967) identified the question above as "the central preoccupation in all of Rapaport's theoretical and empirical efforts" (p. 9). Addressing this paradox within psychoanalytic theory required an account of the roles of both drive and reality in human functioning. For Rapaport (1951), this account centered on the organization and pathology of *thought* in reconciling the inherent conflict between drive and drive restraint. Rapaport was critical of theoretical formulations that placed a one-sided emphasis on drive or on environment, and for that reason he was favorably disposed toward Hartmann's (1939) concept of autonomous ego development and Erikson's (1950) theory of psychosocial development. He facilitated the consolidation of the ego psychology movement by translating Hartmann's work into English, and by providing an illuminating historical introduction to Erikson's selected papers (Rapaport, 1959a).

Rapaport believed that the Rorschach is best employed as one test in a battery of tests, rather than as an all-purpose instrument for assessing personality. He advocated a relatively simple method of Rorschach administration, using as few scoring categories as possible, and conducting only a "minimal inquiry" (Rapaport et al., 1946). His emphasis was on providing both the novice and the experienced tester with a helpful frame of reference derived from *cumulative experience* that would be easily applicable to each new case.

> And only with such an approach could we avoid the temptation—especially for the beginner—to translate a multitude of highly refined scores into "psychological" statements with the help of a source book of interpretations, and then to throw these psychological "dream-book" statements together in an interpretation-hash. (Rapaport et al., 1946, Vol. II, p. 88)

In formulating what happens psychologically when a patient is asked to respond to a Rorschach card, Rapaport relied upon what was known about perceptual and associative processes in the late 1940s. He emphasized that in everyday life, human perceptions may be thought of as varying along a continuum of degrees of "structuredness," depending on the clarity and familiarity of the stimuli. The literature of perception suggested to him that responses to such stimuli involve such processes as memory, concept formation, attention, concentration, and anticipation. *"These considerations may prompt the examiner to see in the subject's reaction to the Rorschach inkblots a perceptual organizing process which has a fundamental continuity with perception in everyday life"* (Rapaport et al., 1946, Vol. II, p. 90; emphasis in original). Despite this continuity, however, the unstructured and novel nature of the Rorschach test situation brings to the fore an organizing aspect of perception and provides unique insights into the respondent's adjustment or maladjustment.

In the procedures followed at the Menninger Clinic, the respondent was handed a Rorschach card and asked, "What could this be?" and "What does this suggest to you?" Clearly there are associative processes involved in responses to the inkblots as stimuli. But again, the novelty and unfamiliarity of the inkblots make it likely that the respondent's *own* associative patterns and difficulties will be brought to the fore in this situation.

The perceptual and associative processes involved in responses to inkblots were also considered in terms of concept formation, memory, attention, concentration, and anticipation. Overall, Rapaport identified three prominent phases in the process leading to a response to a Rorschach inkblot:

... in the first phase, the salient perceptual features of the blot initiate the association process; in the second, this process pushes beyond these partial perceptual impressions and effects a more or less intensive organizational elaboration of the inkblot; in the third, the perceptual potentialities and limitations of the inkblot act as a regulating reality for the association process itself. (Rapaport et al., 1946, Vol. II, pp. 93–94)

The foregoing summary of Rapaport's rationale for administration and interpretation of the Rorschach test is not meant to suggest that Rapaport's approach to this instrument would be more akin to that of a cognitive psychologist than to that of a psychoanalyst. Rather, his approach stems from the perspective of a psychoanalytic ego psychology that is firmly based on the principles of general psychology. Although there are many examples of this interpretive approach in *Diagnostic Psychological Testing* and in other writings of Rapaport (see Gill, 1967), the practicing clinician is likely to find the writings provided by Rapaport's long-time friend and collaborator Roy Schafer to be more accessible.

Roy Schafer

The original two-volume edition of *Diagnostic Psychological Testing* (Rapaport et al., 1946) was devoted in large part to a detailed description of the results of the Menninger Clinic study contrasting the test responses of different diagnostic groups (e.g., schizophrenic, depressive, and neurotic groups) with each other, and with the responses of a control group (54 randomly selected members of the Kansas Highway Patrol). As noted by Holt in his abridged and edited version of *Diagnostic Psychological Testing* (Rapaport, Gill, & Schafer, 1968), the research project itself was statistically and methodologically flawed, and the results are no longer considered to be compelling (e.g., Kleiger, 1993). The original volumes did not include the kind of broad diagnostic summaries or individual case studies that would be of interest to those who wish to learn interpretive procedures. In that respect, Roy Schafer's *The Clinical Application of Psychological Tests* (1948) may be regarded as a much-needed sequel to the original two volumes.

Schafer's book provided: (1) diagnostic summaries of typical patterns of test response in 19 pathological syndromes and in normal records for the Bellevue Scale, a learning efficiency measure, a sorting test, the Rorschach, a word association test, and the TAT; (2) case studies with full protocols of the aforementioned tests for nine pathological syndromes and an inhibited normal subject; and (3) briefer case studies of nine pathological syndromes with full protocols of selected tests. This book remains one of the major pedagogical achievements in the evolution of the psychodynamic paradigm, and for many years it was the "bible" for those seeking instruction in the ego-psychological approach to test interpretation.

Schafer's *Psychoanalytic Interpretation in Rorschach Testing* (1954) provided the first full explication of the contributions of psychoanalytic ego psychology to test theory and interpretation. It begins with a remarkable portrait of the "Interpersonal Dynamics in the Test Situation" based on the transference–countertransference dynamics of the psychotherapeutic relationship. The needs and problems of the tester are considered with reference to unconscious reaction tendencies that may be manifested in aspects of the *role* the tester assumes in his or her relationship with the respondent (e.g., voyeuristic, autocratic, oracular, or saintly). The personality characteristics of the tester that are likely to interfere with effective testing are also considered (e.g., rigid defenses against dependency or hostility, uncertain sense of identity, socially inhibited/withdrawn). The needs and problems of the patient are considered as well, with specific reference to the patient's psychological position, violation of privacy, loss of control, dangers of self-confrontation, regressive temptations, dangers of freedom, and psychosexual orientation toward his or her responses.

The more technical portions of Schafer's (1954) book are devoted to an analysis of the response process in Rorschach testing, thematic analysis of the content of Rorschach responses, and criteria for judging the adequacy of interpretations of Rorschach protocols. The major substantive contribution of the book is to be found in the detailed analysis of the psychoanalytic conceptualization of defense and its application (along with case studies) to repression, denial, projection, and obsessive–compulsive defensive operations. Like his mentor David Rapaport, Schafer is a major systematizer of psychoanalytic theory (e.g., Schafer, 1968, 1976); an innovator in the application of psychoanalytic theory to projective testing (e.g., Schafer, 1967); and, as suggested by Table 1.2, a highly influential mentor within the psychodynamic paradigm.

Joel Allison, Sidney Blatt, and Carl Zimet

. . . our goal is to show how a psychologist working in an ego-psychological framework goes about the process of analyzing a patient's test battery from start to finish and how he synthesizes a rich array of inferences into a meaningful description of personality functioning.

—ALLISON ET AL. (1988, p. vi)

Allison and colleagues' (1988) textbook on the ego-psychological interpretation of the major tests in the Menninger battery provided an updated restatement and extension of the earlier work of Rapaport and colleagues (1946), in light of significant advances in research and interpretation that had occurred since that work (e.g., Holt, 1966). This book has been aptly described as a Rapaport system for beginners (Auerbach, 1999), to emphasize the exceptional accessibility of the material presented. Concise and informative summaries of the administration, scoring, and interpretation of the WAIS, Rorschach, and TAT are provided from an ego-psychological perspective, along with brief case examples. Consistent with the Rapaport–Schafer position, the interpretive emphasis is on test scores, content or themes of response, style of verbalization, and the interpersonal relationship between tester and patient.

Unlike previous textbooks of interpretation, the Allison and colleagues (1988) text is focused almost exclusively on the test protocols of one person ("Mrs. T"), a randomly selected patient. This innovative format imparts a degree of "clinical realism" to the learning experience. Separate chapters focus on the administration, scoring, and interpretation of the WAIS, TAT, and Rorschach, along with brief case examples. The reader is provided with the full protocol of Mrs. T's responses to each of these tests, and with her referral request, preliminary background information, and material elicited during a brief interview preceding formal testing—in other words, the kinds of information typically available to the tester in a psychiatric setting. As the results of each test are summarized, hypotheses are generated for consideration in the subsequent test. Findings from the WAIS, TAT, and Rorschach are then summarized, and a model test report is provided.

The final part of the book presents the results of Mrs. T's retesting after a period of 2½ years, excerpts from a diary she kept during her early hospitalization, an interview with Mrs. T's therapist concerning the usefulness of the test report, and notes on Mrs. T's life following release from the hospital. For more than three decades, this highly informative and clearly written book has served as an excellent introduction to what successive generations of graduate students have referred to as the "ABZs of psychodiagnostic testing."

John E. Exner, Jr.

Exner has almost single-handedly rescued the Rorschach and brought it back to life. The result is the resurrection of perhaps the most powerful psychometric instrument ever envisioned.
—AMERICAN PSYCHOLOGICAL ASSOCIATION,
BOARD OF PROFESSIONAL AFFAIRS (1998, p. 392)

As emphasized in the Introduction, a student's orientation toward research and practice in personality assessment is often influenced by the graduate school he or she attends and by the particular advisor and/or clinical supervisor with whom he or she works most closely. This type of "indoctrination" was almost a necessity for learning the Rorschach during the 1950s, for how else might the student choose among the bewildering variety of scoring and interpretive systems listed in Table 1.3 for the 1920s–1930s through the 1950s? Although there were many exceptions, the choice most frequently narrowed down to one between the "empirical" system of Beck and the rival "clinical" system of Klopfer. And although there was clearly merit to be found in both systems, it behooved graduate students to accept the choice that had been made by their supervisors—with the notable exception of a graduate student named John Exner.

> How many Rorschachs are there really? No one can say but to guess gives rise to alarm. There are five reasonably distinct systems and so it can be argued that there at least five reasonably distinct Rorschachs. But when the potential combinations of these systems are considered, the possibilities become astronomical. (Exner, 1974, p. 14)

In 1954, when he was a second-year graduate student at Cornell University, Exner had the opportunity of spending a summer studying the Rorschach under the close supervision of Samuel Beck in Chicago.[4] During this period, Exner spent many hours in the library studying the Rorschach test.

> One day he came across a copy of Klopfer and Kelley's (1942) book, *The Rorschach Technique*, which he innocently carried along with him to Beck's house for their daily meeting. Noticing the small green book out of the corner of his eye, Beck asked with some initial suspicion, "What's that?" As Exner showed him the book he noticed Beck's suddenly changed demeanor. "Where did you get that book?" he asked, somewhat tersely. "In the library," a shaken Exner replied. "In *our* library?" asked Beck, as if the book itself had intrusively transgressed its boundaries by its mere presence in the University of Chicago library, Beck's library. (Handler, 1996, pp. 651–652)

Exner spent the following summer and one additional summer studying the Rorschach under Bruno Klopfer and assisting Klopfer in his workshops. Having become a close friend of both Beck and Klopfer, and appreciating their distinctive contributions, Exner recalled: "I had hoped because they were so very nice to me, to get them to sit down in a room with a tape recorder and I would interview them about their differences, and maybe they could come together" (quoted in Handler, 1996, p. 652). They both refused, but Beck suggested that Exner write a paper on the *differences* between the two systems. By this time Exner had become familiar with the work of Piotrowski, of Hertz, and of Rapaport and Schafer, and he decided to write a short monograph comparing all five systems. This "short mono-

---

[4] The following biographical information is based on Leonard Handler's (1996) interviews with Exner.

graph" eventually became Exner's *The Rorschach Systems* (1969), which Handler (1996) has described in his article title as "The Book That Started It All."

The initial sources on which Exner based the Comprehensive System, his massive revision and standardization of the Rorschach test, are listed in Table 1.4. In assembling materials for his comparative analysis of Rorschach systems, Exner (1969) relied on his personal contacts with the major systematists themselves to ensure accurate presentation of their approaches. The manner in which the systems were being used was determined in a survey of 395 practicing clinicians (Exner & Exner, 1972). The latter findings were disconcerting. Some 22% of clinicians surveyed had abandoned scoring altogether, and of those who continued to score, 75% did not follow any one system consistently. Exner (1974) concluded that "most 'Rorschachers' solve the dilemma of several systems privately by intuitively adding 'a little Klopfer,' a 'dash of Beck,' a few 'grains' of Hertz, and a 'smidgen' of Piotrowski, to their own experience, and call it *The Rorschach*" (p. x).

Exner also surveyed the practices and opinions of highly experienced Rorschach users, and the views of published authors on research methods and problems, before embarking on the first of what would be an enormous number of empirical studies of scoring procedures for Rorschach protocols.

> The goal of this work is to present, in a single format, the "best of the Rorschach." This system draws from each of the systems, incorporating those features which, under careful scrutiny, offer the greatest yield, and adds to them other components based on more recent work with the test. The product, if successful, should be a method which is easily taught, manifests a high interclinician reliability, and which will stand well against the various tests of validity. It is not based on any particular theoretical position, and hopefully, can be useful to both the behaviorist and the phenomenologist. It is predicated on the notion that the Rorschach is one of the best methods available from which a useful description of the uniqueness of the person can be gleaned. (Exner, 1974, pp. x–xi)

Although several "schools" of Rorschach interpretation have been devised by colorful individuals, there is nothing in the history of the test that can be compared with the Exner phenomenon. Those of us who have had the pleasure of meeting Exner (and this is a very large number of persons) can attest to the fact that he belies the image of the aloof, introverted university professor. His outgoing nature and infectious enthusiasm for developing a uniform and empirically sound Rorschach have enabled him to seek the opinions and learn the practices of hundreds of colleagues, and to enlist hundreds of individuals from diverse backgrounds to conduct the

TABLE 1.4. Original Sources for Exner's Comprehensive System

Method	Focus	Source
Comparative analysis	Five major Rorschach systems	Exner (1974)
Interviews and conversations	Positions and attitudes toward systems	Major systematists themselves
30-item questionnaire	Practice and use of major systems	Exner and Exner (1972)
90-item questionnaire	Practices and opinions	131 experienced ABPP Rorschach users
55-item questionnaire	Rorschach research methods and problems	100 published authors of Rorschach research
Analysis of Rorschach protocols	Study and cross-reference of normative baselines	835 Rorschach protocols from more than 150 psychologists

studies emanating from the Rorschach Workshops over the years. Perhaps of equal importance has been his energetic and unswerving commitment to developing standard, reliable, and empirically based procedures for the administration, scoring, and interpretation of the Rorschach test (Exner, 1969, 1974, 1978, 1986, 1990, 1991, 1993, 1994, 1995b; Exner & Weiner, 1982, 1995).

Over the years, Exner has presented the following, in successive editions: (1) detailed rules for administration, inquiry, scoring, and interpretation; (2) evidence on the reliability and validity for individual scales and summary scores; and (3) normative data from a variety of clinical and nonclinical samples. There is little doubt that Exner's Comprehensive System has become a widely employed system of Rorschach administration and scoring. Surveys of graduate students and predoctoral interns in psychology suggested that when they are taught the Rorschach, most of them are taught the Comprehensive System (e.g., Hilsenroth & Handler, 1995). But ironically, although Rorschach scoring and interpretation can no longer be considered a "seat-of-the-pants" procedure, criticism of the test from other quarters has, if anything, *increased* in recent years (Archer, 1999; Meyer, 1999). Critical opinion on the validity of the Rorschach constitutes one of the grimmest chapters in the history of personality assessment.

THE VALIDITY OF THE RORSCHACH

I would like to offer the reader some advice here. If a professional psychologist is "evaluating" you in a situation in which you are at risk

and asks you for responses to inkblots . . . walk out of that
psychologist's office. Going through with such an examination creates
the danger of having a serious decision made about you on totally
invalid grounds.
                                        —DAWES (1994, pp. 152–153)

Robyn Dawes's strongly held opinion concerning the validity of the Rorschach is not at all unusual. A sampling over the years of critical reviews
(most from the highly respected *Mental Measurements Yearbook* series) reveals many of them to be equally critical:

> What passes for research in this field is usually naively conceived, inade-
> quately controlled, and only rarely subjected to usual standards of experi-
> mental rigor. (Wittenborn, 1949, p. 394)
>   There is no evidence of any marked relationship between Rorschach
> scoring categories combined in any approved statistical fashion into a
> scale, and diagnostic category, when the association between the two is
> tested on a population other than that from which the scale was derived.
> (Eysenck, 1959, p. 277)
>   . . . it seems not unreasonable to recommend that the Rorschach be
> altogether abandoned in clinical practice and that students of clinical psy-
> chology not be required to waste their time learning the technique.
> (Jensen, 1965, p. 509)
>   . . . the monotonous overall conclusions have been that there is little
> evidence to support the claims made for the technique by its proponents.
> The results of the research published subsequent to the last edition of the
> year book have not perceptibly altered this grim picture of the reliability
> and validity of the Rorschach procedure. (Eron, 1965, p. 495)
>   Perhaps the most compelling question that can be asked about the
> Rorschach at this time is whether yet another review of this test is, in
> fact, necessary or even desirable. (Reznikoff, 1972, p. 446)
>   The general lack of predictive validity for the Rorschach raises seri-
> ous questions about its continued use in clinical practice. (Peterson,
> 1978, p. 1045)

But the most damning of all critical judgments is reflected in the fact that
the Rorschach is no longer reviewed in the *Mental Measurements Year-
books* (Dawes, 1994, p. 151).
    Many of the reviews quoted above were, of course, "pre-Exner." Blan-
ket psychometric criticisms of Rorschach research should now be tempered
in light of Exner's subsequent empirical work with Rorschach scoring categories. But the specter of "predictive validity" still looms large:

> Interestingly, the question of establishing the *validity* of the interpretive
> process, the extent to which it results in accurate interpretations, is not ad-
> dressed in Exner's work. Thus, there is no scientific reason to conclude that
> the Comprehensive System is any more valid than the earlier, simple scoring

and interpretation procedures it was designed to replace. (Lanyon &
Goodstein, 1997, pp. 96–97; emphasis in original)

Moreover, the utility of learning the Exner scoring system has been ques-
tioned:

> The Rorschach can be administered and scored in a reliable manner, but the
> training that is necessary to learn how to score reliably the 168 variables of
> the Exner Comprehensive System is daunting at best. (Widiger & Saylor,
> 1998, p. 162)

The last quotation is from a chapter in the 11-volume *Comprehensive Clinical Psychology*—a project that was designed, as the title states, to provide
comprehensive coverage of the entire field of clinical psychology (Bellack &
Hersen, 1998). Perhaps not surprisingly, this massive work does not include a separate chapter on Rorschach testing of adults.

THE COMPREHENSIVE SYSTEM
AND THE PSYCHODYNAMIC PARADIGM

Debate over the Comprehensive System

There are two main reasons why the current widespread acceptance of the
Comprehensive System has not resulted in a consolidation of the Rorschach
within the psychodynamic paradigm: (1) The Comprehensive System de-
emphasizes the "projective" aspects of responses to the cards, and (2) this
system is essentially atheoretical (or at least theory-neutral) in nature. With
respect to projection, Dawes (1994) observed: "The [Comprehensive Sys-
tem] presupposes that the blots actually do look like certain things. Which
is the exact *opposite* of the rationale for the Rorschach" (p. 149; emphasis
in original). Similarly, Shontz and Green (1992) made the point that "It en-
courages the use of the Rorschach as a standardized test rather than as a
minimally structured instrument. . . . Thus, the Exner system may have
transformed the instrument into something that its originator and many of
its users might not wish it to be" (pp. 149–150). With respect to theory, it is
true that some of the scoring categories of Rapaport and Schafer have been
incorporated into the Comprehensive System, but psychoanalytic rationales
for interpretation—or, for that matter, theoretical rationales in general—are
clearly avoided: "In other words, the presence or absence of an underpin-
ning theory is irrelevant, as the data are the data" (Exner, 1997, p. 41).

Exner's (1989) insistence that the Rorschach does not assess projection
has alienated some members of the psychodynamic community (e.g.,
Aronow, Reznikoff, & Moreland, 1995; Kramer, 1991). Aronow, Reznikoff, and Moreland (1994) argue that it was "a fundamental mistake to try

to 'regiment' this clinically sensitive procedure into some sort of inkblot version of an MMPI [the Minnesota Multiphasic Personality Inventory]" (p. 18). On the other hand, major proponents of the Comprehensive System (e.g., Weiner, 1994) have also alienated the more psychometrically oriented members of the Rorschach community by arguing that the Rorschach is not a psychological test, but rather a flexible method of interviewing not constrained by traditional psychometric principles.[5] The Comprehensive System has without doubt improved the psychometric status of the Rorschach as a testing instrument, but in a sense it may now be an instrument without a paradigm. Interestingly, the paradigm with which the Comprehensive System of the Rorschach has been most compared in recent times is the *empirical* paradigm.

The Rorschach and the MMPI

Competition

Parker, Hunsley, and Hanson (1988) conducted a meta-analytic comparison of the Rorschach and the MMPI with respect to their reliability, stability, and validity in 411 published studies and concluded:

> The MMPI and Rorschach are both valid, stable, and reliable under certain circumstances. When either test is used in the manner for which it was designed and validated, its psychometric properties are likely to be adequate for either clinical or research purposes. (p. 373)

This conclusion, together with other promising findings from meta-analyses of the MMPI and Rorschach (Atkinson, 1986) and of the Rorschach alone (e.g., Parker, 1983) appeared to grant equal "status" to the Rorschach and the MMPI as clinical assessment instruments (e.g., Ganellen, 1996a)

Garb, Florio, and Grove (1998) strongly contested the results of meta-analyses that appeared to grant equal status to the Rorschach and MMPI:

> When we reanalyzed the data from the most widely cited meta-analysis [Parker et al., 1988], we found that for confirmatory studies . . . the [MMPI] explained 23% to 30% of the variance, whereas the Rorschach explained only 8% to 13% of the variance. *These results indicate that the Rorschach is not as valid as the MMPI.* (p. 402; emphasis added)

In a paradigm-free "open market," it would appear that the Rorschach test fares less well than the MMPI. But closer examination of the commit-

---

[5] This opinion is specifically disavowed by Exner (1997, pp. 40–41).

ments of the participants in this contest suggests that the market is not entirely "paradigm-free." For example, Paul Meehl (1954), the conceptual architect of the empirical paradigm, was well known for his advocacy of "statistical" (empirical) rather than "clinical" (judgmental) prediction. In the prediction of socially relevant criterion measures (the goal of the empirical paradigm), Meehl was concerned about the fallibility of clinical judgment and decision making, and his concern is still shared by other members of the empirical paradigm who have been strongly influenced by Meehl, such as Garb (1998), Grove (Grove & Meehl, 1996), and Dawes (1994).

In the controversy over statistical versus clinical prediction, it was Robert Holt (1958), a distinguished member of the psychodynamic paradigm, who first presented the strongest case for clinical judgment, and Holt's position is strongly endorsed by the originator of the Comprehensive System:

> Holt also makes a strong argument that prediction, as such, is not an end in itself. Rather, understanding is at least equally important as a scientific goal. Holt could easily have gone one step further to emphasize that understanding is the principal goal of the clinical assessment routine, and that prediction, in many instances, is of somewhat lesser importance. (Exner, 1974, p. 4)

Although the Rorschach Comprehensive System may no longer be affiliated with the psychodynamic paradigm, some of the underlying assumptions of that paradigm concerning the importance of "understanding," as opposed to "predicting," still remain.

Integration

That the two personality tests most frequently employed in clinical assessment (the MMPI and the Rorschach) should be viewed as "competitive" is to lose sight of the fact that the tests arose from quite different paradigms. On the other hand, the fact that they do represent such different paradigms could be fueling the intensity of their competition. In this context, Widiger (2001) has expressed the opinion that this onslaught on the Rorschach is part of a wider professional dispute. He has argued that the Rorschach is being attacked not only because its validity and utility have been exaggerated by its proponents, but also because it is the instrument of, and a symbol for, the psychodynamic perspective. In his opinion, the attack is not simply on the Rorschach; it is on the psychodynamic perspective (and on intuitively oriented practicing clinicians).

In any case, the results of comparative studies have suggested that there is little relation between scores from the Rorschach and from the MMPI, even when the scores purportedly measure the same constructs (e.g., Archer & Krishnamurthy, 1993a, 1993b). On the basis of these and other studies, Archer (1996) asserted: "An extensive literature, spanning 50 years and 45 published investigations, leads to the conclusion that the Rorschach and the MMPI bear little or no meaningful relationship to each other" (p. 504). Although hope has been held out for the "integration" of the Rorschach and the MMPI in personality assessment (e.g., Ganellen, 1996b), and conceptual commonalities between the two instruments have been identified on a high level of abstraction (see Chapter 6), the increasingly atheoretical use of the Rorschach could eventually result in invidious comparisons being made with the ultraempirical and highly successful MMPI-2.

CONTRASTING VIEWS ON THE CURRENT STATUS OF THE RORSCHACH

After over 50 years of disagreement about the utility of the Rorschach, the field of personality assessment still remains strongly divided. Most journals on assessment, and many others, have devoted considerable space to the presentation of extensive and at times even scathing critiques of the validity of the Rorschach (e.g., Burns & Viglione, 1996; Dawes, 1999; Garb, 1999; Garb et al., 1998; Wood & Lilienfeld, 1999; Wood, Lilienfeld, Garb, & Nezworski, 2000; Wood, Nezworski, Garb, & Lilienfeld, 2001; Wood, Nezworski, & Stejskal, 1997; Wood, Nezworski, Stejskal, & Garven, 2001; Wood, Nezworski, Stejskal, Garven, & West, 1999), as well as equally passionate rejoinders (e.g., Acklin, 1999, Exner, 1995a, 1996, 2001; Ganellen, 1996a; Hiller, Rosenthal, Bornstein, Berry, & Brunell-Neuleib, 1999; Meyer, 1997a, 1997b, 2000, 2001; Weiner, 1996, 1999, 2000a, 2000b).

Irving Weiner (1995) has observed that "those who currently believe the Rorschach is an unscientific or unsound test with limited utility have not read the relevant literature of the last 20 years; or, having read it, they have not grasped its meaning" (p. 73). This situation may be due, Weiner (1996) later noted, to the fact that

> the Rorschach will yield valid inferences primarily in relation to conditions and events that are largely determined by known personality characteristics and in which nonpersonality variance plays little part or can be carefully controlled; hence, for example, the predictive validity of Rorschach variables tends to be less extensive than their concurrent validity. (p. 212)

In contrast, Sechrest, Stickle, and Stewart (1998) concluded that the Rorschach may be best characterized as what Richard Feynman (1985) referred to as "cargo cult science":

In the South Seas there is a cargo cult of people. During the war they saw airplanes land with lots of good materials, and they want the same thing to happen now. So they've arranged to make things like runways, to put fires along the sides of the runways, to make a wooden hut for a man to sit in, with two wooden pieces on his head like headphones and bars of bamboo sticking out like antennas—he's the controller—and they wait for the airplanes to land. They're doing everything right. The form is perfect. It looks exactly the way it looked before. But it doesn't work. No airplanes land. So I call these things cargo cult science, because they follow all the apparent precepts and forms of scientific investigation, but they're missing something essential, because the planes don't land. (p. 340)

In the view of Sechrest and colleagues, "use of the Rorschach has failed to demonstrate convincing evidence of validity in decades of attempts to find it. The planes still don't land" (p. 24).

THE THEMATIC APPERCEPTION TEST

Psychoanalytic Theory of Responses to the TAT

Holt (1951) suggested that the seventh chapter of Freud's (1900) *The Interpretation of Dreams* was a fertile source of hypotheses for investigating the processes underlying the production of imaginative stories to TAT cards. The "day residue" of dreams, according to Freud, is an event that has occurred during the preceding day. The theme of this residue leads to a train of associations that touch upon a repressed wish. But the day residue itself is not conflicted, and an elaboration of its theme permits a "partial discharge" of an unacceptable impulse in a form that is *related*, but not *equivalent*, to that impulse. Telling a TAT story may serve the same function. However, the TAT story will not be a direct expression of the unacceptable impulse; it will be a "secondary elaboration" of the underlying theme that "is fashioned into a more or less coherent, usually dramatic form" (Holt, 1951, p. 184).

The TAT and the Menninger Battery

The TAT was devised by Henry Murray, the founder of the personological paradigm (Morgan & Murray, 1935); it has continued to play a central role in that paradigm, in which the primary focus is on the life story of individuals (Cramer, 1996). The test has also played an important role within the psychodynamic paradigm, because it was a central component of the original Menninger battery:[6]

---

[6] David Rapaport and Robert Holt provided input to Murray when he was developing the TAT (Morgan, 1995).

It was our purpose to include a test in our battery which should give us an appraisal of the subject's experiencing of his own world and of himself as a part of it. In a sense, we wanted to obtain thereby a direct picture of the material dealt with by the intellectual conceptual apparatus and personality dynamics of the subject which were incidentally indicated by the other tests. Therefore we had to find a test which would supply us with more than incidental information about these contents and attitudes. . . . Our choice fell on the Thematic Apperception Test. (Rapaport et al., 1946, pp. 396–397)

When respondents are asked to make up imaginative stories from ambiguous pictures of people in a variety of settings and to tell what the characters are thinking and feeling, the *ideational content* of their responses differs qualitatively from that produced in response to the WAIS or to the Rorschach. Whereas the WAIS calls for consensually agreed-upon "knowledge," and the Rorschach appears to call for statements of what the blot "really is," the TAT calls for fantasies and imaginative products that represent a different type of thought:

. . . the characteristics, attitudes, and striving of figures in the TAT stories are all memory products; as such they are subject to the laws of memory organization which order single experiences into patterns conforming with the emotional constellations of the subject's life. This is the theoretical basis for assuming that the TAT stories may allow for inferences concerning the make-up of the subject and his world. (Rapaport et al., 1946, pp. 419–420)

Interpretive Principles

Clinical experience has established a set of normative expectations for the stories produced to each card of the TAT. For example, Card 1 (which depicts a young boy contemplating a violin) "usually elicits the subject's attitude toward duty (compliance, coercion, rebellion) and frequently also gives some inkling as to his aspirations (difficulty, hope, achievement)" (Rapaport et al., 1946, p. 421). Perceptual distortions may be assessed with reference to this normative base (e.g., the respondent fails to notice the violin). Highly normative stories are analogous to "popular" responses to Rorschach cards, and Rapaport and colleagues (1946) consider these to be "clichés" that are not especially revealing, although they suggest that one may infer the "rules" by which the respondent selects clichés from the interrelationships among clichés.

A normative story for Card 1 would describe a boy sitting in front of a violin who does not want to play it and would rather be out playing baseball with his friends; as such, this is not very revealing. On the other hand, a story in which "the child's father is a great musician who has died and the child is holding the violin with the determination to take the place of his father in the musical world and to care for his mother" (Rapaport et al., 1946, p. 415) strongly suggests an Oedipal constellation. Similarly, consider the brief story given by a patient with psychotic depression: "A boy looking at a violin. . . . What led up to it? I guess a string broke, is that it? What the outcome will be? He'll stop playing. (Feel?) He feels sad" (Schafer, 1948, p. 296). Schafer noted that "The theme, stated with simple finality, is that one gives up in the face of even minor difficulty" (1948, p. 299).

As the preceding example suggests, Rapaport and colleagues (1946) emphasized the importance of attending to the *affective tone* of a story, as well as to its content. They also emphasized the importance of assessing strivings and defenses, compliance with instructions, consistency of the stories (both interindividual and intraindividual), and obstacles or barriers. Schafer (1967), in particular, has emphasized the importance of attending to *narrative style*: "A TAT story has this in common with poetry: we cannot grasp its full import if we consider only its content, its narrative detail" (p. 114). Consider the narrative style in a story given to Card 1 by a 52-year-old Hollywood film story editor with a long history of heavy drinking:

> Now from this I'm supposed to tell you what? [Instructions repeated.] He has just finished practicing and . . . and he is sitting there reflecting . . . over his violin . . . on a score which he's just tackled. Is that enough [Make up more of a story.] . . . [How does he feel?] . . . I should say he feels a little . . . hmmm, disturbed, no, not disturbed; well, we'll [mumbles something], we'll say a little disturbed by the fact that he hadn't brought off, what will we say, the Scarlatti exercise to his satisfaction. He is a sensitive, thoughtful child who, like myself, needs a haircut. You can leave that out if you wish. Okay, that takes care of Buster. Oh, you put everything down [noticing verbatim recording]. (Schafer, 1967, p. 116)

Schafer then provided a detailed and insightful analysis of the extent to which this man was acutely aware that *he* was making up a story (1967, pp. 117–128).

In their updated presentation of the Rapaport–Gill–Schafer system, Allison and colleagues (1988) provided the responses of "Mrs. T" to Card 1:

> Uh—this child—uh—[sigh] has been studying music for a few years. He's— he feels very deeply about music. He can hear it—hear lovely sounds in his head, but he can't get them to come out of his violin. At the time of the picture, he's sitting there very unhappy, because he can't create anything himself. And—uh—so he gets up and he—and very frustrated, he smashes his violin. (pp. 110–111)

The authors emphasized the initial passivity and lack of action, which later became an eruption of affect and aggression. They also called attention to the initial ambiguity regarding the sex of the "child" (uncertain sexual identity?) and the subsequent identification of the child as male (belated capacity for facing identity problems?). "Studying music for a few years" was and is normatively less common than the boy's having recently obtained the violin, and this extended time span was seen as emphasizing the boy's failure to "get them to come out of his violin" (depressive tone). This juxtaposition of unhappiness and not being able to get sounds out suggested to these authors a state of tension and "a longing for an active role which is finally and only expressed through violent, volcanic activity" (p. 111).

THE WECHSLER SCALES
Rapaport, Gill, and Schafer

It is not surprising that the intelligence test developed by David Wechsler (1939) should be included in the Menninger battery of the 1940s, since the principal role of psychologists at that time was that of "intelligence testers," and the Bellevue Scale was the state of the art within that realm (as its successors are today). What may be surprising is that Rapaport and colleagues (1946) had concluded, "In our clinical work, the I.Q. level proved to be of almost no diagnostic significance" (p. 51); they chose to emphasize instead the quantitative *interrelations* among subscale scores of this test, as well as the *qualitative* aspects of responses to individual items. They stated their intention "to demonstrate that the different types of maladjustment tend to have different distinguishable and recognizable impairments of test performance" (p. 39).

The rationale for this approach was based on five premises:

[1] ... one must consider not only every subtest score, but every single response and every part of every response as significant and representative of the subject ... [2] one may gain some understanding of the subject by comparing the successes and failures on a given type of test item ... [3] the relationship of the score of one subtest to the scores of other subtests is also representative of the subject ... [4] the relationship of all the Verbal scores to all the Performance scores is significant of the makeup of the subject ... [5] the data to which the above four points refer must be considered in the light of findings of tests other than those of intelligence. (Rapaport et al., 1946, pp. 40–41)

Scatter Analysis

The Wechsler scales appear especially well suited for profile analysis, because all subtest scores are expressed in directly comparable standard scores. From the outset, Wechsler was interested in clinical applications of the Bellevue Scale and its successors that examined indices derived from the interrelations among test scores. For example, he derived an index of "mental deterioration," which was based on the difference in standard scores between subtests that "hold" with age and subtests that "don't hold." Rapaport and colleagues (1946) employed a related method, which became known as "scatter analysis" and which was defined as "the relationship of any two scores, or of any single score to the central tendency of all the scores" (p. 48). In this method, the Vocabulary subtest, because of its centrality and stability, served as a baseline of comparison for the analysis of deviations on other subtests. Configural patterns of this nature were examined in relation to various indices of psychopathology. These analyses yielded findings that were generalized in this form: "An extreme discrepancy between Digits Forward and Digits Backward is in general indicative of psychosis" (p. 193). Such analyses received considerable criticism on psychometric grounds (e.g., Schofield, 1952), and as Anastasi (1976) concluded, "Three decades of research on these various forms of pattern analysis with the Wechsler scales have provided little support for their diagnostic value" (p. 466).

Qualitative Analysis

A less controversial use of the Wechsler scales in psychodiagnostic testing was the analysis of qualitative features of an individual's responses. This involved (1) formulation of the cognitive and emotional demands of an item, and of how the respondent met these demands; and (2) attending to the diagnostic implications of verbalizations (whether right or wrong). For example, the items in the Comprehension subtest were judged to require not only the activation, selection, and organization of information, but the delaying of first impulses as well:

> In the question, "What should you do if, while sitting in the movies, you were the first person to discover a fire?" the impulsive response, "Holler fire!" must be suppressed if a "good response" is to be achieved. Many self-controlling impulsive people will begin, "I won't holler fire, but rather . . . "; others, who are less contained, will say: "I know one shouldn't holler fire but I am afraid that's what I'd do." (Rapaport et al., 1946, p. 112)

Roy Schafer

Unfortunately most research into the clinical usefulness of tests has attempted to correlate test "signs" with diagnoses and not with characteristics of thinking or behavior. . . . This is a fault of the statistical investigations in *Diagnostic Psychological Testing*. It is a roundabout method and can never yield conclusive results.

—SCHAFER (1948, p. 22)

Schafer placed a heavy emphasis on a patient's distinctive style of thinking and problem solving, as revealed in the "verbalized end products" (1948, p. 17) of thought initiated by the variety of problem situations found in the subtests of the WAIS. He viewed such thought processes as involving past intellectual achievements (and liabilities), and the application of these achievements to the succession of challenges represented by the different problem situations. They also, he believed, reflect the effectiveness of the patient's "characteristic-adjustment efforts" (1948, p. 18).

A response to the Comprehension item concerning being lost in the forest in the daytime may be technically correct but may also be diagnostically revealing of the patient's characteristic efforts at adjustment, as in the following response to this item given by an obsessive–compulsive patient:

> "If I were lost in the forest in the daytime I might follow the sun . . . or go by the moss on the north side of the trees . . . or maybe follow a stream. Do I have a compass? If I had one I'd . . . (etc.)." (Which would you do?) "It depends on the terrain: if . . . (etc.)." (Schafer, 1948, p. 25)

Schafer's sequel to *Diagnostic Psychological Testing* (1948) solidified the psychodynamic paradigm by presenting concrete case studies that illustrated the value of qualitative analysis of intelligence test protocols, and by deemphasizing the controversial scatter-analytic findings of the Menninger research project.

Allison, Blatt, and Zimet

A concise and updated presentation of the Rapaport–Schafer position on interpreting the WAIS within the psychodynamic paradigm was presented by Allison and colleagues (1988). On the basis of their combined clinical and research experience (e.g., Blatt, Allison, & Baker, 1965) and their familiarity with developments in the Menninger approach to WAIS interpretation (e.g., Mayman, Schafer, & Rapaport, 1951), these authors provided a useful overview of interpretive principles. Table 1.5 is an attempt to summarize, in highly abbreviated form, the overall structure of Allison and colleagues' presentation. They began by noting that both the Rorschach and the TAT are presented in such a manner as to encourage the respondent to give free rein to imaginative flights of fancy and free association. In contrast, the WAIS presents the respondent with a number of different types of structured situations to which he or she must respond in an organized and realistic fashion, *without* being influenced by distracting unconscious materials or by defensive operations called forth by such materials. Each subtest of the WAIS may be classified with respect to the psychological function required by the task, and unusually high or low scores on a given subtest (with reference to the baseline of Vocabulary) may be interpreted as reflecting either facilitating or inhibiting influences of psychodynamic factors on the acquisition or performance of the task required by the subtest.

In this context, Vocabulary (which correlates about .85 with Full Scale IQ) represents the breadth of concepts, ideas, and experience acquired in a lifetime. "The acquisition of these concepts and their availability to memory is contingent both on innate ability and on an enriched early life experience" (Allison et al., 1988, p. 24). Because of its demonstrated temporal stability and relative resistance to neurological impairment and psychological disturbance, Vocabulary serves as a baseline against which deviations in other subtests may be evaluated. Like Vocabulary, Information calls for the wealth of available information acquired by innate ability and life experience, but this subtest is more vulnerable to defensive processes. Highly driven efforts to acquire a great store of information reflect "intellectual ambitiousness" (high score in relation to Vocabulary). Repressive tendencies to block out memories have long been known to be associated with an impoverished store of information. Conversely, individuals with obsessive–compulsive tendencies will tend to obtain a relatively high score on this subtest.

"Mrs. T," the patient whose protocols were interpreted most completely by these authors, obtained a Full Scale IQ of 120 on the WAIS, reflecting her superior intellectual potential. Her elevated score on Comprehension suggested social conventionality and good judgment. The authors qualified this conclusion, however:

> With Comprehension higher than Information, a predominantly hysterical organization or character structure would be indicated. This interpretation follows from the notion that her relatively reduced fund of information stems from the use of repression as a major defense mechanism and the counterbalancing by high Comprehension indicates an outwardly directed orientation towards social conventionality and conformity. (Allison et al., 1988, p. 61)

CURRENT TRENDS WITHIN THE PSYCHODYNAMIC PARADIGM

Within the last three decades, theory and method within the psychodynamic paradigm of personality assessment have evolved into an object relations perspective that is highly compatible with contemporary formulations of social cognition, information processing, attachment research, and ego development (see Westen, 1990, 1998). Sidney Blatt and his associates at Yale have been primarily responsible for this paradigm shift. From the early 1950s until his untimely death in 1960, Rapaport contributed to the devel-

TABLE 1.5. Clinical Interpretation of the WAIS Subtests

WAIS subtest	Psychological function	Interpretation
Vocabulary	Breadth of concepts, ideas, and experience	Baseline to which other tests may be compared
Information	Wealth of available information	Intellectual ambitiousness (high); especially hindered by repression (low)
Comprehension	Grasp of social conventionality and social judgment	Hyperconventionality and naiveté (high); impairment of judgment (low); diminished interest in social interaction (low)
Similarities	Abstractness of verbal concept formation	Obsessive and paranoid modes of thought (high); impaired thought processes (low); organic impairment (low)
Digit Span	Rote memory and recall (attention)	Lack of anxiety, blandness, *belle indifference*; anxiety, intrusion of drive derivatives (low); brain damage (low)
Arithmetic	Concentration and use of prior skills	Narcissistic and hysterical persons avoid active, effortful ideation and the elaboration of internal experience (low)
Picture Arrangement	Capacity to anticipate social events and their consequences and to plan effective courses of action	Cautious, guarded, hyperalert paranoids, glib psychopaths (high)
Picture Completion	Visual organization and capacity to observe inconsistencies and incongruities	Hyperalert and hypervigilant paranoids (high); obsessive–compulsives (high); concerns over body intactness and passivity (low)
Object Assembly	Capacity to grasp a whole pattern by anticipating interrelations of parts	Concerns over bodily integration and intactness (low); blocking on specific item—e.g., "hand" (concerns over aggression and masturbation) (low)
Block Design	Concept formation task involving both analysis and synthesis	Blandness and lack of anxiety (high); schizoids (high); organic impairment (low)
Digit Symbol	Capacity to utilize energy in a simple task	Overcompliant striving and need for achievement (high); depressive lack of energy output (low)

Note. Data from Allison, Blatt, and Zimet (1988, pp. 23–33).

opment of ego psychology and its application to personality assessment; from the early 1970s until the present, Blatt has contributed to the development of object relations theory and its application to current personality assessment methods.

Within the context of a developmental theory of internal representations of both self and others, meaningful contrasts have been made between self-definition and interpersonal relatedness (Blatt & Blass, 1996)—constructs of far-ranging theoretical significance (see Chapter 6). These constructs have been coordinated with issues of separateness and attachment (Blatt & Blass, 1990), narcissism and object love (Erlich & Blatt, 1985), and self-criticism and dependency (Blatt, Quinlan, Chevron, McDonald, & Zuroff, 1982). The theory has also been applied to specific developmental pathologies, such as schizophrenia (Blatt & Wild, 1976), depression (Blatt & Zuroff, 1992), and "borderline" conditions (Blatt & Auerbach, 1988), as well as to topics as diverse as therapeutic change (Blatt & Ford, 1994) and modes of representation in art (Blatt with Blatt, 1984).

> The study of the representation of the human form on the Rorschach is an ideal data base for assessing an individual's representational world—his conception of people, including himself, and their actual and potential interactions. The representation of people, that is, object representations, have both structure and content. (Blatt & Lerner, 1983b, p. 8)

The structural aspects of object representations are emphasized in the Rorschach scoring system developed by Blatt, Brenneis, Schimek, and Glick (1976), which provides a developmental analysis of object representations in terms of such categories as differentiation, articulation, and integration of object and action. The content and affective themes of object representations are emphasized in the Rorschach scoring system developed by Mayman (1967), which emphasizes phenomenological dimensions such as affect states, ego states, experience of self, and sense of identity. A useful comparison of the research programs of Blatt at Yale and Mayman at the University of Michigan was provided by Blatt and Lerner (1983a, pp. 234–239). Both programs employed the Rorschach, TAT, and dreams in the assessment of object representations.

An object relations scoring system for the TAT has been developed by Westen (1991), in which stories are rated for complexity of representations of people, affective tone of relationship paradigms, capacity for emotional investment, and understanding of social causality. A similar scoring system has been developed for the Picture Arrangement subtest of the WAIS (Westen, 1991). In sum, the three major instruments of the original Menninger battery continue to show promise under a revised conceptual orientation that is most compatible with current thinking in personality, social, clinical, and developmental psychology.

2

The Interpersonal Paradigm

Scientific psychiatry has to be defined as the study of
interpersonal relations, and this end calls for the use of the
kind of conceptual framework that we now call *field theory*.
—SULLIVAN (1953b, p. 368)

METAPSYCHOLOGICAL CONSIDERATIONS:
I. THE NATURE OF INTERPERSONAL FIELDS

The Field Concept in Physics

Faraday's Fields

In 1821, Michael Faraday began a series of experiments suggesting that the
results of previous experiments on electricity and on magnetism could be
incorporated within a single unified theory. He demonstrated that (1) a
changing magnetic field can create an electric current, and (2) a changing
electric current can create another electric current. These findings, together
with an earlier finding that (3) a steady electric current can produce a magnetic field, suggested a possible unified theory of electricity, magnetism, and
possibly light—a theory that was not easily reconciled within the old physics.

> Faraday pondered on the idea of action at a distance, and there grew in his
> mind the idea that, surrounding a magnet or charged body, there was an in-
> visible, immaterial "sea," an entity that exists in space, rather like the
> waves that spread out from a stone thrown into a pond. (Silver, 1998, p. 91)

Maxwell's Equations

In 1864, James Clerk Maxwell summarized existing knowledge of "electro-
magnetism" in a series of differential equations that provided a quantitative
expression of electric and magnetic fields. Einstein and Infeld (1938) later

characterized Maxwell's equations as "the most important event in physics since Newton's time, not only because of their wealth of content, but also because they form a pattern for a new type of law ... representing the *structure* of the field" (p. 143; emphasis added). From these equations, Maxwell predicted that electromagnetic waves should travel through space at the speed of light, and this prediction was confirmed by Hertz in 1888. The excitement generated by the concept of an invisible and immaterial "force field" determining the interactions among material objects extended well beyond the discipline of physics.

The Field Concept in Psychology

Psychological Proponents of Field Theory

Within experimental psychology, the field-theoretical approach to understanding human behavior was championed by the influential Gestalt school of thought (Koffka, 1935; Kohler, 1929; Wertheimer, 1912), and this approach was extended to social psychology by Kurt Lewin (1939). J. R. Kantor (1924–1926) had earlier founded his school of interbehavioral psychology, which was heavily influenced by the field-theoretical ideas of the physics of his day (Kantor, 1953). The field-theoretical perspective in physics was also highly influential in the theoretical formulations of Harry Stack Sullivan (1940), whose interpersonal theory of psychiatry eventually provided the conceptual foundation for the interpersonal paradigm (Wiggins & Trobst, 1999).

Interactionism and Interpersonalism

In considering the influence of physical field theory on psychological theorizing, it is useful to make a distinction between "interactionism" and "interpersonalism." The interactionist perspective, as presented by Lewin (1946), focuses on the manner in which behavior is determined by the interaction between a person and the environment in which the person is situated: $B = f(P, E)$. In its modern form, this perspective assesses the relative contributions of person and situation by calculating the relative variance contributions to behavior of person, situation, and the statistical interaction of person and situation (Endler, 1975). Contemporary interactionism is based on an analysis-of-variance model for conducting empirical research, and as such does not claim to be a theoretical perspective (Endler, 1983).

The interpersonalist perspective, as presented by Sullivan (1953a), focuses on the interrelation between two persons within a common environment: $B = f[E(P_1 \leftrightarrow P_2)]$. Sullivan's form of radical interpersonalism may be difficult to comprehend on first exposure, because of our ingrained "individualist language" (1953a, p. 50) for describing personality as reflecting attributes of a discrete individual who is separate from others and from a shared social environment. Theorists within the interpersonal paradigm have attempted to operationalize Sullivan's view of personality in ways that avoid this individualistic bias by defining personality as: "nothing more (or less) than the patterned regularities that may be observed in an individual's relations with other persons, who may be real in the sense of actually being present, real but absent and hence 'personified,' or 'illusory' " (Carson, 1969a, p. 26).

Within Sullivan's radical interpersonalism, dyadic relationships with others constitute the environment, and a person's recurrent patterns of such relationships over time constitute his or her "personality." He stated: "In extreme abstract, the theory holds that we come into being as persons as consequence of unnumbered *interpersonal fields of force* and that we manifest intelligible human processes only in such interpersonal fields" (Sullivan, 1948a, p. 3; emphasis added). Thus personality was for Sullivan (1948a) "the hypothetical entity which we posit to account for interpersonal fields" (p. 6).

METAPSYCHOLOGICAL CONSIDERATIONS: II. THE INDIVIDUAL AND SOCIETY

In addition to emphasizing dyadic interpersonal force fields, Sullivan placed a heavy emphasis upon the cultural and societal contexts in which these interactions occur, in light of the new perspectives on the relation between the individual and society that were emerging in the fields of psychiatry, sociology, and cultural anthropology during the 1920s and 1930s. Although acknowledging the discoveries of Freud (e.g., Breuer & Freud, 1893–1895) as providing the initial impetus for his own investigations, Sullivan (1953b, pp. 16–26) also acknowledged the influence of three additional "tributaries" outside the psychoanalytic tradition: (1) the emphasis upon the integrated psychobiological *individual* as the central unit of study (Meyer, 1907; White, 1922); (2) the emphasis upon the *reflected appraisals* of significant others as determinants of the individual's self-view (Cooley, 1930; Mead, 1934); and (3) the emphases upon the potency of *culture* in shaping individual lives (Benedict, 1934; Lapsley, 1999; Sullivan, 1948b) and upon the importance of *language* within both interpersonal and cultural contexts (Sapir, 1935).

The Metaconcepts of Agency and Communion

Because of its origins in the conceptualizations of Sullivan, the interpersonal paradigm of personality assessment is best understood as a broadly based interdisciplinary effort to understand the individual in relation to society. For that reason, it is helpful to summarize the conceptual foundations of this paradigm with reference to the manner in which David Bakan's (1966) meta-concepts of "agency" and "communion" may be applied to related conceptualizations within a variety of disciplines, as outlined in Table 2.1.

"Agency" refers to the condition of being a differentiated individual, and it is manifested in strivings for mastery and power, which enhance and protect that differentiation. "Communion" refers to the condition of being part of a larger social or spiritual entity, and it is manifested in strivings for intimacy, union, and solidarity within that larger entity. These two "meta-concepts" (concepts about concepts) underlie—at different levels, in different ways, and in different disciplines—the distinctions made in the rows of Table 2.1.

Conceptions of Agency and Communion within Disciplines

Hogan (1996) considered it axiomatic that "people always live in groups, [that] every group has a status hierarchy [and that] people need social acceptance—which facilitates group living and enhances individual survival" (p. 165). Redfield (1960) considered "getting a living" and "getting along" to be the common challenges provided by all societies. The classic distinction between "instrumental" and "expressive" roles in society was made by Parsons and Bales (1955) with reference to the division of labor required to meet these two challenges. From an evolutionary perspective, successful competition for a reproductive advantage over members of one's own sex requires the negotiation of status hierachies (for men) and the formation of reciprocal alliances (for women) (Buss, 1991). From cross-cultural psychology, we know that "individualistic" cultures are those in which personal goals are pursued that benefit individuals, and that "collectivist" cultures are those in which collective goals (ones that benefit the group) are pursued (Triandis, 1990).

Psychodiagnostic work within the interpersonal paradigm focuses upon the recurrent interpersonal situations that characterize the life of an individual. It is assumed that the agentic and communal challenges of group living are reflected in the character and quality of an individual's pattern of dyadic interactions as well. Thus Sullivan (1948a) maintained that interpersonal transactions are motivated primarily by the desire to avoid anxiety due to loss of self-esteem (agency), and by the desire for interpersonal security (communion). Baumeister's (1990) more recent version of this dynamic distinguishes different forms of "social exclusion" that may give rise to agentic and communal anxiety (see Wiggins & Trapnell, 1996).

The social exchange theory of Foa and Foa (1974) defines "status" (esteem, regard) and "love" (acceptance, liking) as the principal interpersonal resources that are exchanged (given or denied) in interpersonal transactions. For example, a dominant individual tends to grant love and status to

TABLE 2.1. Conceptual Foundations of the Interpersonal Paradigm

	Agency	Communion	Discipline	Author
Group living	Hierarchical organization	Group cohesiveness	Personality psychology	Hogan (1996)
Common challenges	Getting a living	Getting along	Anthropology	Redfield (1960)
Division of labor	Instrumental roles	Expressive roles	Sociology	Parsons and Bales (1955)
Reproductive problems	Negotiating status hierarchies	Forming reciprocal alliances	Evolutionary psychology	Buss (1991)
Cultural alternatives	Individualism	Collectivism	Cross-cultural psychology	Triandis (1990)
Psychodynamic goals	Self-esteem	Security	Psychiatry	Sullivan (1953b)
Social exclusion	Agentic anxiety	Communal anxiety	Social psychology	Baumeister (1990)
Resource exchange	Status	Love	Social psychology	Foa and Foa (1974)
Interpersonal coordinates	Dominance	Affiliation	Clinical psychology	Leary (1957)

self, and to grant love but *not* status to others. This explicit theory of social exchange allows one to predict the empirical interrelations among interpersonal dispositions (e.g., dominance, hostility) in terms of the similarity of resource patterns among different dispositional variables (Foa, 1965). When the intercorrelations among dispositional variables are subjected to a principal-components analysis, a two-dimensional circular structure emerges, the coordinates of which were first labeled "dominance" and "affiliation" (Leary, 1957). Although the interpersonal circumplex was originally seen as a convenient scheme for classifying interpersonal dispositions (LaForge, 1977), it is now regarded by many as providing both the conceptual and empirical foundations of the interpersonal paradigm of personality assessment.

THE INTERPERSONAL CIRCUMPLEX

Louis Guttman and the Structure of Mental Abilities

Guttman's (1954) "radex" model was developed in the context of data on human abilities, in which various tests of ability were conceived of as differing along the two dimensions of complexity and kind. The vertical dimension, called a "simplex," orders tests in terms of increasing complexity, as would be found in tests of addition, subtraction, multiplication, and division. Thus, for example, abilities at a higher order of complexity (e.g., division) presuppose or include abilities at lower orders of complexity (addition, subtraction, multiplication). One must be able to add in order to learn subtraction; one must understand multiplication in order to grasp division. The simplex model is perhaps most familiar in the context of attitude measurement, in which "Guttman scales" are frequently employed. These scales have the property that endorsement of an item at a given level of intensity entails endorsement of all items at lower levels of intensity.

Guttman's (1954) horizontal dimension is called a "circumplex," and it describes the circular ordering that exists within tests of different content at the same level of complexity. Thus one may select a test of verbal ability, a test of numerical ability, and a test of spatial ability, all of which are at the same level of difficulty or complexity:

> The new hypothesis is that the different kinds of abilities should have an order among themselves, but not of such a nature that there is a ranking from highest to lowest. Is it possible to have an ordering without a head and foot to it? Yes, quite simply, by having it *circular*. Then the order has neither beginning nor end. . . . A system of variables which has a circular law of order is a circumplex. (p. 325; emphasis in original)

Guttman did not himself apply the circumplex model to interpersonal behavior. But the model was "waiting in the wings" for another discovery that was made in a quite different context.

The Kaiser Foundation Group and the Structure of Interpersonal Behavior

We can safely conclude that the use of objective systems of this sort for categorizing interpersonal behavior will make public, reliable, and communicable the complexities of human relationship which have previously remained intuitive, subjective, and speculative.
                                                                —LEARY (1950, p. 77)

In 1947, a University of California faculty member (Hubert Coffey) and three graduate students (Mervin Freedman, Timothy Leary, and Abel Ossorio) initiated a psychodiagnostic investigation of patients who were undergoing group psychotherapy at a Unitarian church in Berkeley (Coffey, Freedman, Leary, & Ossorio, 1950). The same team later studied psychiatric patients in group psychotherapy at the Kaiser Foundation Hospital in Oakland, California (Leary, 1957). Direct observations of interpersonal behavior in group psychotherapy, individual interviews, and a broad array of psychodiagnostic testing procedures were all employed in "an attempt at systematization and operational definition of the concepts of Harry Stack Sullivan" (Freedman, 1985, p. 623). In seeking to understand the interrelations among the many different kinds of ratings obtained in this study, the investigators noticed some interesting psycholinguistic features of the ratings:

> . . . what you actually *do* in the social situation as described by a verb (e.g., *help*) can be related to your description of yourself as described by the attribute *helpful* and to your description of your dream-self or fantasy-self (also attributive, *helpful* or perhaps *unhelpful*). (Leary, 1957, p. 63; emphasis in original)

This principle of psychological synonymy was useful in reducing a list of several hundred terms to a list of 16 "generic interpersonal themes" (Leary, 1957, pp. 62–66).

From its inception, the Kaiser Foundation study included a large number of personality variables, of which 16 were eventually emphasized. These variables were measured from a variety of perspectives—a procedure that would later be called "multitrait–multimethod" (Campbell & Fiske, 1959). The challenge was to find a common structural model that would permit meaningful comparisons both within and between methods of measurement. In the construction and conceptualization of rating scales, Leary originally had a quasi-circular model in mind (LaForge, 1985, p. 615), but the circular model that was eventually decided upon was done so on the basis of empirical data: "A close-fought battle with empirical fact, not lofty considerations of symmetry, produced the sixteen categories. In the closing stages, the circle emerged" (LaForge, 1977, p. 8). However, once the model appeared, Leary (1957) was able to state clearly the basic conceptual assumptions that have guided all subsequent work within the interpersonal paradigm:

> In surveying the list of more or less generic interpersonal trends, it became clear that all had reference to a *power* or *affiliation* factor. When dominance–submission was taken as the vertical axis and hostility–affection as the horizontal, all of the other generic interpersonal factors could be expressed as combinations of these four *nodal points*. The various types of nurturant behavior appeared to be *blends* of strong and affectionate orientations toward others. Distrustful behaviors seemed to blend hostility and weakness. (p. 26; emphasis added)

Classification of Interpersonal Behavior

Leary's (1957) description of the circular model (presented in Figure 2.1) provides a prescient summary of some of the major conceptual and empiri-

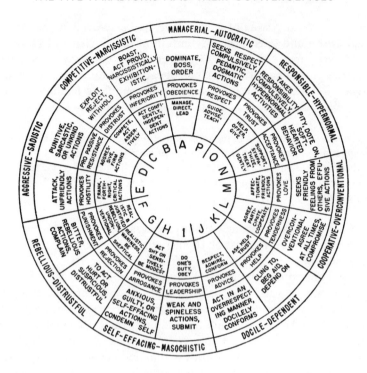

FIGURE 2.1. Leary's conception of the interpersonal circle. From Leary (1957, p. 65). Copyright 1957 by Ronald Press. Reprinted by permission.

cal issues that have come to be associated with contemporary circumplex measurement of interpersonal behavior; it also provides an introduction to some notational and terminological conventions that have since become standard. I first consider Leary's description of the contents of this figure, and then elaborate on their implications for interpersonal assessment.

1. In the inner ring of this circle, the 16 generic interpersonal themes are assigned alphabetic designations in a counterclockwise direction: P, A, B, C . . . O.

2. Moving outward to the next ring, we find the characteristic "mechanisms" or "reflexes" (traits) associated with each 16th (e.g., P = guide, advise, teach; A = manage, direct, lead).

3. The next outer layer specifies the reaction that is provoked in others by these mechanisms (e.g., P provokes respect; A provokes obedience).

4. The next layer illustrates extreme or rigid expression of mechanisms (e.g., extreme P = seeks respect compulsively, pedantic, dogmatic actions; extreme A = dominate, boss, order).

5. In the outermost layer, the categories have been combined into eight sectors: PA, BC, ... NO. The label of each "octant" reflects, successively, the adaptive and maladaptive forms of each mechanism: PA, Managerial–Autocratic; BC, Competitive–Narcissistic; ... NO, Responsible–Hypernormal.

I now elaborate on each of these points:

1. The issue with respect to the 16 generic interpersonal themes designated by the category labels in the inner ring of the circle is whether or not they constitute a "basic level" of categorization. A basic level is one in which the categories carry the most information, possess the highest cue validity, and are most clearly differentiated from one another (Rosch, Mervis, Gray, Johnson, & Boyes-Braem, 1976; Wiggins, 1980a). Leary (1957) clearly opted for an 8-category system (PA, BC, ... NO), whereas LaForge (1977) just as clearly preferred a 16-category system (P, A, ... O). The number of categories employed in interpersonal circumplex interpretation has varied from 4 (Carson, 1969a) to 36 (Benjamin, 1974), and the optimal number of categories depends very much on the substantive domain being scaled and on the discriminative capabilities of the raters and respondents.

2. In the recent history of personality psychology, concepts of "traits" and "motives" have increasingly converged (Winter & Barenbaum, 1999).

3. Sullivan's notion of "complementarity" in interpersonal relationships is based on the notion that certain patterns of response tend to "elicit" predictable responses in others, based on their respective locations within the interpersonal circle. These responses may or may not be desirable for the relationship.

4. The assumption that abnormal or "disordered" behavior is an exaggeration of normal adaptive behavior is axiomatic in the interpersonal paradigm.

5. These labels provide dimensional descriptions of the preceding point. Thus "Managerial" is used to describe the adaptive and effective expression of strength and leadership in interpersonal situations, whereas "Autocratic" describes the domineering, overambitious, and maladaptive expression of the same trait.

6. Virtually all types of interpersonal relatedness are included somewhere within the interpersonal circle. All forms of relating to one another can be represented in terms of the two fundamental dimensions of agency and communion that define the interpersonal circle.

HISTORICAL DEVELOPMENT
OF THE INTERPERSONAL PARADIGM

The conceptual and empirical results of the Kaiser Foundation research project first appeared in a series of doctoral dissertations from the University of California (Freedman, 1950; LaForge, 1952; Leary, 1950; Ossorio, 1950). These results were soon published in a series of classic papers on the interpersonal dimension of personality (Freedman, Leary, Ossorio, & Coffey, 1951; LaForge, Leary, Naboisek, Coffey, & Freedman, 1954; LaForge & Suczek, 1955), followed shortly thereafter by Leary's (1957) canonical formulation of the interpersonal paradigm in personality assessment. It is difficult to overestimate the achievements of the originators of the interpersonal paradigm. Within a decade, the basic concepts of Sullivan had been successfully operationalized with reference to a two-dimensional circumplex model. Within this model of interpersonal behaviors and dispositions, patterns of dyadic interactions could be understood at several different levels of measurement. Given these achievements, and the posthumous publication of Sullivan's major works during the same decade (Sullivan, 1953a, 1953b, 1954, 1956), one might have reasonably anticipated a groundswell of interest in this promising new paradigm for personality assessment in the decades that followed.

For a variety of personal reasons, the originators of the interpersonal paradigm chose not to continue their project: " . . . the conspicuous lack of implementation of the original scheme for systematization suggest[s] that the system is in danger of 'dropping out' along with its celebrated principal investigator" (Wiggins, 1968, p. 322). As is well known, in 1960 Leary ingested a "magic mushroom" that changed his life and the lives of a substantial number of others during the 1960s and 1970s (Leary, 1983). The coincident rediscovery of behaviorism within clinical psychology, attacks on the psychometric-trait viewpoint (e.g., Mischel, 1968), and a focus upon mechanistic models of person–situation interaction all contributed further to an atmosphere that was inhospitable to the further development of the interpersonal paradigm. Nevertheless, the interpersonal paradigm remained viable during the ensuing four decades— not as the result of the intensive efforts of a single research team, but as a more broadly based enterprise involving collaboration among a much larger group of investigators, many of whom were not personally acquainted with one another (Wiggins, 1985).

Ten years after the first interpersonal circumplex was described (Freedman et al., 1951), Foa (1961) noted a convergence of thinking among several investigators with respect to the circumplex as a common structural representation of interpersonal behavior. Two decades later, I was able (Wiggins, 1982) to identify 20 circumplex models that had been independently constructed, all of which employed agentic and communal axes. By 1996, Kiesler was able to identify 21 different domains or content areas in which comparable two-dimensional circular representations had been reported (e.g., parent–child interactions, vocational behavior).

Notable contributions during the 1960s included the conceptualization of both maternal and child behavior within an interpersonal circumplex framework (Schaefer, 1961); a psychometrically sophisticated replication of the circumplex within a clinical population (Lorr & McNair, 1963); and a highly influential integration of the circumplex with the clinical, social, and experimental psychology of that time (Carson, 1969a). Alternative conceptual formulations of the interpersonal model were presented in the 1970s (e.g., Benjamin, 1974; Kiesler, 1979; Wiggins, 1979), and during the 1980s, the model was applied to psychotherapy (e.g., Anchin & Kiesler, 1982), complementarity (e.g., Kiesler, 1983), and interpersonal problems (e.g., Horowitz, Rosenberg, Baer, Ureno, & Villasenor, 1988). Among the contributions of the 1990s were an updated and psychometrically sound version of the original interpersonal checklist (Wiggins, 1995), a comprehensive exposition of contemporary interpersonal theory and research (Kiesler, 1996), and a presentation of the impressive variety of contexts in which the interpersonal circumplex model has been applied (Plutchik & Conte, 1997).

In 1994, a symposium in honor of Timothy Leary was held at the annual meeting of the American Psychological Association, at which many of the aforementioned authors paid tribute to the originator of the interpersonal paradigm (see Strack, 1996). On this occasion—his first attendance at a meeting of the Association in 30 years—Leary remarked: "I must say that I do not take it personally. All of us involved in this project are celebrating ourselves and our charming underground community of dedicated interpersonal researchers" (Leary, 1996, p. 301).

REPRESENTATIVE ASSESSMENT INSTRUMENTS

Interpersonal Adjective Scales

The Interpersonal Adjective Scales (IAS; Wiggins, 1995) evolved from a psychological taxonomy of trait-descriptive terms that was developed within the framework of a larger program of collaborative research on language and personality (Goldberg, 1977). Within a representative pool of trait-descriptive adjectives selected from an unabridged dictionary, an "interpersonal domain" was distinguished from other domains, such as characterological, temperamental, and cognitive domains (Wiggins, 1979). Approximately 800 interpersonal adjectives were assigned to Leary's (1957) original categories of the interpersonal circumplex on both conceptual and empirical grounds. By means of computer-based multivariate procedures, it was found that scales based on the original categories failed to meet certain circumplex criteria that could be better met with scales based on the revised categories that now constitute the IAS (Wiggins, 1995). The IAS consists of 64 adjectives that respondents rate for self-descriptive accuracy on an 8-point Likert scale ranging from "extremely inaccurate" to "extremely accurate." Eight scales, of eight items each, assess the interpersonal dispositions listed in the second column of Table 2.2. For example, the PA octant includes items such as "dominant," "forceful," and "assertive."

Inventory of Interpersonal Problems

Horowitz (1979) transcribed statements of problems expressed by psychiatric outpatients in the course of videotaped intake interviews. In classifying these statements, a distinction was made between interpersonal problems (e.g., "It is hard for me to let other people know when I am angry") and noninterpersonal problems (e.g., "I have difficulty falling asleep at night"). The interpersonal problems were further subdivided into those involving inhibition ("It is hard for me to . . . ") and those involving excess ("I . . . too much"). The resultant statements were employed as items in the construction of the Inventory of Interpersonal Problems (IIP). This inventory requires respondents to indicate the extent to which each of 127 statements is problematic on a 5-point Likert scale ranging from "not at all" to "extremely" (Horowitz et al., 1988).

We (Alden, Wiggins, & Pincus, 1990) developed a Circumplex version of Horowitz's inventory (IIP-C) consisting of eight scales, with eight items each, that assess the interpersonal problems listed in the third column of Table 2.2. The PA scale includes such items as "I try to control other people too much." The IIP has more recently become available as a commercial

TABLE 2.2. Octant Scales from Four Interpersonal Assessment Instruments

	Interpersonal Adjective Scales (IAS)	Inventory of Interpersonal Problems (IIP)	Impact Message Inventory (IMI)	Support Actions Scale—Circumplex (SAS-C)
PA	Assured–Dominant	Domineering	Dominant	Directive
BC	Arrogant–Calculating	Vindictive	Hostile–Dominant	Arrogant
DE	Cold-hearted	Cold	Hostile	Critical
FG	Aloof–Introverted	Socially Avoidant	Hostile–Submissive	Distancing
HI	Unassured–Submissive	Nonassertive	Submissive	Avoidant
JK	Unassuming–Ingenuous	Exploitable	Friendly–Submissive	Deferential
LM	Warm–Agreeable	Overly Nurturant	Friendly	Nurturant
NO	Gregarious–Extraverted	Intrusive	Friendly–Dominant	Engaging

test (Horowitz, Alden, Wiggins, & Pincus, 2000) that has been standardized on a representative U.S. sample of 800 adults. In its 64-item version (IIP-64), this instrument is identical to the IIP-C (Alden et al., 1990), which had been previously demonstrated to be a promising clinical instrument (e.g., Gurtman, 1995; Wiggins & Trobst, 1997a). The new manual (Horowitz et al., 2000) reports additional evidence of the clinical utility of the IIP-64.

Impact Message Inventory

The Impact Message Inventory (IMI; Kiesler, 1987; Kiesler & Schmidt, 1993) is a highly original and promising method of assessment that is based on Kiesler's (1988) theory of interpersonal communication in psychotherapy. The theory postulates that disordered individuals are unaware of the unintended, inappropriate, and ambiguous messages they repetitively "send" to others, and that they are thereby confused and distressed by the pattern of negative responses they consistently evoke or "pull" from others. The IMI attempts to identify the location within the interpersonal circumplex of these patterns of negative response evoked in *others*, as a means of gaining insight into a client's maladaptive transactional behavior. This instrument has been the focus of a considerable amount of empirical research (Kiesler, 2001).

Items were generated from a content analysis of free responses to 15 interpersonal vignettes that described characters enacting 15 different interpersonal styles, similar to those found in the second column of Table 2.2. Respondents were asked to imagine themselves in the company of each of these characters and to record their covert reactions using the stem *"He makes me feel . . . "*. Content analysis of responses suggested three categories of covert reaction: (1) direct feelings, (2) action tendencies, and (3) perceived evoking messages. The Octant Version of the IMI (Kiesler & Schmidt, 1993) consists of six items for each of the target stimuli listed in the fourth column of Table 2.2. For each octant, there are two items for each of the three categories of covert reaction to the target stimulus. Thus the PA scale includes two items each for direct feelings (e.g., "bossed around"), action tendencies (e.g., "I want to tell him to give someone else a chance to make a decision"), and perceived evoking messages (e.g., "He thinks he's always in control of things"). Respondents (e.g., a psychotherapist) are asked to imagine themselves in the company of a particular person (e.g., a psychotherapy patient) and to indicate the extent to which they experience the covert reactions on a 4-point scale. Covert reactions to a target person (e.g., feeling "bossed around") are thus revealing of the personality of that target person (e.g., rigidly dominant [PA]).

Support Actions Scale—Circumplex

The Support Actions Scale—Circumplex (SAS-C; Trobst, 1999, 2000) is an individual-differences measure of dispositions to provide (or not to provide) esteem (status) and emotional (love) support to those in need of help or assistance. On the basis of the general logic of the interpersonal circumplex and the facet-analytic theory of Foa and Foa (1974), three expert judges devised items to measure the postulated eight categories of support listed in the final column of Table 2.2 (Trobst, 2000). Representative items include the following: PA, "Give advice"; BC, "Persuade them to change their behavior"; DE, "Remind them that whining doesn't help"; FG, "Remain detached while listening to their problem"; HI, "Avoid being directive"; JK, "Not argue with them"; LM, "Give them a hug"; and NO, "Check up on them frequently." Successive pools of these items were administered to samples of undergraduates with instructions to rate, on a 7-point Likert scale, the degree to which they characteristically or typically performed these actions when a friend or family member was in need of support. The resultant circumplex structure of the SAS-C is comparable to the best structures reported in the literature. The SAS-C has been used in the study of physically ill recipients of social support and their support providers, and has been found to be related to personality characteristics (Trobst, 2000) and marital satisfaction (e.g., Trobst & Hemphill, 2000).

INTERPRETIVE PRINCIPLES

Among the most valuable features of the circumplex model is the opportunity it provides for interpreting interpersonal variables with reference to the geometric properties of a circle (LaForge et al., 1954). The variables of traditional multiscale inventories are typically displayed as "factor lists" (Hogan, 1983), in which the ordering and interrelations among variables lack both conceptual and interpretive significance. In contrast, the trigonometric procedures that can be applied to the variables of an interpersonal circumplex permit descriptions and diagnostic inferences that cannot be generated from traditional scale analyses (Wiggins, Phillips, & Trapnell, 1989).

Some general principles of circumplex interpretation may be illustrated with reference to the IAS profile of a 33-year-old male bank manager displayed in Figure 2.2. At the bottom of the figure are T-scores on the octant variables, expressed with reference to an appropriate normative group (Wiggins, 1995, pp. 70–71). These scores have been plotted on shaded sectors of the circle, and they are interpreted as representing eight vectors in two-dimensional space. The mean or "average directionality" of these vectors is of critical diagnostic significance, because it determines the typo-

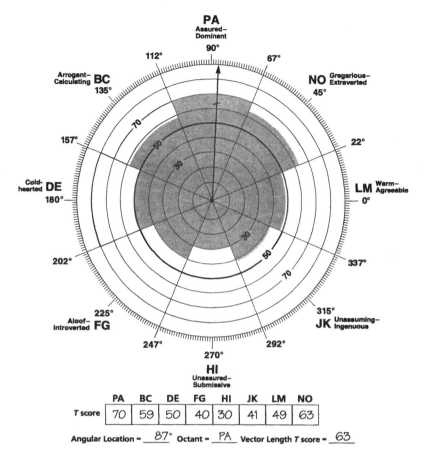

	PA	BC	DE	FG	HI	JK	LM	NO
T score	70	59	50	40	30	41	49	63

Angular Location = __87°__ Octant = __PA__ Vector Length T score = __63__

FIGURE 2.2. IAS profile of a 33-year-old male bank manger. Adapted and reproduced by special permission of the Publisher, Psychological Assessment Resources, Inc., 16204 North Florida Avenue, Lutz, FL 33549, from the Interpersonal Adjective Scales—Revised, by Jerry S. Wiggins. Copyright 1995 by PAR, Inc. Further reproduction is prohibited without permission from PAR, Inc.

logical category to which this man will be assigned. By trigonometric procedures, this average directionality was determined to be 87°, which falls near the midpoint of the Assured–Dominant (PA) category. This angular location is considered to be representative of individuals classified as pure PA "types." Had the location been at 110°, a more hostile manifestation of dominance (BC) would have been suggested; had it been at 65°, a more affiliative expression of dominance (NO) would have been suggested.

The general shape of the profile in Figure 2.2 closely resembles the "characteristic configuration" of IAS profiles, which is found in the average profiles of subjects in all IAS typological groups (Wiggins et al., 1989). The characteristic configuration of an IAS profile is one in which the principal elevation occurs on the defining octant (in this case, PA), with secondary and approximately equal elevations occurring on adjacent octants (BC and NO), and diminishing and approximately equal elevations occurring on subsequent pairs of octants (DE and LM, FG and JK), down to a highly truncated "opposite" (to the principal) octant (HI). Thus, across interpersonal situations, we would expect this man to behave frequently in a forceful, assertive, dominant, and self-confident manner (PA); to behave somewhat less frequently in aggressive (BC) and gregarious (NO) ways; to behave seldom, if ever, in a submissive (HI) fashion; and so forth.

The "vector length" of an interpersonal profile is a measure of "deviance" in both a statistical and a psychiatric sense. In the former sense, vector length is the standard deviation of the eight interpersonal variables, which indicates the "intensity" or clarity with which a pattern of interpersonal behavior is expressed. In the latter sense, high-variance profiles are found most often in psychiatric groups. The length of the arrow indicating angular location in Figure 2.2 is the vector length of the profile, which is approximately 1.6 standard deviations above that of the normative group. This would suggest that the pattern of interpersonal behaviors described above would be expressed vigorously, although not necessarily rigidly or intemperately.

Once it has been established that this individual's profile is representative of those obtained by Assured–Dominant (PA) types, and that this pattern of behavior is expressed in a differentiated fashion, interpretation proceeds with reference to the empirical literature of the interpersonal paradigm that has examined both the PA dimension and the characteristics of PA types (e.g., Kiesler, 1996). This would include the literatures of other circumplex instruments that have studied this dimension in such contexts as interpersonal problems (the IIP-C) and impact messages (the IMI).

DEFINING AND EVALUATING
CIRCUMPLEX STRUCTURE

A circumplex structure can be defined and evaluated by a number of different but complementary methods. Guttman (1954) originally defined the circumplex as a particular *pattern* of correlations when he demonstrated that the intercorrelations of tests of mental abilities have this distinctive pattern. In the same year, LaForge and colleagues (1954) independently identified "a two-dimensional array in ordinary Euclidian space [in which] conventional trigonometric and analytic formulas relate . . . the variables" (p. 140). More recent accounts have emphasized the two principal components that underlie the intercorrelations among interpersonal variables (e.g., Wiggins, Steiger, & Gaelick, 1981). That these two principal components clearly reflect the metaconcepts of agency (power, control, dominance) and communion (intimacy, nurturance, love) has allowed for an unusually close relationship between theory and measurement in the interpersonal paradigm (Wiggins, 1991). This close relationship makes it possible to introduce the variables of the paradigm and their underlying measurement model at the same time.

Principal-Components Representation

Figure 2.3 illustrates the circumplex formed by a principal-components analysis[1] of the intercorrelations among the eight scales of the IAS (Wiggins, 1995) in a sample of 2,988 university students. The IAS scales were constructed according to the general logic of the classification scheme employed by the Kaiser Foundation group (see Figure 2.1), although a number of substantive modifications were made in light of empirical findings (Wiggins, 1979). One advantage of principal-components analysis is that it presents a clear picture of the extent to which the scales of a given circumplex measure conform to the underlying logic of the interpersonal circumplex. Thus the first principal component is clearly defined by the LM octant at one end and the DE octant at the other; the second principal component is equally well defined at the poles of the orthogonal PA–HI coordinate. The eight variables (octants) can be seen to be evenly spaced around the circle formed by these coordinates of nurturance (horizontal) and dominance (vertical). This finding is compatible with the assumption that the off-quadrant variables of BC, FG, JK, and NO may be interpreted as "blends" of the two principal components; for example, JK is a blend of warmth and submissiveness, and NO is a blend of dominance and warmth.

Correlational Representation

The location of the eight variables in Figure 2.3 is determined by their correlations with one another, which conform to an expected pattern. Thus the Assured–Dominant (PA) variable is strongly *negatively* correlated with the Unassured–Submissive (HI) variable, which lies at the opposite pole of the vertical axis. The PA variable is *uncorrelated* with both the Cold-hearted (DE) and Warm–Agreeable (LM) variables, which are aligned at right angles to the dominance axis. And, as expected, the PA variable is moderately positively correlated with the nearby Arrogant–Calculating (BC) and Gregarious–Extraverted (NO) variables. PA is moderately negatively correlated with the more distant Aloof–Introverted and Unassuming–Ingenuous (JK) variables.

The pattern of correlations just described should hold for *all* of the

---

[1] The essentials of factor analysis are discussed in Chapter 4.

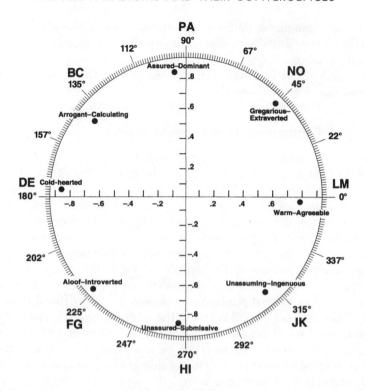

FIGURE 2.3. Circumplex structure of the IAS scales (*n* = 2,988). Adapted and reproduced by special permission of the Publisher, Psychological Assessment Resources, Inc., 16204 North Florida Avenue, Lutz, FL 33549, from the Interpersonal Adjective Scales—Revised, by Jerry S. Wiggins. Copyright 1995 by PAR, Inc. Further reproduction is prohibited without permission from PAR, Inc.

octant variables. That is, there should be strong negative correlations with polar opposite variables; zero correlations with variables at right angles ("orthogonal") to the variable itself; and moderate positive and negative correlations with adjacent and more distant pairs of variables, respectively. Table 2.3 presents the general pattern of intercorrelations among variables within what Guttman (1954) called a "circulant correlation matrix." In that table, the correlation of a variable with itself is assumed to be 1.00, and that value appears in every cell of the principal diagonal. Note also that, in theory, successive diagonals all have the same values, which decrease as indicated by the inequality symbols.

In the IAS data obtained from 2,988 university men and women that formed the basis for Figure 2.3, the obtained correlations in each of the diagonals specified in Table 2.3 were used to obtain ordinary least-squares estimates of population correlation coefficients for elements in each diagonal

TABLE 2.3. Representation of a Circulant Correlation Matrix

Variable	1	2	3	4	5	6	7	8
1	1.00							
2	ρ_1	1.00			where $\rho_1 > \rho_2 > \rho_3 > \rho_4$			
3	ρ_2	ρ_1	1.00					
4	ρ_3	ρ_2	ρ_1	1.00				
5	ρ_4	ρ_3	ρ_2	ρ_1	1.00			
6	ρ_3	ρ_4	ρ_3	ρ_2	ρ_1	1.00		
7	ρ_2	ρ_3	ρ_4	ρ_3	ρ_2	ρ_1	1.00	
8	ρ_1	ρ_2	ρ_3	ρ_4	ρ_3	ρ_2	ρ_1	1.00

Note. From Wiggins, Steiger, and Gaelick (1981, p. 267). Copyright 1981 by Lawrence Erlbaum Associates, Inc. Reprinted by permission.

(Steiger, 1980). These population correlation coefficient estimates are presented in Table 2.4.

One method for evaluating the circumplexity of a measuring instrument is that of comparing the estimated population correlation matrix with the empirical correlation matrix obtained within a given sample of respondents (Wiggins et al., 1981). The empirical correlation matrix obtained from the Wiggins (1995) study of university students is shown in Table 2.5. Subtraction of the elements in Table 2.5 from those in Table 2.4 yields a residual correlation matrix that indicates the differences between the obtained correlation matrix and the estimated population correlation matrix. As can be seen from inspection, these differences are small; their absolute mean value is .04 (Wiggins, 1995).

TABLE 2.4. Estimated Population Correlation Coefficients for IAS Data

Variable	PA	BC	DE	FG	HI	JK	LM	NO
PA	1.00							
BC	.42	1.00			where .42 > .03 > −.36 > −.73			
DE	.03	.42	1.00					
FG	−.36	.03	.42	1.00				
HI	−.73	−.36	.03	.42	1.00			
JK	−.36	−.73	−.36	.03	.42	1.00		
LM	.03	−.36	−.73	−.36	.03	.42	1.00	
NO	.42	.03	−.36	−.73	−.36	.03	.42	1.00

Note. From Wiggins (1995, p. 48). Adapted and reproduced by special permission of the Publisher, Psychological Assessment Resources, Inc., 16204 North Florida Avenue, Lutz, FL 33549, from the Interpersonal Adjective Scales—Revised, by Jerry S. Wiggins. Copyright 1995 by PAR, Inc. Further reproduction is prohibited without permission from PAR, Inc.

TABLE 2.5. Obtained Correlation Coefficients for IAS Data

Variable	PA	BC	DE	FG	HI	JK	LM	NO
PA	1.00							
BC	.39	1.00						
DE	.14	.49	1.00					
FG	−.33	.09	.46	1.00				
HI	−.71	−.24	.00	.50	1.00			
JK	−.44	−.75	−.34	.04	.40	1.00		
LM	.08	−.32	−.70	−.36	.11	.31	1.00	
NO	.42	.01	−.37	−.78	−.45	−.03	.43	1.00

Note. From Wiggins (1995, p. 48). Adapted and reproduced by special permission of the Publisher, Psychological Assessment Resources, Inc., 16204 North Florida Avenue, Lutz, FL 33549, from the Interpersonal Adjective Scales—Revised, by Jerry S. Wiggins. Copyright 1995 by PAR, Inc. Further reproduction is prohibited without permission from PAR, Inc.

Multiple Perspectives

Principal-components analyses and correlational analyses do not exhaust the available methods for defining and evaluating circumplexity. In recent years, a number of new methods for evaluating circumplexity have been introduced (e.g., Browne, 1992; Browne & Cudeck, 1992; Davison, 1994; Fabrigar, Visser, & Browne, 1997; Gurtman, 1994; Tracey & Rounds, 1997); these differ in the ways in which a circumplex is defined and evaluated. In light of these differences in conceptualization and analysis, Gurtman and Pincus (2000) have suggested that multiple perspectives be applied in a given circumplex analysis, in order to more fully understand the specific strengths and weaknesses of the measures under investigation. Their own analyses are particularly germane to the present discussion, because they applied three quite different methods of circumplex evaluation to the IAS data set based on 2,988 students that we have been considering. The methods described by Gurtman and Pincus and applied to the IAS data set were the spatial representation model (Shepard, 1978), the circulant correlation model (Wiggins et al., 1981), and the "circular-order" model of analysis developed by Tracey and Rounds (1997). This last model involves highly fine-tuned criteria of circumplexity:

> As applied to the IAS, perfect fit to the circular model requires that (a) correlations of scales adjacent on the circle (e.g., Assured–Dominant [PA] and Arrogant–Calculating [BC]) be of greater magnitude than are correlations for scales more than one step away, (b) correlations of scales two steps apart on the circle (e.g., PA and Cold-hearted [DE]) be greater than for scales more than two steps apart (e.g., PA and Aloof–Introverted [FG]) and (c) correlations of scales three steps (e.g., PA and FG) away exceed those for

scales opposite on the circle (e.g., PA and Unassured–Submissive [HI]). For an 8 × 8 matrix of correlations, the test of the circular order model would involve 288 order predictions, each involving a comparison between two correlations. (Gurtman & Pincus, 2000, pp. 378–379)

Although this is a rather stringent set of structural criteria, all 288 of these predictions were confirmed in the IAS data set.

CLASSIFICATION OF PERSONALITY SCALES WITH THE INTERPERSONAL CIRCUMPLEX

I originally developed the IAS as a theory-driven taxonomy for the classification of trait descriptive adjectives within the interpersonal domain (Wiggins, 1979). The longer-range goal of this research was to provide a taxonomic framework within which we could classify some of the literally hundreds of personality scales that have been developed within the fields of personality, social, and clinical psychology. During the subsequent decade, various scales and inventories believed to be "interpersonal" in nature were administered, along with the IAS, to approximately 2,000 university students (Wiggins & Broughton, 1991).

The manner in which we determined what Gurtman (1991) has called the "interpersonalness" of a given personality scale can be understood with reference to Figure 2.4. Assume that a particular personality scale has been administered to a group of respondents, along with the IAS. The scale of interest is scored, as are the eight octants of the IAS, which are expressed as standard scores. The next step is to compute factor scores for each respondent on the two coordinates of Love (LOV; Factor I) and Dominance (DOM; Factor II). In the case of a well-structured circumplex, such as the IAS, the computation of factor scores is a relatively simple procedure:

LOV = .3[(LM – DE) + .707(NO – BC – FG + JK)]

DOM = .3[(PA – HI) + .707(NO + BC – FG – JK)]

In Figure 2.4, it can be seen that factor scores for both LOV and DOM range from –1 to +1. Each subject has a factor score on LOV (x) a factor score on DOM (y), and a raw score on the outside variable of interest (v). The correlation between x and v gives the distance from the origin of the variable along the horizontal axis ($x = Rxv$); the correlation between y and v locates the variable on the vertical axis ($y = Ryv$). The angular displacement of the variable from the x axis is given by ($\theta = \tan^{-1}(y/x)$, an operation that can be performed on most scientific calculators; this value is referred to as the "angular location" of the outside variable. The length of the vec-

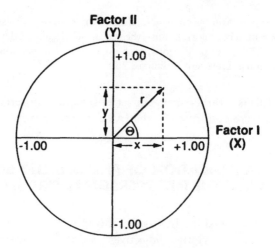

FIGURE 2.4. Projection of an outside variable onto coordinates of the interpersonal circumplex. From Wiggins and Broughton (1991, p. 348). Copyright 1991 by John Wiley and Sons. Reprinted by permission.

tor associated with the outside variable is given by $r = (x^2 + y^2)^{1/2}$; this value is referred to as the "vector length" of the variable.

Our geometric taxonomy of personality scales involved the classification of 172 such scales in terms of their angular location and vector length when projected upon the IAS (Wiggins & Broughton, 1991). The classification was divided into eight sections that reported the angular location and vector length of each projected scale for each of the eight octants of the IAS. A fragment of this taxonomy is illustrated in Table 2.6. The Unassuming–Ingenuous (JK) octant of the IAS occupies a sector ranging from 292° to 337°. In Table 2.6, the angular location of each scale that fell in this sector is displayed, along with the author(s) of the scale, the inventory from which it came, the name given to the scale by its author(s), and the vector length of the scale's projection.

The Unassuming–Ingenuous (JK) scale from the IAS is highlighted to serve as a marker variable for this octant, and it is located at the midpoint of the JK octant (315°) with a substantial vector length (.82). There is considerable convergence among scales from Gough and Heilbrun's Adjective Check List (.76), Campbell's Murray Need Scales (.38), Stern's Activities Index (.29), and Edwards's Personal Preference Schedule (.28) on the common construct of "deference," which is a word that frequently comes to mind with reference to the unassuming–ingenuous individual (Wiggins, 1995, pp. 25–26). The related construct of "abasement" appears in scales from the inventories of Campbell (.41) and Jackson (.27). Less central, but still related to the unassuming–ingenuous personality, are the constructs of

TABLE 2.6. Classification of Personality Scales within the Unassuming–Ingenuous (JK) Octant of the IAS

Angle	Author(s)	Inventory	Scale	Vector length
296°	Edwards (1959)	Personal Preference Schedule	Deference	.26
302°	Campbell (1959)	Murray Need Scales	Deference	.38
—	Jackson (1987)	Personality Research Form	Harm Avoidance	.27
—	Campbell (1959)	Murray Need Scales	Abasement	.41
303°	Gough & Heilbrun (1980)	Adjective Check List	Deference	.76
314°	Jackson (1987)	Personality Research Form	Abasement	.34
315°	**Wiggins (1979)**	**Interpersonal Adjective Scales**	**Unassuming–Ingenuous**	**.82**
318°	Gough & Heilbrun (1980)	Adjective Check List	Self-Control	.55
326°	Stern (1970)	Activities Index	Deference	.29
328°	Strack (1991)	Personality Adjective Check List	Dependent Personality	.35

Note. From Wiggins and Broughton (1991, p. 357). Copyright 1981 by John Wiley and Sons. Reprinted by permission.

"self-control" from the Adjective Check List (.55) and "harm avoidance" from the Personality Research Form (.27).

As we noted in an earlier paper,

> Investigations of the relationships between the IAS and other existing measures from the same (interpersonal) or different domains (e.g., temperament) serve two related purposes: (1) the conceptual meaning of a given measure or set of measures . . . may be clarified by establishing its location within the IAS circumplex space or (2) the nomological network within which the IAS variables are embedded may be enriched by establishing the external correlates of the IAS. (Wiggins & Broughton, 1985, p. 3)

AXIOMS OF CONTEMPORARY INTERPERSONAL THEORY

Contemporary theory and research within the interpersonal paradigm are concerned with a wide range of topics that are approached from a number of somewhat differing viewpoints using different measurement procedures (see Kiesler, 1996). Nevertheless, two widely accepted principles seem to be subscribed to by most, if not all, workers in the field. These principles stem directly from Sullivan's notion of "interpersonal force fields," and from his emphasis on "security" and "self-esteem" as the principal sources of satisfaction in interpersonal relations.

Interpersonal Force Fields

In the following quotations, Kiesler (1996) provides an exceptionally succinct statement of several interrelated principles concerning the dynamics of interpersonal behavior that are central to the interpersonal paradigm:

> *Interpersonal theory asserts that each of us continually exudes a force field that pushes others to respond to us with constricted classes of control and affiliation actions; thereby we pull from others complementary responses designed to affirm and validate our chosen style of living and being.* (p. 85; emphasis in original) . . . The abnormal individual imposes an extreme and intense force field on his or her interpersonal transactions. (p. 128)

Although stated somewhat differently by different interpersonal theorists, the central idea of complementarity here is that during interactions, Person A (perhaps unknowingly) attempts to "elicit" behavior from Person B that is compatible with Person A's preferred definition of an interpersonal situation with respect to the dimensions of control (agency) and affiliation (communion). It has also been suggested that persons tend to elicit behaviors opposite to them on the interpersonal circle when their behavior is within the realm of the dimension of agency (e.g., dominance begets submission, and submission begets dominance), whereas behaviors within the realm of communion tend to elicit similar behaviors (e.g., love begets love, and hate begets hate). For example, Person A may wish to define the situation as one in which Person A him- or herself is important and likeable, and Person B is a likeable but unimportant person. To the extent that Person B responds with behavior that conforms to Person A's definition of the situation, the relationship between Person A and Person B is said to be complementary (Carson, 1979). The strength and determination with which Person A tends to impose his or her force field on all partners at all times is an index of the maladaptive nature of Person A's recurrent patterns of interpersonal situations.

Social Exchange

Whereas the notion of "interpersonal force fields" emphasizes the strength and flexibility of interpersonal transactions, the idea of "social exchange" specifies the *content* of these transactions. Interpersonal transactions may be thought of as occasions for exchange in which participants give social resources to or take them away from each other. Foa and Foa (1974) have provided a theory of social exchange that emphasizes the development of cognitive categories of social perception with respect to directionality (accepting or rejecting), object (self or other), and resource exchanged (love or status). Foa (1965) had earlier applied this facet-analytic approach in a social exchange analysis of Leary's circumplex model of interpersonal behavior. I (Wiggins, 1982) later applied a slightly modified version of Foa's circumplex analysis in the development of the IAS, and this is shown in Table 2.7a.

Although the resources exchanged in interpersonal transactions may include money, goods, services, and information, the resources of status (agency) and love (communion) are considered to be the coins of the realm of interpersonal exchange (Foa & Foa, 1974). In Table 2.7a, the facet elements of giving (+1) and denying (−1) of love and status to self and to other are specified for each of the eight variables of the IAS. Thus the Assured–Dominant (PA) variable is defined as the granting of status and love to self, and the granting of love but *not* status to the other. The Arrogant–Calculating (BC) variable is defined as the granting of status and love to the self, and the denial of both status and love to the other. Examination of the rows of Table 2.7a reveals that each row differs from the preceding row in *one* element (BC differs from PA in not granting love to the other, DE differs from BC in not granting love to self, etc.). Note also that the first variable (PA) and last variable (NO) differ from each other on one element (PA does not grant status to other). To the extent that these facet assignments are in fact true, the relationship among the eight variables will necessarily be circular (Foa, 1965).

When the entries in Table 2.7a are treated as standard scores ($M = 0$, $SD = 1$), the relation between any two variables may be obtained by summing the cross-products of their respective row elements. Thus the relation between PA and BC is $(+1 \times +1) + (+1 \times +1) + (+1 \times -1) + (-1 \times -1) = 2$. The sums of the cross-products for all combinations of the eight variables are presented in Table 2.7b. Dividing the elements in Table 2.7b by the number of "observations" (i.e., 4) yields the correlation matrix shown in Table 2.7c. Extracting and rotating two principal components from this matrix (see Chapter 4) yields the factor matrix in Table 2.7d. Figure 2.5 presents a plot of this solution in which the black squares indicate the location of the eight variables. It can be seen from this figure that the eight variables fall at the center of each of the eight categories and are close to the perimeter of the interpersonal circle. This perfect, evenly spaced circumplex is the standard against which interpersonal assessment instruments are evaluated.

THE NATURE OF INTERPERSONAL SPACE

Although the basic geometry of interpersonal space is well established and may be analyzed by a variety of methods (Gurtman & Pincus, 2000), the

TABLE 2.7. Derivation of the Interpersonal Circumplex

a. Facet composition of interpersonal variables

	Self		Other	
	Status	Love	Love	Status
PA	+1	+1	+1	-1
BC	+1	+1	-1	-1
DE	+1	-1	-1	-1
FG	-1	-1	-1	-1
HI	-1	-1	-1	+1
JK	-1	-1	+1	+1
LM	-1	+1	+1	+1
NO	+1	+1	+1	+1

b. Sums of cross-products (ΣXY)

	PA	BC	DE	FG	HI	JK	LM	NO
PA	4							
BC	2	4						
DE	0	2	4					
FG	-2	0	2	4				
HI	-4	-2	0	2	4			
JK	-2	-4	-2	0	2	4		
LM	0	-2	-4	-2	0	2	4	
NO	2	0	-2	-4	-2	0	2	4

c. Correlation matrix ($\Sigma XY/N$)

	PA	BC	DE	FG	HI	JK	LM	NO
PA	1.00							
BC	.50	1.00						
DE	.00	.50	1.00					
FG	-.50	.00	.50	1.00				
HI	-1.00	-.50	.00	.50	1.00			
JK	-.50	-1.00	-.50	.00	.50	1.00		
LM	.00	-.50	-1.00	-.50	.00	.50	1.00	
NO	.50	.00	-.50	-1.00	-.50	.00	.50	1.00

d. Rotated factor matrix

	I	II	h^2
PA	.92	.00	.85
BC	.65	-.65	.85
DE	.00	-.92	.85
FG	-.65	-.65	.85
HI	-.92	.00	.85
JK	-.65	.65	.85
LM	.00	.92	.85
NO	.65	.65	.85
% variance	42.5%	42.5%	85%

Note. PA, Assured–Dominant; BC, Arrogant–Calculating; DE, Cold-hearted; FG, Aloof–Introverted; HI, Unassured–Submissive; JK, Unassuming–Ingenuous; LM, Warm–Agreeable; NO, Gregarious–Extraverted. Adapted from Wiggins and Trapnell (1996, p. 122). Copyright 1996 by The Guilford Press. Adapted by permission.

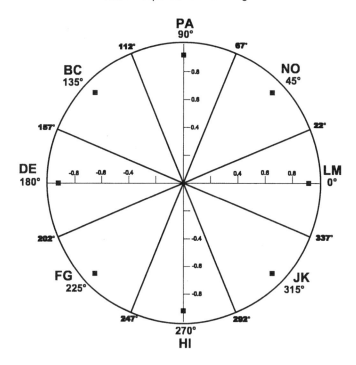

FIGURE 2.5. A plot of the factor matrix solution presented in Table 2.7d, representing ideal circumplex structure.

boundary conditions of its applications are less well established (Wiggins & Trobst, 1997b). In measuring interpersonal dispositions ("traits"), for example, the fit between the circumplex model and interpersonal theory is so close that one can hardly distinguish the theory from the model (Wiggins et al., 1989). But the precise relations between interpersonal dispositional space and the many circumplex structures obtained for other "spaces," such as interpersonal problems (Alden et al., 1990), covert reaction tendencies (Kiesler & Schmidt, 1993), and emotions (e.g., Plutchik, 1997), has only begun to be investigated.

Conceptually, it might be helpful here to think of multiple interpersonal "fields," but the mathematical and empirical work still remains to be done. A recent comparison of two different circumplex spaces suggests that much can be learned from such comparisons. For example, in a recent study, Trobst (2000) examined the relations between interpersonal traits as measured by the IAS and social support behaviors as measured by the SAS-C. When scales from either of these two measures were projected onto the space of the other, the "dominance" axis of the projected measure collapsed. This structural finding suggests that whereas dispositional nurturance (IAS) and nurturant social support style (SAS-C) are closely related, dispositional dominance and dominant social support style are largely unrelated. Additional analyses demonstrated that in comparison with individuals of other personality "types," dispositionally nurturant individuals reported performing more of *all* potentially helpful behaviors, including relatively dominant actions (e.g., giving advice), and less of *all* "unhelpful" behaviors (e.g., reminding them that whining doesn't help). Metaphorically speaking, the "force field" of a social support *context* appears to perturb the usual structure of a dispositional "field."

CLINICAL APPLICATIONS OF THE INTERPERSONAL CIRCUMPLEX

Psychiatric Diagnosis

The recent revival of interest in the application of circumplex models to the formal diagnostic categories of the American Psychiatric Association is not without historical precedent. For many years, the interpersonal paradigm has been recommended either as a *supplement to* the *Diagnostic and Statistical Manual of Disorders* (DSM) criteria (e.g., Benjamin, 1993, 1996; Kiesler, 1986; Leary, 1957; Plutchik & Conte, 1986; Plutchik & Platman, 1977; Wiggins, 1982), or as a *replacement for* that diagnostic system (e.g., Adams, 1964; Carson, 1996; McLemore & Benjamin, 1979). Over 40 years ago, Leary (1957) proposed an equivalence between the typological categories of the circumplex and the diagnostic categories of DSM-I: PA, compulsive personality; BC, narcissistic personality; DE, psychopathic personality; FG, schizoid personality; HI, obsessive personality; JK, dependent personality; LM, hysteric personality; and NO, "hypernormal" (psychosomatic) personality. The categories, labels, and criteria of DSM have changed since that time, as have the descriptive labels attached to interpersonal categories, but Leary's prescience in these matters should be evident.

The definition of the personality disorders in terms of personality traits by the American Psychiatric Association (1980), and the availability of new instruments and techniques for assessing personality disorders, have resulted in an increased understanding of this diagnostic axis. For example, the DSM-III and DSM-III-R personality disorder categories have been shown to be well captured by the two-dimensional structures of the IAS (e.g., Wiggins & Pincus, 1989, 1994) and the IIP-C (e.g., Pincus & Wiggins, 1990; Soldz, Budman, Demby, & Merry, 1993). Similarly, clinicians' ratings of DSM-III personality disorder categories have been found to be well captured by an interpersonal circumplex model (e.g., Blashfield, Sprock, Pinkston, & Hodgin, 1985; Plutchik & Conte, 1986). And Benjamin (1993, 1996) has provided detailed and perceptive descriptions of procedures for the diagnosis of DSM-III-R and DSM-IV personality disorders within the framework of her variant of the interpersonal circumplex model.

Psychotherapy

The interpersonal paradigm originated in the context of psychotherapy and, perhaps more than any other paradigm, has contributed to an understanding of the therapeutic process itself (e.g., Anchin & Kiesler, 1982; Benjamin, 1993, 1996; Kiesler, 1988; Safran & Segal, 1990; Sullivan, 1953b). The most notable contribution of the paradigm to psychotherapy has been the circumplex structural model, which provides a framework for representing dyadic interactions in the therapeutic relationship. A number of different assessment devices based on the interpersonal circumplex, and variants of that model (Benjamin, 1974), have proven useful in studies of psychotherapy process and outcome (Kiesler, 1992). The IIP has been employed in the prediction of response to treatment (Alden & Capreol, 1993; Horowitz, Rosenberg, & Bartholomew, 1993; Mohr et al., 1990), the development of therapeutic alliance (Muran, Segal, Samstag, & Crawford, 1994), and prediction of continuation in psychotherapy (Horowitz et al., 1988).

Henry (1996) has made a case for the Structural Analysis of Social Behavior (Benjamin, 1974) as a common metric for programmatic psychotherapy research. Kiesler, Schmidt, and Wagner (1997) have stressed the conceptual advantages of the IMI in analyzing the psychotherapeutic relationship. And Kiesler (1996) has also emphasized the potential of the revised Check List of Psychotherapy Transactions (Kiesler, Goldston, & Schmidt, 1991) for measuring the interpersonal behavior of interactants in the therapy relationship. In sum, such studies constitute an impressive empirical literature that attests to the heuristic potential of the interpersonal circumplex model in psychotherapy research.

OVERVIEW

The field-theoretical perspective in physics influenced the theoretical formulations of Harry Stack Sullivan, whose interpersonal theory of psychiatry eventually provided the conceptual foundation for the interpersonal paradigm. In the 1950s, Timothy Leary and other members of the Kaiser Foundation research group in Oakland, California, attempted to operationalize Sullivan's ideas with reference to the coding of interpersonal interactions among patients in psychotherapy groups. The system that emerged identified an array of interpersonal behaviors that were ordered in circular fashion around the two coordinates of power and affiliation. Leary's

(1957) seminal formulation of this interpersonal system of personality diagnosis launched the interpersonal paradigm in personality assessment.

As Gurtman (1992) has emphasized, the interpersonal circumplex itself functions as a nomological net within which the construct validity of other interpersonal measures may be evaluated. We (Wiggins & Broughton, 1985, 1991) had similarly emphasized the integrative function of the circumplex model in providing a single framework for interpreting personality scales from a variety of research traditions in personality, clinical, and social psychology. Circumplex representations of the interpersonal field have proven to be of considerable heuristic value in both the conceptualization and measurement of a variety of interpersonal phenomena, as is evident from the approximately 1,000 references that appear in Kiesler's (1996) magisterial survey of that literature. Research topics to which the model has proven particularly applicable include complementarity (e.g., Kiesler, 1983), nonverbal behavior (e.g., Gifford, 1991), manipulation tactics (e.g., Buss, Gomes, Higgins, & Lauterbach, 1987), agentic and communal situations (e.g., Moskowitz, 1994), and attachment styles (e.g., Bartholomew & Horowitz, 1991).

Although Guttman's (1954) circumplex model was originally developed to capture the structure of mental abilities, it has proven especially valuable as a model of interpersonal behaviors. The circumplex has provided both a conceptual and a computational model of interpersonal assessment. In conceptualization, the model may be used to describe the manner in which interpersonal behavior is influenced by the underlying coordinates of agency and communion. In computation, the model permits the rigorous analysis of patterns of both test and person variables in psychodiagnostic work. Although once considered an "underground movement" running counter to the mainstream, the interpersonal paradigm of personality assessment must now be counted among the major paradigms on the contemporary scene.

3

The Personological Paradigm

How shall a psychological life history be written?
—ALLPORT (1967, p. 3)

HISTORICAL OVERVIEW OF THE PERSONOLOGICAL PARADIGM

Dramaturgical Origins of the Paradigm

All the world's a stage,
And all the men and women merely players;
They have their exits and their entrances,
And one man in his time plays many parts.
—SHAKESPEARE, *As You Like It*
(ca. 1599, Act II, Scene 7)

In his classic textbook on personality, Allport (1937) noted that the Latin word *persona* originally denoted the theatrical mask first used in Greek drama and adopted about 100 B.C. by Roman players. Current usage of the word "personality" may be traced to the phrase *per sonare* (to sound through): "According to this theory the term had reference to the large mouth of the mask or perhaps to a reed device inserted into it for projecting the voice of the actor" (Allport, 1937, p. 26). As the English word "personality" evolved over time, a distinction was made between a person as he or she appears to others (the mask) and the "true" personal qualities of the person beneath the mask (the player)—a distinction that has also proved useful in the classification of personality theories (Monte, 1999). In more recent times, the dramaturgical metaphor was employed literally by Goffman (1959) to emphasize that people's everyday behavior in the presence of others involves dramatic performances designed to create a particular impression; this idea has proven fruitful in the sociology of everyday life (e.g., Brissett & Edgley, 1975).[1]

Harold Bloom's (1994) magisterial summary and evaluation of the "Western canon" in literature concludes that William Shakespeare *is* this canon: "Shakespeare . . . had no true precursor in the *creation of character*, except for Chaucerian hints, and has left no one after him untouched by his *ways of representing human nature*" (p. 524; emphasis added). In his more recent book *Shakespeare: The Invention of the Human*, Bloom (1998) has argued that Shakespeare, in effect, "invented" personality as we know it, stating that he

> went beyond all precedents (even Chaucer) and invented the human as we continue to know it. A more conservative way of stating this would seem to me a weak misreading of Shakespeare: it might contend that Shakespeare's originality was in the *representation* of cognition, personality, character. But there is an overflowing element in the plays, an excess beyond representation, that is close to the metaphor we call "creation." (p. xviii; emphasis in original)

Early Modern Period

As the citations in Table Int.3 of the Introduction might suggest, the personological paradigm and the psychodynamic paradigm have common origins. The elaborations of the nature of "character" by Freud (1908) and Abraham (1921) were among the first to suggest a constellation of enduring and determining tendencies that give rise to distinctive personality types—as seen, for example, in the "anal character." In this context, the psychodynamic paradigm provided an explanation of the origins and course of neurotic symptoms within an explicit conceptual framework (the psychoanalytic theory of neuroses). As in other psychiatric approaches, the vehicle for communicating this explanation was the "case history."

In contrast, the origins of the personological paradigm reside in Freud's (1910) biographical analysis of the life and works of Leonardo da Vinci, Jones's (1910) analysis of the Oedipus complex in Shakespeare's character Hamlet, and Abraham's (1911) analysis of the life of the Swiss painter Giovanni Segantini. These works are now considered to be psychobiographies because they involve *"the explicit use of systematic or formal psychology in biography"* (Runyan, 1982, p. 202; emphasis added).The systematic framework applied to these biographies need *not* have been psychoanalysis, although some of the advantages of psychoanalysis for this purpose continue to be evident (e.g., Anderson, 1981).

---

[1] Although not acknowledged as such, remarkably similar ideas were proposed earlier by the English humorist Stephen Potter (1950).

In the 1930s, there were a number of attempts to apply formal psychological and sociological principles to life history materials, the most notable being that of Dollard (1935). However, this decade is more memorable for the appearance within it of two milestone works that signaled the emergence of the modern personological paradigm in personality assessment. The origins of the contemporary personological paradigm, and in fact the origins of academic personality psychology itself, can be traced most directly to Harvard University in the 1930s. At that institution, Gordon Allport (1937) wrote the first textbook on personality, defined the person as the basic unit of observation, and established personality psychology as an academic discipline (Craik, Hogan, & Wolfe, 1993). He subsequently emphasized the use of personal documents in psychobiography (Allport, 1942, 1965) and spent a lifetime pondering the question of "How shall a psychological life history be written?" (Allport, 1967, p. 3). At the Harvard Psychological Clinic, Henry Murray (1938) introduced a multiform organismic method for studying "lives in progress" (White, 1952), in which an interdisciplinary team of investigators applied a variety of assessment procedures to the study of individuals over the course of their lives. A variant of this procedure was employed during World War II in the selection of intelligence agents and saboteurs (Office of Strategic Services [OSS] Assessment Staff, 1948), and subsequently this approach spawned a variety of successful peacetime assessment programs (e.g., MacKinnon, 1975; Stern, Stein, & Bloom, 1956).

Murray's enduring contributions to the personological paradigm go well beyond those just mentioned. During his 60 years at Harvard, Murray was a source of personal inspiration for an extraordinarily talented and diverse group of students, colleagues, and visitors who have continued to apply and expand his personology over the years. Early associates at the clinic included Samuel Beck, Erik Erikson, Jerome Frank, Daniel Levinson, Donald MacKinnon, Silvan Tomkins, and Robert White. Dan McAdams and William McKinley Runyan are more recent products of this Harvard tradition.[2]

During the war years of the 1940s, the social relevance of the study of lives became evident in the work of the originators of the personological paradigm. Allport, Bruner, and Jandorf (1941) solicited over 200 life histories from former residents of Germany on the topic of "My life in Germany before and after January 30, 1933." All documents were content-analyzed by a team of psychologists and sociologists according to a fixed schedule.

---

[2] Although the personological tradition had its origins at Harvard University, it should be noted that none of the faculty members (Allport, Erikson, McClelland, Murray, White) had tenured positions in the Department of Psychology, which was not at all favorably disposed toward personality study (McClelland, 1996).

Allport and his colleagues noted that "perhaps the most vivid impression gained by our analysts from this case-history material is of the extraordinary continuity and sameness in the individual personality" (1941, p. 7).

In his characteristically scholarly fashion, Allport (1942) later described 21 different purposes for the use of personal documents in psychological research. And Murray, together with his wartime staff, published the details of the OSS assessment program for the selection of overseas intelligence agents (OSS Assessment Staff, 1948)—a classic account of a milestone study within the personological paradigm (Wiggins, 1973b).

The Postwar Era

There was a decline of interest in the study of individual persons and lives during the 1950s and early 1960s—during which time the research agendas set forth by Allport and Murray were set aside in favor of psychometric issues and the experimental study of specific processes. Nevertheless, during this so-called "dark era" of personality psychology, those most closely associated with the original paradigm continued to provide the foundation for what would be its full flowering in the 1980s. McClelland's (1951) textbook provided a canonical introduction to the paradigm for advanced students of psychology. The assessment studies of Stern and colleagues (1956) demonstrated the utility of Murray's multiform assessment strategy within an educational setting. And Erikson's (1958) psychobiography of the young Martin Luther introduced the paradigm to a broader readership of both scholars and laypersons.

By the 1960s, psychobiography had become a major focus within the personological paradigm, and its differences from the traditional psychodynamic case study were becoming more evident. During this decade, three of the most influential figures in the history of the personological paradigm published virtuoso psychobiographical studies. Allport (1965) provided a psychobiography of "Jenny," based on her long-term correspondence with friends of her son. Murray's (1967b) earlier psychobiographical essay on Herman Melville became more widely available at this time. And Erikson's (1969) Pulitzer Prize-winning psychobiography of Gandhi set a new standard for psychohistorical studies. In the 1960s, Erikson's writings (e.g., 1968) and the works of those he influenced (e.g., Keniston, 1965) were also viewed as "relevant" by a younger generation in search of identity.

The next decade was characterized by further elaborations of the methods and concepts of the personological paradigm. Block's (1971) comprehensive longitudinal study of personality development introduced sophisticated methods and concepts that captured the development of personality patterns over time. Levinson's (1978) study of 40 American men between the ages of 35 and 45 identified distinctive developmental periods or "seasons" within what had been previously classified as global "early adulthood." And Tomkins (1979) provided a summary of his script theory, which describes the manner in which narrative "scripts" enable people to make sense of the affectively tinged "scenes" of their life stories. Tomkins's concepts occupy a central analytical role in contemporary psychobiography (Carlson, 1998).

Contemporary Period

During the period extending from the 1980s to the present, the personological paradigm has become an increasingly coherent and distinctive discipline with its own concepts and methods, and with its own place among related areas of scholarly investigation. This coming of age is nowhere better illustrated than in the work of William McKinley Runyan. Runyan's *Life Histories and Psychobiography: Explorations in Theory and Method* (1982) provided a scholarly but accessible introduction to the "descriptive, conceptual, and interpretive issues in the study of individual lives" (p. viii); it became an instant classic. In his more advanced edited book on *Psychology and Historical Interpretation* (Runyan, 1988a), he made a convincing argument for the place of psychology (not just psychoanalysis) among the more established disciplines of history, biography, and literature (Runyan, 1988b). As a further indication of this coming of age, McAdams and Ochberg (1988) provided a collection of essays on psychobiography and life narratives that were meant to emphasize the increased methodological rigor and conceptual pluralism characterizing this discipline.

The appearance of three influential books by major contemporary psychobiographers in the 1990s illustrates both the diversity and the established nature of the paradigm today. The long-awaited book by Alexander (1990), *Personology*, is a modern textbook in the tradition of Murray. McAdams's *The Stories We Live By* (1993), a lucid presentation of the narrative life history school of personology, is the focus of much current empirical research. And Elms's *Uncovering Lives: The Uneasy Alliance of Biography and Psychology* (1994) shares the wisdom of a psychobiographer in the practice of his trade. It is somewhat paradoxical that the personological paradigm is among both the oldest and the newest of approaches to personality assessment. Although it has origins in common with the psychodynamic paradigm, the distinctiveness of the personological approach is now clearly apparent.

CASE STUDIES AND PSYCHOBIOGRAPHIES

Table 3.1 provides selected examples of the variety of purposes the case study method served in the 20th century. From that table, it can be seen that within the first decade, the psychoanalytic method of studying lives

TABLE 3.1. Milestones in the Historical Development of Case Studies and Psychobiographies

Author and subject	Category	Description
Freud's (1905) "Dora"	Clinical patient	A case of hysteria in an 18-year-old woman, illustrating the sexual basis of the illness.
Freud's (1910) Leonardo	Historical figure	This first psychobiography analyzed the original "Renaissance man."
Jones's (1910) Hamlet	Literary character	Oedipal themes in Shakespeare as revealed in his most famous character.
Murray's (1938) "Earnst"	Representative subject	One of the participants in the Harvard Psychological Clinic's assessment program.
White's (1943) "Joseph Kidd"	Longitudinal analysis	Comparative longitudinal study of a college student interviewed until the age of 54.
McClelland's (1951) "Karl"	Didactic use of case study	Teaching concepts of personality with reference to a single life.
Allport's (1965) "Jenny"	Use of personal documents	Analysis of mother's letters to the former college roommate of her son and the roommate's wife.
Erikson's (1969) Gandhi	Historical event	Pulitzer Prize-winning psychobiography of the originator of militant nonviolence.
Alexander's (1990) Harry Stack Sullivan	Comparative biography	Psychobiographical essay on the "missing years" in published Sullivan biographies.
Robinson's (1992) Henry A. Murray	Biography of the founder	In-depth study of Murray's heretofore "secret life."
Nasby and Read's (1997a, 1997b) Dodge Morgan	Extraordinary people	Multimethod case study of a sailor who completed a solo circumnavigation of the globe in 150 days.

was applied to psychiatric patients, historical figures, and literary characters. In subsequent decades, beginning with the work of Murray (1938) and extending to that of Alexander (1990), both conceptual frameworks and psychobiographical methods multiplied to encompass the broad range of subject matters to which case studies and psychobiographies are now applied. The studies from 1905 to 1990 are briefly described in the next section on classic studies. The work of Robinson (1992) and that of Nasby and Read (1997a, 1997b) are described in later sections.

CLASSIC STUDIES IN PSYCHOBIOGRAPHY

Freud's (1905) "Dora"

The first published psychoanalytic case study was conceived and written during a particularly tumultuous time for Sigmund Freud. In 1896, Freud had suggested to the Viennese Society for Psychiatry and Neurology that neuroses are caused by the sexual seduction of children by adults—a proposition that was broadly dismissed by Krafft-Ebing and others as "a scientific fairy tale." Four years later, it appeared to Freud that his masterpiece, *The Interpretation of Dreams* (1900), would also be neither understood nor appreciated. In 1900, an 18-year-old woman ("Dora") who exhibited classical hysterical symptoms and a likelihood of having earlier been sexually abused was referred to Freud. Because Dora appeared to be an exemplar of his sexual seduction theory, Freud decided to publish her case history as an adjunct to *The Interpretation of Dreams* entitled "Dreams and Hysteria." When Dora abruptly terminated her analysis after 11 weeks, Freud (1905) could publish only a "Fragment of an Analysis of a Case of Hysteria."

Freud's case histories were meant to provide an evidentiary basis for the propositions of psychoanalytic theory, which at that time rested largely on Freud's self-analysis and his undocumented clinical experience. But given Freud's (1905) heretical assumption that the sexuality of the hysteroid patient "provides the motive power for every single symptom, and for every single manifestation of a symptom" (p. 115), he did not anticipate that his documentation of the sexual details of Dora's case would be well received: He noted that "whereas before I was accused of giving no information about my patients, now I shall be accused of giving information about my patients which ought not to be given" (p. 13). Nevertheless, Freud met these anticipated reactions head on, declaring that

> sexual questions will be discussed with all frankness, the organs and functions of sexual life will be called by their proper names, and the pureminded reader can convince himself from my description that I have not hesitated to converse upon such subjects in such language even with a young woman. (pp. 15–16)

Perhaps more impressive than Freud's candor, during this era when Victorian mores still predominated, was his willingness to admit that Dora's premature termination of the analysis was largely due to his own failure to recognize and deal with the negative transference recognizable in the first dream reported by Dora (p. 118). Freud also chided himself for failing to recognize the unconscious homosexual component in Dora's mental life (p. 120).

Over the years, critics of Freud have found other shortcomings in his interpretations of the Dora case, including the most recent feminist charge that Freud betrayed Dora's hope of establishing a relationship of trust and mutual respect with an authoritative adult by demanding that she take personal responsibility for the sexual conduct of an older male who had been trying to seduce her since she was 14 (Lakoff & Coyne, 1993). The fact that Freud's case study of Dora, and his subsequent studies of "Little Hans," the "Rat Man," "Schreber," and the "Wolf Man," continue to be read and discussed today attests to their seminal role in the historical development of the case history as a tool for studying lives.

Freud's (1910) Leonardo da Vinci

Freud's study of the psychosexuality of Leonardo da Vinci is generally considered to be the first psychobiography. From a letter he wrote to Jung on October 17, 1909, it is clear that this project was part of a concerted effort to subsume an ever-increasing number of fields within the framework of the psychoanalytic movement:

> I am glad you share my belief that we must conquer the whole field of mythology. . . . We must also take hold of biography. I have had an inspiration since my return. The riddle of Leonardo da Vinci's character has suddenly become clear to me. That would be a first step in the realm of biography. (McGuire, 1974, p. 255)

It was assumed by Freud that direct contact with the subject in psychoanalysis is not necessary to reconstruct the psychodyamics of critical themes in a subject's life—in this case, a subject who had lived almost 500 years earlier. And Freud's efforts in this regard were a brilliant success in many respects. Freud's (1910) insightful analysis of the artist and his paintings was, and to a large extent still is, regarded as a milestone achievement by biographers and art historians.

The bulk of Freud's evidence for the origins of themes of homosexuality and infantile dependency in the life and work of Leonardo came from an early memory reported by the subject:

> It seems that it had been destined before that I should occupy myself so thoroughly with the vulture, for it comes to my mind as a very early memory, when I was still in the cradle, a vulture came down to me, opened my mouth with his tail and struck me many times with his tail against my lips. (Leonardo da Vinci, quoted in Freud, 1910, p. 82)

The psychobiography of historical figures opened up a new scholarly medium, which cut many ways; thus, it is not unprecedented today to write psychobiographies of psychobiographers. For example, Alan Elms's (1988) essay "Freud as Leonardo: Why the First Psychobiography Went Wrong" examines Freud's "obsession" with the Leonardo project and identifies a major scholarly error in Freud's analysis that was probably "overdetermined" by Freud's identification with his subject. It seems that Freud relied upon an erroneous German translation of the word "vulture" from the original Italian version that, in effect, vitiated Freud's entire argument (Elms, 1988, pp. 26–29).

Perhaps more importantly, Elms (1988) has used Freud's psychobiography to illustrate several important guidelines for psychobiographical research. These include "the rejection both of pathography and of idealization and the avoidance both of arguments built upon a single clue and of strong conclusions based upon inadequate data" (p. 19), all of these being guidelines that Freud himself clearly violated in his work on Leonardo. In general, contemporary psychobiographies of historical figures are now much more sophisticated (see Craik, 1988, and Runyan, 1988a).

Jones's (1910) Hamlet

Hamlet and Oedipus

Jones's paper on Hamlet was among the first psychobiographies of a literary character to be published in a psychological journal. It was based on Freud's earlier interpretation of Hamlet's hesitation to avenge the death of his father at the hands of his uncle (Claudius), who subsequently marries his father's wife (Gertrude). Having recently discovered the universal and timeless gripping power of Sophocles's *Oedipus Rex*, in which the protagonist slays his father and marries his mother (without any awareness that he has committed patricide and is living in an incestuous relationship), Freud saw the same myth to be the basis of Hamlet's dilemma. Moreover, he argued that Shakespeare was not consciously aware of the Oedipus myth; he contended in an October 15, 1897, letter to Wilhelm Fliess that Shakespeare "was impelled to write [Hamlet] by a real event because his own unconscious understood that of the hero"(Masson, 1985, p. 272). In other words, Shakespeare had an "Oedipus complex."

Freud and Shakespeare

Freud's subsequent influence on literary theory and criticism may be found in Bloom's (1994) summary and evaluation of the "Western canon" in literature. As discussed earlier in this chapter, Bloom considers the canon to have begun with Shakespeare, who "invented" the human. On the more contemporary scene, Bloom considers "the strongest modern writers" to be "Freud, Proust, and Joyce" (p. 471). Bloom further concludes that "Freud is essentially prosified Shakespeare" (p. 371).

Freud's life and work provide a convincing illustration of Bloom's (1973) earlier concept of the "anxiety of influence." Freud read Shakespeare in English throughout his life: "Freud found himself quoting (and misquoting) Shakespeare in conversation, in letter writing, and in creating for psychoanalysis a literature of its own" (Bloom, 1994, p. 372). And yet, according to Bloom, Freud was intellectually threatened by the genius of Shakespeare and could not bear to recognize the source of his own "prosified Shakespeare." Given that Oedipus was totally unaware of his patricidal and incestuous misdeeds,

> Why didn't Freud call it the Hamlet complex? . . . the Hamlet complex would have drawn the menacing Shakespeare too closely into the matrix of psychoanalysis; Sophocles was far safer and also offered the prestige of classical origins. (Bloom, 1994, pp. 380–381)

Murray's (1938) "Earnst"

The case of "Earnst," which appears in Murray's seminal *Explorations in Personality* (1938), has the distinction of being associated with the research project that consolidated the personological paradigm in personality assessment. Although Earnst may be said to be "representative" of the 50 Harvard men who participated in the milestone assessment study conducted at the Psychological Clinic in the 1930s, his published case study was primarily meant to be representative and illustrative of the multimethod, multiple-observer *procedures* used in that study.

> If we have made any contribution to personology it is probably to be found in our general plan of action: numerous sessions, of which as many as possible are controlled experiments, conducted by different examiners who work independently until at a final session they meet to exchange their findings and interpretations. (Murray, 1938, p. 705)

Earnst arrived at the Harvard Psychological Clinic for a preliminary interview in which the purpose of the study was explained, his willingness to participate in approximately 36 hours of assessment over 3–4 months was established, and his first assignment of writing an autobiography was given. On his next visit, he was interviewed by a "diagnostic council," the five members of which interviewed him on such topics as interests, social experiences, and attitudes. Subsequent individual interviews with different members of the council explored more specific topics, such as family relations and sexual development. Impromptu conversations with staff members over the 3 months of assessment provided additional data.

The variety and sheer number of psychological tests and experimental procedures administered to Earnst by staff members was, and probably still is, unparalleled in the history of assessment. Psychological tests included the Thematic Apperception Test (TAT), the Rorschach, and a 600-item personality questionnaire. Experimental procedures provided measures of such variables as aesthetic appreciation, hypnotizability, level of aspiration, repression, memory for failures, reaction to frustration, violation of prohibitions, and sensory–motor learning. Although some of the experimental procedures are no longer employed, others are clearly recognizable today. For example, the "social interaction" procedure clearly anticipated the social psychology of the 1970s:

> The [subject] . . . was informed upon entering that he would have to wait a short while for the [experimenter]. He was then conducted into a room in which he could be observed through a one-way screen. In this room he found another student, presumably also waiting. In reality, the latter was an assistant of the [experimenter] and was acting according to definite instructions. (pp. 599–600)

Upon conclusion of the testing and experimental procedures, a biographer was selected for Earnst (Robert W. White). The biographer was the member of the diagnostic council whose task was to integrate all of the observations and interpretations that had been made in the course of the 3-month assessment into a "portrait" of Earnst, which stressed the "unity thema" in Earnst's life. A meeting of the full diagnostic council was then called, in which the biographer outlined his conclusions and each member of the council reported his own findings based on testing and interview sessions with Earnst. After approximately 4 hours of discussion, ratings were made on the major variables of assessment and resolved by majority vote. Robert White's summary and the reports of other members of the diagnostic council are reported and discussed in "The Case of Earnst" (Murray, 1938, pp. 604–702).

Murray's (1938) assessment of the worth of these procedures was characteristically modest:

> We came to view our work as a mere point of departure and the Clinic as an *anlage* [plan, layout] of some future institute where more exhaustive studies could be made. Such an institute might eventually bring about a unification of the various schools of psychology. (p. 34)

White's (1943) "Joseph Kidd"

There is perhaps no better exemplar to be found of Henry Murray's grand scheme for studying personality than the writings of Robert W. White. White extended Murray's procedures to include *comparative* longitudinal studies of the natural growth of personality over periods extending from late adolescence to middle age. He did so within a broad theoretical context that emphasized the social, biological, and developmental determinants of personality. White's approach allowed him to study both the organization and growth of personality in a manner not possible with "clinical case records taken at a time when the patient, overwhelmed by difficulties, is preoccupied with the problem of getting well" (White, 1975, p. vi).

The "lives in progress" of "Joseph Kidd," "Hartley Hale," and "Joyce Kingsley" were presented and compared in three successive editions of White's (1952, 1966, 1975) classic book over a period of 23 years.[3] Joseph Kidd was 18 years old when he, like Earnst, was a paid subject in the Harvard Psychological Clinic's assessment program (White, 1943). Interview and autobiographical material obtained from Kidd during his college years was supplemented by test results (e.g., the TAT, the Wechsler–Bellevue, self-ratings of social skills and attitudes). Letters were exchanged with Kidd during his wartime service; upon his return, he agreed to be interviewed at widely separated intervals, the last of which occurred when he was 54 years old.

White's presentation of the life of Joseph Kidd is a perceptive and fascinating account of the course of a "normal" life (i.e., Kidd was neither a famous person nor a psychiatric patient). White's interpretations of the social, biological, and developmental forces that shaped Kidd's life have a compelling realism seldom encountered in introductory textbooks. This realism is accentuated by the *comparative* framework of the text, which at several points contrasts the life of Joseph Kidd (a businessman) with those of Hartley Hale (a physician and scientist) and Joyce Kingsley (a housewife and social worker). For example,

> Because [Kidd] was late both in marrying and in finding a vocation, his present position in life is in some respects comparable to that of Hartley Hale at thirty-three, and it is interesting that in both cases, though obviously for different reasons, the interests of career tend to take precedence over those of family. (White, 1975, p. 199)

These and other features of this excellent textbook tend to support White's (1975) pedagogical assumption that "the initial facts of personality are the lives of people, and lives cannot be adequately understood unless they are described at considerable length" (p. vi).

McClelland's (1951) "Karl"

As noted in the Introduction, providing students with specific exemplars of previously successful applications of a paradigm is part of the educational process that ensures the continuity of the paradigm over time. Murray's

---

[3] An additional comparative study of "John Chatwell" and "Harold Merritt" is presented in White (1963a).

Explorations in Personality (1938) has no doubt served that function for some relatively advanced practitioners, although it was not written as a textbook. McClelland's *Personality* (1951), on the other hand, is a proto-typical example of a textbook designed to provide the advanced psychology student with exemplars of and "hands-on" experience with the person-ological paradigm.

> I have chosen a single individual, Karl, whose behavior will be studied each time a new theoretical construct is introduced. After all, the proof of the pudding is in the eating. . . . It is for this reason also that I have made a practice of having each student analyze his own case as we have proceeded from one theoretical construct and method of measurement to another. (McClelland, 1951, pp. xiii–xiv)

"Karl" was a 24-year-old college student for whom extensive biographi-cal and autobiographical material were available, and for whom an extraor-dinary number of test, interview, and performance measures had been col-lected. These measures included, among others, the Strong (1943) Vocational Interest Blank; measures of physique (described by a fraternity friend, a teacher, and a psychiatrist) and measures of temperament (Sheldon & Stevens, 1942); the Rorschach (interpreted by J. D. Holzberg); the TAT (Murray, 1943); the "Big Five" personality trait dimensions (Fiske, 1949)[4]; perfor-mance tests (Cattell, 1946); and measures of status and roles (Linton, 1945).

Test forms and test results were reproduced in the text and in the in-structor's manual in such a way that the reader was provided with both test data and an opportunity to predict test performance. In addition, portions of biographical materials were withheld to provide a "prediction question-naire," the use of which taught the student that "prophetic infallibility is beyond the reach of social scientists" (OSS Assessment Staff, 1948, p. 8). The rich diversity of concepts and methods covered in this text reflected McClelland's self-proclaimed "eclecticism," which encouraged the integra-tion of the personological paradigm with concepts and methods from other paradigms. The contemporary counterpart of McClelland's *Personality* (1951) is McAdams's introductory personality textbook, *The Person* (1994)— which has achieved substantial integration of other paradigms within the framework of the personological perspective, and which is more sharply fo-cused on narrative life history per se.

Allport's (1965) "Jenny"

Allport (1942) was a long-standing advocate of the use of personal docu-ments in research on personality, and he himself contributed substantially

---

[4] As will become evident in Chapter 4, this was a remarkably prescient selection of trait dimensions.

to this tradition with the publication of *Letters from Jenny* (Allport, 1965). The letters that were the focus of Allport's study were written during the years 1926–1937 by "Jenny" to "Glenn" and his wife, "Isabel"; they mainly concerned Jenny's son, "Ross," who had been Glenn's roommate in college.[5] These fascinating letters "tell the story of a mother–son relationship and trace the course of a life beset by frustration and defeat" (Allport, 1965, p. v).

Allport's analyses of these documents is deservedly considered to be a milestone contribution to psychobiographical work. In his characteristically broad and integrative approach, Allport interpreted the letters from a variety of theoretical perspectives, including those of learning theory and the theories of Jung, Adler, and Freud. He also used several different methods of analysis, including trait ratings by judges and a computer-based analysis of the co-occurrence of significant themes.

Erikson's (1969) Gandhi

This is the man who has stirred three hundred million people to revolt, who has shaken the foundations of the British empire, and who has introduced into human politics the strongest religious impetus of the last two hundred years.
                                                                —ROLLAND (1924, p. 5)

While on a visit to the city of Ahmedabad in India, Erik Erikson became intrigued with an event that had happened there in March 1918. On that earlier occasion, a 48-year-old man named Mohandas Gandhi (the title "Mahatma," by which he later became known, was bestowed on him as a mark of respect by his followers) had resolved a labor dispute between workers and mill owners by vowing to cease eating until workers had received their promised 35% increase in wages. Realizing that he was staying on the estate of the mill owner who had opposed Gandhi, and that many of his new acquaintances had known Gandhi in those days, Erikson "decided to reconstruct what in this book we will call the Event as a focus for some extensive reflections on the origins in Gandhi's early life and work, of the method he came to call the 'truth force' " (1969, p. 10).

Erikson's (1963) psychosocial theory of personality development and identity formation emphasizes the mutually formative interplay between the developing individual and the cultural and historical forces of society. Erikson's virtuosity as a psychobiographer is beautifully illustrated in his 1969 book *Gandhi's Truth*, in which he interwove materials from interviews with those who knew Gandhi, from Gandhi's autobiography and collected works, and from a variety of historical sources, to provide a psycho-

---

[5] In a clever piece of detective work, Winter (1993) was able to establish clearly that "Glenn" and "Isabel" were in fact Gordon and Ada Allport.

logical analysis of Gandhi as a person and a characterization of the nature and origins of militant nonviolence.

Alexander's (1990) Harry Stack Sullivan

In Chapter 6 of his classic textbook on *Personology*, Alexander (1990) introduced an innovative method for conducting psychobiographical studies that, for lack of a better label, might be called "psychodyamic metabiography." This approach frames a specific incident or time period in a subject's life and attempts to resolve inconsistencies in existing published (and unpublished) accounts of that incident or time period. The analysis is conducted with reference to the biographers themselves, and the professional and interpersonal circumstances under which they wrote their biographies, in relation to all that is known (or suspected) about the focal incident or time period.

Alexander (1990) believed that an understanding of a personality theory is enhanced by an understanding of the life and personality of the theorist (see Stolorow & Atwood, 1979). To this end, his textbook included psychobiographical studies of three theorists whose work had influenced his own: Freud, Jung, and Sullivan. The frame of investigation for Sullivan's life was the so-called "missing years" (1909–1911) in biographical accounts of Sullivan—the years in which Sullivan "disappeared" and for which no definitive documentation was available. The principal question posed by Alexander (1990) concerning these missing years was "how Sullivan, with little or no formal training in psychiatry, began a program almost immediately in his first psychiatric post which used methods hitherto unknown in the psychiatric community" (p. 56).

The published biographies considered by Alexander were written by (1) A. L. Chapman (1976), a psychiatrist; (2) Kenneth Chatelaine (1981), a psychologist; and (3) Helen Swick Perry (1982), Sullivan's definitive biographer and principal editor in the preparation of his posthumous books. Despite the wealth of material available in these substantial works, "There are large gaps in the story pertaining to the development of [Sullivan's] personality, his sexual development, and his career development" (Alexander, 1990, p. 201). The manner in which Alexander filled these gaps, the provocative hypotheses developed from them, and the broad and humane contexts in which hypotheses were evaluated have all the impact of a fictional thriller.[6] Sullivan's homosexuality and his "inability to achieve heterosexual

---

[6] When I first encountered a draft of this chapter of Alexander's book, I was familiar with the works of Sullivan in general and the biographies of Chapman and Perry in particular. As a consequence, my own "peak experience" while reading Alexander's chapter could be attributed to familiarity with the subject matter. However, the very positive reactions of graduate students to this chapter leads me to recommend this work strongly to all who might be interested in psychobiography.

gratification was viewed by him as a *failure in ultimate development*" (Alexander, 1990, p. 256; emphasis in original). Alexander used the concept of "scripts" (Tomkins, 1979) to integrate this hypothesis with Sullivan's academic failures: "This [inability to achieve heterosexual gratification] together with failures in academic achievement form a scriptlike pattern" (p. 256). He continued:

> In the first instance, there is a failure connected with intellectual achievement, or, analogously, failure to live up to an expected role that was conferred by such an achievement. This failure is then followed by disquieting negative affect (of different descriptions at different times) which culminates in silence and/or disappearance. The sequence is continued by a new attempt to reestablish self-esteem. During the nine-year period in question, we have three instances in which the same script was lived out. (Alexander, 1990, p. 256)

CHARACTERISTICS OF A MORE RECENT PSYCHOBIOGRAPHICAL STUDY

There is little doubt that the more recent case study of Nasby and Read (1997a, 1997b) is a milestone in the historical development of the personological paradigm that will have a solidifying effect on that paradigm:

> Nasby and Read's study of Dodge Morgan deserves to take a prominent place among a small number of seminal case studies in the history of personality psychology. . . . It is a model of how lives should be studied. (McAdams & West, 1997, p. 759)

This study is highly deserving of such accolades because it was, among other things, opportunistic, methodologically pluralistic, and paradigmatically pluralistic.

Opportunism

"Opportunistic" research capitalizes on once-in-a-lifetime situations in which it is possible to conduct meaningful naturalistic research that would not be possible in the laboratory or clinic (Campbell & Stanley, 1966). When Dodge Morgan, at the age of 54, was planning to complete a nonstop solo circumnavigation of the earth in his sailboat, *American Promise*, his wife saw an opportunity to create some benefit to others from what she saw otherwise as a "personal, even selfish pursuit" (Lehman, 1986, p. 55). Morgan eventually agreed to take an extensive battery of psychological tests before, after, and *during* each day of the voyage (the last being provided in dated, waterproof packets aboard the boat). Nasby capitalized on this opportunity by designing and implementing a study of unprecedented rigor and scope, and by devoting more than a decade of his own "life story" to this enterprise.

Methodological Pluralism

An unusual variety of methods and concepts were brought to bear on the subject of this case study (Craik, 1997). The principal focus was upon the life story of Dodge Morgan, and this was obtained from both biographical and autobiographical sources covering the period from early childhood to the end of the voyage. Standardized tests administered before and after the voyage included measures of "personality traits, needs and motives, emotional predispositions and states, interpersonal adjustment, and cognitive aptitudes and abilities" (McAdams & West, 1997, p. 758). During the voyage, daily tests of mood and cognitive functions were self-administered. The different methods employed have historically been associated with different paradigms of personality assessment, such as the multivariate (Personality Research Form; Jackson, 1984), the interpersonal (Affect Grid; Russell, Weiss, & Mendelsohn, 1989), and the personological and psychodynamic (TAT; Murray, 1943) paradigms.

Paradigmatic Pluralism

Perhaps the most outstanding feature of this case study was the manner in which different paradigms were employed and compared in the evaluation of Dodge Morgan's personality. The basic design of the study was one in which hypotheses generated from the life story model (McAdams, 1993) were compared with those generated from the five-factor model (McCrae & John, 1992) with respect to the psychological effects of the journey upon Dodge Morgan (see Nasby & Read, 1997b, pp. 907–908). The interpretive frameworks of the personological paradigm and the multivariate paradigm were enriched by interpretations from the perspective of the psychodynamic paradigm (e.g., Blatt, 1992). In addition, alternative interpretations from the perspective of the interpersonal paradigm were solicited (Wiggins, 1997) and an historical perspective achieved by Craik's (1997) direct comparison of the life story of Dodge Morgan with that of an earlier voyager (Slocum, 1900) and with Murray's (1938) classic study of Earnst.

CONCEPTUAL FRAMEWORKS
OF THE PERSONOLOGICAL PARADIGM

Murray's Theory of Personality

"Murray's conception of personality still awaits its final exposition by his own pen," as White (1963b, p. 3) noted in his preface to *The Study of*

Lives, a collection of papers presented to Murray on his 70th birthday by 18 former students and colleagues (White, 1963c). This, as Robinson (1992) has reminded us, is but one of many tasks that remained unfinished by Murray, including his 1,000-page biography of Melville. But a perusal of the broad range of conceptual accomplishments of the distinguished contributors to *The Study of Lives* quickly dispels the notion that Murray was not influential in the realm of personality theory, however unready Murray was to provide a formal statement of his own theory. When called upon to do so by Sigmund Koch for a volume in the canonical series *Psychology: A Study of a Science*, Murray (1959) submitted a paper entitled "Preparations for the Scaffold of a Comprehensive System." In it, he admitted that

> setting up a logically articulated skeleton of the whole—was so much more difficult that, despite an extension of time as well as every possible guidance and encouragement from a most charitable Director, I was unable to arrive at a satisfactory set of basic propositions before the date line. In short, I proved unequal to the set standard. (p. 9)

Nevertheless, the "intellectual autobiography" that Murray finally submitted in lieu of a formal statement of his theory is a valuable source of information for those interested in the development of Murray's thinking and the diverse origins of his ideas.

Murray's personology provided a set of orienting attitudes (rather than an explicit theory) that guided the multiform (many assessors, many tests), organismic (holistic) approach to the study of lives over time. In *Explorations in Personality*, he introduced a number of concepts that have subsequently proven useful in guiding the study of lives. By taking the life cycle of the individual as the largest unit of study, Murray was committed to studying personality "the long way" (White, 1981), and he introduced units of time varying in duration and complexity from the "proceeding" (single episode) to the "unity-thema" (central life motif). A thema may be understood in terms of the interaction of "needs" (for which Murray developed his famous taxonomy) and "press" (environmental facilitation or obstruction of a need). The TAT (Murray, 1943) was developed as a projective measure of need–press interaction and has been utilized in large-scale studies of needs for achievement (McClelland, 1961), power (Winter, 1973), and intimacy (McAdams, 1989). Although grand in scope, Murray's theorizing is not explicit enough to generate predictions that would permit the testing of its basic assumptions:

> It is as though the theory says so much that no single thing is said with a salience and conviction that makes it stand out from the rest of the theory, or that makes the theory itself stand out from others. (Hall & Lindzey, 1978, p. 237)

Erikson's Psychosocial Theory of Development

Erik Erikson's (1963) ego-psychological theory of personality development provided a more explicit account of the stages of development over the entire life span than had been provided by classical psychoanalysis. Moreover, Erikson's central "epigenetic principle" of maturation involved two assumptions that were meant to encompass both personality development *and* the structure of society:

> (1) that the human personality in principle develops according to steps predetermined in the growing person's readiness to be driven toward, to be aware of, and to interact with, a widening social radius; and (2) that society, in principle, tends to be so constituted as to meet and invite this succession of potentialities for interaction and attempts to safeguard and to encourage the proper rate and the proper sequence of their enfolding. (p. 270)

The principal differences between Erikson's "psychosocial" account of personality development and Freud's "psychosexual" theory may be illustrated with reference to Erikson's eight developmental stages, which are listed in Table 3.2. Although Erikson acknowledged the biological contribution of Freud's five stages of psycho*sexual* development (the second column), his own emphasis was upon the psycho*social* implications of these maturational changes, both for the developing individual and for the societal institutions that accommodate the role to be enacted at each stage of development (the third column).

Comparison of the second column with the third immediately suggests Erikson's conviction that significant changes do take place in personality after the age of 17, and that social institutions foster such changes. The bipolar, psychosocial "crises" listed in the fourth column reflect the positive (or negative) outcomes associated with resolving (or not resolving) the psychosocial challenges presented by each stage. Successful positive development at each stage imparts a new strength to the individual (e.g., trust, identity, generativity) and provides a corresponding virtue for society (e.g., hope, fidelity, care).

It has been observed that Freud was a "father figure" for Erikson (e.g., Gardner, 1999), and Erikson was understandably deferential toward his mentor to the end. Nevertheless, his theory represents a radical departure from classical psychoanalysis. Erikson's theory of development is a theory of *ego* development, in which the ego is granted full autonomy and the classical account of the influence of parents on psychosexual development is replaced by an emphasis on the historical/cultural matrix in which the ego develops. Rather than emphasizing unconscious mental life and the childhood traumas that bring about psychopathology in adulthood, Erikson stressed the positive ego qualities that emerge upon successful resolution of psychosocial crises and that lead to growth and mastery. Perhaps most im-

TABLE 3.2. Erikson's Stages of Development

Age	Psychosexual	Psychosocial	Crisis	Virtue
0–1	Oral	Infancy	Trust vs. mistrust	Hope
1–3	Anal	Early childhood	Autonomy vs. shame, doubt	Will
3–5	Phallic	Play age	Initiative vs. guilt	Purpose
5–12	Latency	School age	Industry vs. inferiority	Competence
12–17	Genital	Puberty and adolescence	Identity vs. role confusion	Fidelity
17–22		Young adult	Intimacy vs. isolation	Love
25–65		Middle adult	Generativity vs. stagnation	Care
65+		Maturity	Ego integrity vs. despair	Wisdom

Note. Data from Erikson (1963, p. 27).

portantly, Erikson's theory is a truly *psychosocial* theory of personality development. His theory informed his own classic psychobiographies (e.g., those of Martin Luther [Erikson, 1958] and Gandhi [Erikson, 1969]), as well as contributing to more recent psychobiographical efforts (e.g., Stewart, Franz, & Layton, 1988).

McAdams's Theory of Identity Development

In a book entitled *The Stories We Live by: Personal Myths and the Making of the Self* (1993), Dan McAdams has presented a neo-Eriksonian theory of identity development—one that is enriched by more contemporary concepts such as "image," "prototype," and "script," and that is guided by the metatheoretical concepts of "agency" and "communion" (Bakan, 1966). This work has been hailed as "the most original and important new book on personality theory since George Kelly's *Psychology of Personal Constructs*" (Hogan, 1994, p. 356). The heuristic potential of McAdams's conceptual framework is suggested by the quality and quantity of critical response it has elicited from personality psychologists representing diverse theoretical perspectives (see McAdams, 1996, and the peer commentary therein). Although McAdams's framework is more formal, explicit, and testable than earlier efforts, its roots in the formulations of Allport and Murray are easily traceable (see McAdams, 1994).

McAdams's (1993) basic premise is that each of us creates, consciously or unconsciously, a personal myth that is a "patterned integration of our remembered past, perceived present, and anticipated future" (p. 12). The two superordinate content themes of such narratives are agency and communion (Bakan, 1966). On the level of personality assessment, these themes are best exemplified in measures of power/achievement and intimacy/love, respectively. During Erikson's first stage of development (see Table 3.2), relationships with parents contribute to a sense of hope (or despair) in the infant. This, in turn, contributes to the "narrative tone" of later personal myths (optimism vs. pessimism). During the second stage of development, children learn the "images" (emotionally charged symbols) of stories in their culture, and these images become incorporated within their personal myths. During the school-age period, children come to understand the intentional and goal-directed nature of stories, and they begin to develop their own patterns of power and intimacy motivation; images become transformed into "themes." Adolescence is a critical period for identity formation, and it is during this period that adolescents become "self-conscious myth makers." In this period, the questioning of conventions and associated philosophical ruminations provide an "ideological setting" for the development of future personal myths based on agentic and communal superordinate themes.

McAdams's formulations of Eriksonian concepts such as "generativity" are not restricted to specific stages, but are seen as developing over the life span and as subjects for empirical investigation (e.g., McAdams & de St. Aubin, 1992; McAdams, de St. Aubin, & Logan, 1993). His conceptual and empirical utilization of the metaconcepts of agency and communion are highly sophisticated (e.g., McAdams, 1985b), and his interview procedures (described in the next section) are especially promising.

ASSESSMENT METHODS

In what is now widely recognized as the definitive general treatise on life histories and psychobiography, Runyan (1982) observed:

> It should be clear that there is no single life history method, any more than there is a single personality research method, and that life histories may be studied through phenomenological self-reports, archival research, prospective longitudinal research, and experimental research. (p. 6)

Personality assessment psychologists from Murray to McAdams have recognized the need for methodological pluralism (Craik, 1986) in the study of lives, and for that reason the "boundaries" of the personological paradigm have historically been somewhat more permeable than those of the other paradigms considered in this book. Nevertheless, it would be inaccurate to characterize this paradigm as "eclectic," because the diversity of methods employed reflects the different levels of analysis encompassed by the term "life history," rather than the selective use of theories and methods to "explain" a given life.

Following Kluckhohn and Murray (1953), Runyan (1982) distinguished three levels of generality in the social sciences: the universal (general laws of human behavior), the group (differences in sex, socioeconomic status, culture), and the individual (distinctive, distinguishing characteristics of a particular person). He then surveyed attempts to establish acceptable criteria for interpretations at each level. Although personologists in general, and clinicians in particular, are primarily concerned with the individual, an awareness of the larger enterprise portrayed by Runyan would help to clarify the nature and broaden the goals of individual personality assessment.

The 25 different assessment procedures employed for the study of individuals at the Harvard Psychological Clinic (Murray, 1938) were indeed "multiform" in terms of both the methods themselves and the assessors who employed them—for example, autobiography (Murray), hypnosis (White), level of aspiration (Frank), dramatic productions (Erikson), and Rorschach (Beck). Perhaps of greater interest to the contemporary clinician is the case study method in which some form of *interview* is employed, with all the attendant advantages and limitations of retrospective, introspective, and qualitative methods (see Runyan, 1982, Ch. 8). The procedures employed by McAdams (1993, Ch. 10) provide an excellent example of a theory-driven approach to the interview.

McAdams's theory of identity formation is based on the idea that we humans come to know ourselves through the creation of mythic life stories that are patterned integrations of our remembered past, perceived present, and anticipated future. The purpose of an interview is to identify the personal myth that an individual has been living—and, in some cases, to change the myth that has shaped and given meaning to an individual's life. The interview begins with the following request:

> I would like you to begin by thinking about your life as if it were a book. Each part of your life composes a chapter in the book. . . . Please divide your life into its major chapters and briefly describe each chapter. . . . Think of this as a general table of contents for your book. (McAdams, 1993, p. 256)

In the ensuing 1½ to 3 hours, the interviewee identifies key events, significant people, future scripts, stresses and problems, personal ideology, overall life theme, and other life story constructs clearly specified in McAdams's theory.

INTERPRETIVE PRINCIPLES

The variety of personality research methods for studying an individual's life history is reflected in a similar variety of interpretive principles associated with different methods. In this context, the interpretive principles elucidated by Alexander (1990) would appear to be "mainstream" in the sense that they evolved directly from the framework of Murray and his coworkers (see especially Tomkins, 1947, 1979) at the Harvard Psychological Clinic.

In analyzing data from directed interviews or autobiographical essays, Alexander (1990) looks for recurring dynamic sequences (scripts, themes, guiding messages) that may be revealed by "letting the data speak" or by "asking the data a question." In the former method, the typically large data set may be reduced by identifying "significant" material according to nine criteria of salience. These criteria have already become more or less canonical: "When I first saw Irv Alexander's list of criteria, it made immediate sense to me, in terms of its individual items and as a whole list. Virtually every example I've noted had already arisen in my own work" (Elms, 1994, p. 247).

Letting the Data Speak

Alexander's (1990) nine criteria for identifying the "significance" of material are as follows:

1. *Primacy* (that which occurs first). In both Freudian and Adlerian perspectives, significance is attached to early memories and experiences, and to the first statements of a patient in analysis. It is also a widespread convention in narratives, myths, and folk tales to allude to the "point" of the story early.

2. *Frequency* (that which occurs often). "When someone tells us the same message about himself repeatedly but short of monotony we are likely to assign importance to that message" (Alexander, 1990, p. 15). That which occurs frequently is often the expression of obvious, conscious value schemas. However, when the unit of analysis is changed to that of frequency of dynamic sequences, the significance may be less obvious to the subject. For example, if the theme "trying to help a friend" is frequently followed by a negative outcome, an aspect of the subject may be revealed that is not immediately apparent to the subject.

3. *Uniqueness* (that which is unusual or odd). Uniqueness is a probabilistic concept, the baseline for which can be either normative or idiographic. Thus uniqueness may be important when a described emotional reaction to an event differs markedly from normative expectations or from the subject's typical emotional reactions to similar events. Uniqueness may also be important when the mode of expression differs markedly from the subject's usual language. "The sudden appearance of street parlance in an otherwise formal presentation might be such a sign" (Alexander, 1990, p. 16).

4. *Negation* (that which is denied or disavowed). "When a biographical subject tells you who he or she is . . . you obviously should pay atten-

tion. But when the subject tells you who she or he *isn't*, you should pay at least as much attention, and sometimes even more" (Elms, 1994, p. 246; emphasis in original). In Freud's (1925b) original example,

> You ask who this person in the dream can have been. "It was not my mother." We emend this: so it *is* his mother. . . . A negative judgment is the intellectual substitute for repression; its "No" is the hall-mark of repression, a certificate of origin—like, let us say, "Made in Germany." (pp. 235–236; emphasis in original)

5. *Emphasis* (that which is either overemphasized or underemphasized). "Overemphasis can usually be detected when the hearer or reader begins to wonder why so much attention is focused on something considered to be a commonplace. . . . Underemphasis would be inferred when the question is raised as to why so little attention is paid to something which seems important" (Alexander, 1990, p. 18).

6. *Omission* (that which is missing by normative standards or by implication). "This is the Sherlock Holmes rule: Sometimes we should ask more questions when a dog doesn't bark than when it does" (Elms, 1994, p. 246). One of Alexander's subjects wrote an autobiographical essay in which all family members were clearly identified and interactions with all but one were described. "The omission in imagery or affect in general, or specific affects, would lead to a search for the particular circumstances which govern relevant affective experiences and their consequences" (Alexander, 1990, p. 20).

7. *Error or distortion* (factual errors and Freudian slips). Alexander (1990) provided an example of an undetected factual error in a subject's autobiography: "I came from a family of tall people; my father is 6-5, my brother is 6-4, my mother is 9-5, and I am the runt at 5-8" (p. 21). (In comparison with his possibly overvalued mother, the subject may have perceived himself as a runt.) Examples of "parapraxes" (slips of the tongue, slips of the pen, misreadings) abound in Freud's *The Psychopathology of Everyday Life* (1901), although the play on words involved is often untranslatable from the German.

8. *Isolation* (that which does not "fit" and non sequiturs). "If in reading or listening, one finds oneself asking the question, 'Where did that come from?' or 'That doesn't seem to follow,' it is highly likely that important personal material is contained in the communication" (Alexander, 1990, p. 21). Detection of isolation is often difficult because of our strongly ingrained tendency to "read in" missing or incongruous elements in social communication.[7] Thus "As a young child my parents were never terribly

---

[7] Alexander's example of reading a long set of essay exams for the "right" answer will strike a chord in many readers.

happy about my eating habits. By the time I was ten I was sent off to a private school where I did well in my subjects. Now as an adult I eat everything" (Alexander, 1990, p. 22) may appear to make sense if one makes the causal attribution that the subject was sent to private school to remedy his eating habits, but closer examination suggests an isolation involving adoption of parental norms.

9. *Incompletion* (that which is not finished or lacks closure). "The person you are studying starts a story but stops in the middle. The person starts a story and then changes the subject, subtly or not. The person starts a story and finishes it, but omits something important from the middle" (Elms, 1994, p. 247). Incompletion in each of these examples signals material of dynamic significance to the storyteller and raises questions of what it was that might provide closure to the stories.

Asking the Data a Question

The method of "asking the data a question" is similar to that employed in the analysis of TAT protocols for such predetermined categories as "power motivation" (Winter, 1973). The database of interview material is reduced by selecting every sequence or incident related to a specific question posed by the investigator, such as themes related to power. When applied to interview material, this method retains the "projective" advantage of addressing issues that the storyteller did not consciously intend to describe or deal with, while circumventing such problems as the identification of the "hero" of the narrative (Alexander, 1990).

CURRENT TRENDS IN PSYCHOBIOGRAPHY
Psychoanalytic Literary Criticism

Sigmund Freud has been dead for 60 years and yet his reburial rituals continue unabated. These contemporary self-styled demolition "experts" are not psychoanalytic clinicians, but rather emerge from college philosophy and English departments.
—LIFF (1998, p. 785)

Freud's influence on literary criticism was somewhat curtailed by the so-called "New Criticism" of the early part of the 20th century, which initiated a trend toward the rejection of the traditional historical-biographical approach in favor of a more rigorous and "objective" textual explication. However, a number of prominent critics resisted this trend, and Lionel Trilling was one of the more influential among them (Wellek & Warren, 1963). Although Trilling was associated with the leftist *Partisan Review*, which was the house organ for New York intellectuals during the 1930s and 1940s, he was more moderate in his political views (Phillips, 1983). Yet there was nothing moderate about his position on the centrality of Freudian thought to literary criticism:

> The Freudian psychology is the only systematic account of the human mind which, in point of subtlety and complexity, of interest and tragic power, deserves to stand beside the chaotic mass of psychological insights which literature has accumulated through the centuries. (Trilling, 1950, p. 32)

Trilling was a polymathic literary critic, novelist, and Freudian scholar, the last being evident in his receipt of an award from the American Psychoanalytic Association for his one-volume abridgment of Jones's (1953–1957) biography of Freud (Trilling & Marcus, 1961). Trilling's work helped forge stronger ties between the liberal intellectual tradition of literary criticism and the psychoanalytic community.

Frederick Crews, a professor of English at the University of California, is a more contemporary example of the psychoanalytic literary critic. Although originally one of Freud's more ardent disciples in the literary realm, he became increasingly disillusioned with psychoanalytic theory (e.g., Crews, 1980, 1988). Crews's most recent writings have done more to discredit psychoanalytic theory and practice than those of any other individual. In fact, Crews was the principal initiator of the "Freud wars." In a 1993 article in *The New York Review of Books*, Crews wrote highly favorable reviews of a number of books that were extremely critical of Freud's work; he concluded that "Without significant experimental or epidemiological support for any of its notions, psychoanalysis has simply been left behind by mainstream psychological research" (p. 55). Richard Webster (1997) later observed:

> But one suspects that the real offence was caused not so much by the contents of Crew's piece as by the place in which it had been published. For the *New York Review of Books* had come to be regarded by many as the house magazine of a particular section of the American liberal intelligentsia who were deeply sympathetic to psychoanalysis. That Frederick Crews's critique of Freud should be featured so prominently there was what really hurt. (p. 10)

In the same journal, Crews (1994) subsequently offered a scathing treatment of the psychoanalytically based "recovered memory" movement, which helped fuel the fires of the "memory wars." These and other criticisms were made more widely available both in the mass media (e.g., Gray, 1993) and in scholarly books (e.g., Crews, 1995, 1998; Forrester, 1998). In *Unauthorized Freud*, Crews (1998) provided introductions to an anthology of critical papers in which it is argued, inter alia, that Freud invented the data on which his theories were based, misrepresented the outcomes of treatments based on these theories, and intruded in patients' lives in ways that were deleterious to their well-being. Although the smoke has not yet cleared from these two battles, it would appear that the current intellectual *Zeitgeist* is no longer as favorably disposed toward orthodox psychoanalytic theory in the study of literature or psychology.

Psychobiographies of Psychobiographers

Every great man nowadays has his disciples, and it is always Judas who writes the biography.
—WILDE (1887, p. 949)

The reflexive nature of psychobiographical studies has been mentioned earlier. Freud was the first psychobiographer to write his own biography (Freud, 1925a); other studies of Freud's life have ranged from Jones's (1953–1957) hagiography, to more critical appraisals (Roazen, 1968), to what many consider the standard modern biography (Gay, 1988). Stolorow and Atwood (1979) have explored the ways in which a theory of personality is influenced and colored by the subjective world of the theorist. They presented psychobiographical analyses of Freud, Jung, Reich, and Rank as illustrations of their theory of "intersubjectivity." A similar approach has been taken by more recent psychobiographers (e.g., Alexander, 1990; Elms, 1994).

Henry A. Murray, the founder of the personological tradition, wrote a brief autobiography, "The Case of Murr" (1967a); this emphasized his feelings of maternal rejection, which created a "marrow of misery and melancholy" he spent his life overcoming. Brief psychobiographical essays on aspects of Murray's life have also been written (Anderson, 1988; Elms, 1987). More recently, however, Forrest Robinson (1992), a professor of literature and American studies at the University of California–Santa Cruz, has written an extraordinary in-depth biography of Murray called *Love's Story Told*, which has sent shock waves through the entire personological community. Runyan, a student of Murray and a recipient of the Henry A. Murray Award, has stated that this book "may well be the most intimate and personally revealing biography of a psychologist yet written" (Runyan, 1994, p. 701). He also noted:

> In talking about the book with friends and colleagues, particularly those who knew Murray or his work, I was struck by the wide array of responses to the story, ranging from fascination and rapt absorption to curiosity and intellectual puzzlement to disgust or moral disapproval. (p. 701)

In addition to revealing new aspects of Murray's near-obsession with the life and work of Herman Melville, Robinson (1992) discussed his extraordinary sexual, spiritual, and intellectual relationship with Christiana Morgan, his mistress for more than 40 years.[8] That Robinson's book is so thoroughly documented, beautifully crafted, and ultimately convincing makes it understandably difficult to assimilate for those who thought they knew Murray well. Although the eventual impact of this book on the personological community is hard to estimate, it may have set a new standard of excellence for professional psychobiographers. And Murray, who was a willing participant in Robinson's study, would certainly have approved of that.

APPLICATIONS AND CURRENT STATUS

In recent years, there appears to have been a "back to basics" movement in personality assessment research (Wiggins & Pincus, 1992); this has rekindled interest in the fundamental assumptions of several paradigms, including the personological:

> Once again, it is okay to study the 'whole person'. Better, contemporary personologists insist, as did pioneers like Gordon Allport, that such an endeavor is the personologist's *raison d'être*. (McAdams, 1988, p. 1)

Although there is currently more research and theoretical writing on psychobiography and life narratives than has appeared at any other time period, this state of affairs cannot be attributed solely to cumulative progress within the personological paradigm itself. Concurrent developments within cognate areas of the social and behavioral sciences would seem to have been of at least equal importance.

Runyan (1982) summarized the development and then-current status of life history research in anthropology, sociology, political science, medicine, and (of course) history itself (see Runyan, 1988b). On a more basic theoretical level, Sarbin (1986) has proposed that narrative be considered the root metaphor of psychology (Pepper, 1942). In reading McAdams's (1994) scholarly textbook on personality psychology, one can discern the potential implications of a "narrative psychology" applied to various broad issues of contemporary concern, such as human cognition (e.g., Bruner, 1986), cultural studies (e.g., Howard, 1991), psychotherapy (e.g., Spence,

---

[8] Morgan was Murray's coauthor of the TAT, principal author of some of the first publications concerning the TAT (e.g., Morgan & Murray, 1935), and illustrator for some of the original TAT cards (Morgan, 1995).

1982), education (e.g., Coles, 1989), mental health (e.g., Pennebaker, 1992), and the postmodern condition (e.g., Gergen, 1992). Within the field of psychology itself, active programs of research on the longitudinal development of normal adult personality (e.g., Block, 1993), developmental psychopathology (e.g., Cicchetti & Toth, 1995), life span developmental psychology (e.g., Baltes, Reese, & Lipsett, 1980), and long-term stability and change in personality (West & Graziano, 1989) have contributed additionally to the creation of an intellectual climate in which the personological paradigm is likely to continue to flourish.

In terms of clinical applications, it should be borne in mind that the personological tradition has tended to focus on relatively normal, nonclinical samples, and that within this tradition life histories have been viewed either as relatively veridical accounts of what has happened in a person's life (Runyan, 1982) *or* as imaginative reconstructions of the past (McAdams, 1993). It is also important to recognize that personality assessment within the personological paradigm occurs on a different level than traditional psychodiagnostic assessment does (Alexander, 1990). Whereas personological assessment attempts to understand current personality functioning in terms of an individual's own life history, traditional psychodiagnostic assessment is concerned with determining an individual's membership in a group or class of individuals that differs from other groups in terms of psychopathology.

> A major difference between the two approaches is that the results of the former [personological] can easily be directed toward answering the questions intended by the latter [psychodiagnostic]. The reverse is, unfortunately, a low probability event in anything other than a global sense. To designate someone as obsessive or hysteric, or depressive, or schizophrenic will place the focus on particular salient aspects of functioning but say little about the dynamics in that individual leading to that particular form of functioning. (Alexander, 1990, p. 7)

OVERVIEW

From its dim origins in ancient Greek drama to the highly technical concerns of present-day psychobiographers, the personological paradigm has been concerned with the question "How shall a psychological life history be written?" Freud's classic case histories were meant to illustrate the singular advantage of psychoanalytic theory in identifying the origins of character in the lives of patients, historical figures, and literary characters. The roots of the personological paradigm of personality assessment may be traced to Harvard University during the 1930s, where Allport first defined the field of personality psychology and Murray introduced the multiform organismic method for studying "lives in progress." Although Murray's method of assessment was adopted by the OSS during World War II, and Erikson's postwar psychobiographies of Luther and Gandhi were well received, the study of life histories and psychobiography was not generally viewed as an internally coherent and distinctive paradigm prior to the publication of Runyan's (1982) *Life Histories and Psychobiography*. Since that time, there has been an unprecedented revitalization of interest in the paradigm (e.g., Alexander, 1990; Elms, 1994; McAdams, 1985b, 1993), both within and outside the field of personality assessment.

4

The Multivariate Paradigm

As I watched Spearman's research, and later Thurstone's, in describing the structure of abilities by use of factor analysis, it had taken no unusual imagination to propose unraveling the structures of temperament and motivation by the same instrument.

—CATTELL (1984, p. 124)

ORIGINS OF THE MULTIVARIATE PARADIGM

The English Eugenicists

The idea that variations in human characteristics have an evolutionary origin was suggested at the end of the 18th century by Erasmus Darwin (1731–1801) in his work on the laws of organic life (1794–1796), and it later bore fruit in the empirical researches of two of his grandsons, Charles Darwin (1809–1882) and Sir Francis Galton (1822–1911). That Galton (1869) was uniquely qualified to conduct research on "hereditary genius" is suggested by the accomplishments and eminence of the Darwin family and by the fact that Galton was, by any criteria, a "genius" himself.[1] Galton coined the term "eugenics" (from the Greek *eugenes*, "well-born") for the field of study examining the inheritance of desirable characteristics, especially intelligence; the purpose of this work was to improve the species by selective breeding. It is unfortunate that the term "eugenics" has subsequently become associated with racist political movements advocating the achievement of "racial purity" through sterilization and genocide. In con-

---

[1] Among many other things, Galton invented the "Galton whistle" for high-pitched tones, the method of word association, test batteries of mental and physical characteristics (administered at the 1893 Chicago World's Fair with "feedback" provided to participants), the twin study method in inheritance studies, a procedure for classifying fingerprints, a rotary steam engine, a printing telegraph, and instruments for automatic weather recording.

123

trast, the field of study founded by Galton has evolved primarily into the quantitative assessment of individual differences and the study of their origins.

University College London was founded by the liberal political philosopher Jeremy Bentham ("the greatest good for the greatest number") and other democratically inclined scholars from Oxford and Cambridge. Unlike Oxford and Cambridge, University College had no religious entrance requirements and was therefore known to some as the "godless institution of Gower Street." Within this setting, the radical ideas of Darwin were given serious consideration. In 1904, Galton endowed a permanent chair in eugenics at University College and appointed the mathematician Karl Pearson (1857–1936) as its first professor. Charles Spearman (1863–1945), the eminent statistician and investigator of mental abilities, was at University College at this time. Also there was Ronald A. Fisher, who is now known to psychologists primarily for his development of the analysis of variance (Fisher, 1937), but is more renowned in general for providing the mathematical foundation for the field of population genetics (Fisher, 1930), which synthesized Darwin's theory of evolution with Mendelian genetics (Huxley, 1942).

Correlation and Factor Analysis

Galton's (1885) paper on "Regression towards Mediocrity in Hereditary Stature" was an attempt to predict the physical characteristics of offspring from knowledge of their parents' physical characteristics. He found that children tended to "revert toward the mean"; for example, taller-than-average parents tended to have children who were shorter than they were. The same phenomenon, he later found, was true of inherited mental abilities as well. Galton (1888) subsequently developed a statistical method for analyzing the "co-relations" between twin pairs on measures of mental abilities. Pearson's (1896) product–moment correlation coefficient (r) was named in honor of Galton's "reversion," which is now called "regression." Spearman (1904) applied his newly developed method of factor analysis to correlation matrices and identified a general factor of intelligence (g) that, together with more specific factors (s), appeared to underlie various tests of mental abilities.

In more contemporary terms, Spearman had observed that the correlations among virtually all extant measures of mental ability (e.g., associational fluency, eduction of figural relations) were positive in nature, and he developed the statistical technique of "factor analysis" to express the relations among test variables by a single factor. "Factors" are statistical abstractions that summarize the relations among test scores in terms of underlying or "latent" variables, which may be thought of as operating at several levels. For example, the Intelligence Quotient (IQ) can be considered a general higher-order factor that summarizes relations between Verbal and Performance major group factors, which in turn summarize relations among multiple minor group factors (see Vernon, 1950). A brief digression on the essentials of factor analysis would appear to be helpful at this point.

ESSENTIALS OF FACTOR ANALYSIS

The close relationship between factor analysis and the multivariate paradigm has given rise to an interpretive language that is not easily comprehended by those working outside the paradigm. Although the mathematical foundations of this language are necessarily abstract, the basic principles are fairly easily grasped in their concrete applications. The material that follows is based in part on the excellent chapter by Goldberg and Digman (1994), and is meant as an introduction to their more advanced introduction.

For a number of reasons, the adjective is considered by some to be the preferred part of speech for initiating a study of personality attributes (see Saucier & Goldberg, 1996b, pp. 30–33). A great deal of social information is conveyed when people describe themselves or others as "extraverted," "tender-hearted," "organized," "anxious," or "philosophical." To calibrate these descriptions, we might ask respondents to indicate how accurately they (or others) are described by each of these adjectives on an 8-point scale ranging from "extremely inaccurate" to "extremely accurate." And that is what Wiggins and colleagues did when we asked 484 respondents to describe themselves on a list of adjectives, 15 of which appear in the first column of Table 4.1.

Intercorrelation Matrix

Our interest here is in identifying the significant dimensions along which individuals differ from one another and in capturing the structure of these differences in terms of the covariation among personality attributes. The basic unit of analysis for expressing the manner in which personality attributes covary in self-report is still the correlation coefficient developed by Galton and Pearson. In Table 4.1, self-ratings on each adjective have been correlated with self-ratings on all other adjectives. It should be stated at the outset that *all of the information regarding the structure, content, and interpretation of this set of self-ratings is contained in this table of intercorrelations.* Although it is conceded that "You only get out of a factor analysis what you put into it," it is also true that the information research-

TABLE 4.1. Correlations among 15 Trait-Descriptive Adjectives (n = 484)

	1	2	3	4	5	6	7	8	9	10	11	12	13	14
1. Organized														
2. Neat	.66													
3. Tidy	.65	.85												
4. Tender-hearted	.12	.11	.13											
5. Gentle-hearted	.10	.07	.08	.71										
6. Soft-hearted	.03	.02	.01	.58	.55									
7. Anxious	.03	.05	.02	−.02	.02	.17								
8. Tense	.06	.04	.04	−.11	−.07	.02	.65							
9. Worrying	.07	.09	.08	.01	.03	.15	.67	.60						
10. Outgoing	.16	.13	.18	.13	.14	.09	−.12	−.15	−.08					
11. Cheerful	.17	.15	.13	.39	.40	.23	−.19	−.27	−.14	.49				
12. Extraverted	.10	.10	.10	.17	.14	.08	−.16	−.19	−.12	.70	.45			
13. Philosophical	.03	.01	−.01	.13	.07	.12	.02	.02	.01	.12	.07	.13		
14. Abstract-thinking	.01	.01	−.01	−.00	.02	.01	.01	−.03	−.04	.18	.11	.15	.53	
15. Inquisitive	.06	.02	.01	.15	.14	.11	−.10	−.09	−.04	.22	.22	.27	.33	.34

ers get out of a factor analysis allows them to see what they have put into it in new and meaningful ways.

It can be seen from the table that persons who described themselves as "neat" tended to describe themselves as "tidy" (r = .85), which is hardly surprising. These unsurprising correlations are printed in bold, and, as can also be seen in the table, these larger correlations appear in five groups or clusters along the main diagonal of the correlation matrix. There may also be potentially important information in the 90 correlations that are not printed in bold, but there is no need to concern ourselves with the entire 15 × 15 intercorrelation matrix. Instead, we tell our computer program to take out or "extract" five independent factors (i.e., principal components) from this matrix, and then examine the results in Table 4.2.

Unrotated First-Order Factors

The first column in Table 4.2 presents the correlations (i.e., factor loadings) of each adjective with Factor I. What the computer program tries to do here is to extract the variance that all 15 adjectives have in common; as a consequence, first factors tend to be larger than subsequent factors. How large this first factor is can be determined by squaring and summing the factor loadings in the first column, and that value turns out to be 3.35. Dividing this value by the number of variables (3.35/15 = .223) tells us that the first factor accounts for 22.3% of all the variance in the original correlation matrix. This percentage is not very large, and it suggests that there is remaining variance that is unique to the remaining clusters of adjectives.

To reiterate, the loadings in Column I are the correlations of each adjective with the first factor, and if we wished to predict a respondent's score on Factor I (i.e., factor score), we would use a regression equation in which the respondent's ratings on each of 15 adjectives would be weighted by the coefficients in Column I and then summed. In other words, a factor is a weighted linear composite of variables. Factor II in Column II represents the computer's efforts to extract another factor that is unrelated (i.e., uncorrelated) with the variance accounted for by Factor I. Factor III is extracted so as to be uncorrelated with the first two factors, and so forth until we obtain five uncorrelated (i.e., orthogonal) factors, which together account for 74% of the variance in the original correlation matrix.

Information concerning the individual items is contained in the rows of Table 4.2. Squaring and summing the values in rows of the table yield the "communalities" (h^2) for each item. These communality values are equivalent to the squared multiple correlation of a given item with the remaining 14 items in the pool. Thus the communality value of .87 for "tidy" indicates that this item is highly predictable from the total pool of items. The item "inquisitive," on the other hand, is relatively independent of the other items ($h^2 = .47$).

TABLE 4.2. Unrotated Factor Matrix

	I	II	III	IV	V	h^2
1. Organized	.43	.53	−.47	−.01	−.15	.72
2. Neat	.43	.60	−.54	−.03	−.17	.86
3. Tidy	.44	.60	−.55	−.05	−.13	.87
4. Tender–hearted	.62	.09	.45	−.42	−.18	.79
5. Gentle–hearted	.58	.10	.48	−.42	−.12	.77
6. Soft–hearted	.42	.18	.59	−.31	−.12	.66
7. Anxious	−.25	.69	.42	.19	.22	.80
8. Tense	−.33	.67	.29	.24	.20	.74
9. Worrying	−.19	.70	.37	.17	.25	.74
10. Outgoing	.65	−.13	−.08	.27	.55	.82
11. Cheerful	.72	−.16	.05	−.07	.27	.61
12. Extraverted	.63	−.21	−05	.25	.54	.79
13. Philosophical	.29	−.02	.28	.60	−.42	.70
14. Abstract–thinking	.27	−.10	.17	.69	−.33	.70
15. Inquisitive	.43	−.15	.15	.45	−.20	.47
% variance = 74.0	22.3	17.2	14.2	11.8	8.5	

Rotated First-Order Factors

After all this, it is disappointing to learn that the factor matrix in Table 4.2 does not make a great deal of sense and is thus not very interpretable to the unpracticed eye. For example, Factor I would be easily interpretable if "outgoing," "cheerful," and "extraverted" had very large loadings (say, in the .80s) and the remaining 12 adjectives all had near-zero loadings. In other words, if we were able to *max*imize the *vari*ance in the first column by making some loadings close to 1.00 and the remainder close to .00, we would be in business. And the "varimax" rotation procedure developed by Kaiser (1958) does just that. To say that varimax rotation involves the multiplication of the "unrotated matrix" in Table 4.2 by an optimal "transformation matrix" is not to explain the procedure. But if one can accept on faith that there is no cheating going on and that the resultant rotated factor matrix in Table 4.3 preserves *all* of the information in Table 4.2, then one can appreciate why so many researchers use this procedure without fully understanding all of its details.

Table 4.3 presents one version of the "Big Five" lexical model of personality attributes, which is discussed in detail in this chapter. The factors have been interpreted as reflecting Conscientiousness, Agreeableness, Neuroticism, Extraversion, and Openness to Experience. Even Big Five advocates admit that "it will rarely be useful to apply factor analysis to sets of less than 50 variables" (Goldberg & Digman, 1994, p. 218), but Wiggins and colleagues did pretty well with the 15 single adjectives that were used for illustrative purposes only. Administering 8-point rating scales to 484 cooperative respondents helped, as did the psychometric potency of the Big Five model itself.

Comparing Table 4.2 with Table 4.3 shows that the proportion of variance accounted for by the factors (22.3%, 17.2%, etc.) has been "spread out" to account for the distinctive substantive contributions of each of the five factors. It would be easier to see the variance contributions of each item if the factor loadings in Table 4.3 were squared. Thus, for example, the sum of the squared factor loadings of Row 1 yields a communality value (h^2) of .72. This tells us how much variance the adjective "organized" has in common with the other 14 adjectives. More technically, .72 is the squared multiple correlation of "organized" with all five factors. And, as before, the sum of the squared factor loadings in Column I tells us how much of the variance (16.5%) in the original correlation matrix is accounted for by the Conscientiousness factor.

What does it mean when we say that the factor solution in Table 4.3 accounts for 74% of the variance in the original correlation matrix? To answer this, we have to square the entire matrix in Table 4.3; that is, we have to multiply the factor matrix by itself. Without worrying too much about

TABLE 4.3. Rotated Factor Matrix

	Consc. (I)	Agree. (II)	Neuro. (III)	Extra. (IV)	Open. (V)	h^2
1. Organized	**.84**	.05	.03	.08	.04	.72
2. Neat	**.93**	.03	.04	.05	.01	.86
3. Tidy	**.93**	.04	.04	.08	−.03	.87
4. Tender-hearted	.10	**.88**	−.07	.10	.06	.79
5. Gentle-hearted	.05	**.87**	−.03	.12	.02	.77
6. Soft-hearted	−.04	**.80**	.15	.03	.07	.66
7. Anxious	.01	.06	**.89**	−.09	−.00	.80
8. Tense	.04	−.09	**.84**	−.14	−.00	.74
9. Worrying	.06	.06	**.86**	−.03	−.02	.74
10. Outgoing	.11	.03	−.04	**.89**	.13	.82
11. Cheerful	.12	.38	−.21	**.65**	.16	.61
12. Extraverted	.03	.04	−.08	**.87**	.13	.79
13. Philosophical	.00	.10	.05	−.01	**.83**	.70
14. Abstract-thinking	−.01	−.06	.01	.08	**.83**	.70
15. Inquisitive	.02	.11	−.10	.23	**.63**	.47
% variance = 74.0	16.5	15.7	15.3	14.1	12.4	

Note. These factors are not ordered in the traditional "Big Five" order, but rather by the percentage of variance accounted for by each factor in this solution.

the arithmetic of matrix multiplication, let us accept that a factor matrix multiplied by itself produces the original intercorrelation matrix itself, or at least in this case, 74% of it (i.e., an approximation matrix). If we subtract our approximation matrix from the original matrix, we would obtain a "residual matrix," which tells us exactly what we are *not* accounting for by a five-factor orthogonal solution.

Armed with all of the foregoing information, we might regret that we included, for example, "cheerful" and "inquisitive"—which in hindsight appear to be ambiguous, because they have more than one meaning and as a consequence have secondary loadings on more than one factor. But the present set of 15 adjectives was assembled for illustrative purposes only and need not concern us further. In fact, this example of a factor analysis bears little resemblance to the data that are actually employed in factor analyses of multivariate personality inventories. A more realistic example would have been one in which an investigator had developed 15 scales with approximately 20 items per scale, measuring nonredundant aspects of personality, such as 15 of Murray's (1938) needs.

Higher-Order Factors

The five orthogonal factors displayed in Table 4.3 are uncorrelated, in part because we made them so by performing a varimax rotation procedure that did its best to make the large factor loadings as close to 1.00 as possible and the small factor loadings as close to .00 as possible. There are other rotational procedures that will attempt to "fit" the rotated matrix to any pattern we wish. For example, just as the Greek mythological robber, Procrustes, chopped up travelers to make them "fit" the length of his bed, the Procrustes rotation (Hurley & Cattell, 1962) will attempt to "fit" factors to any pattern desired.

When factors such as those in Table 4.2 are allowed to be correlated with each other, it is possible to form an intercorrelation matrix of factors and then to "factor the factors." The resultant "superfactors" are called "second-order" or "higher-order" factors, and the original factors are then referred to as "primary" or "first-order" factors. Most of the multivariate inventories to be considered in this chapter are "hierarchical" in nature; this means that they contain a number of relatively narrowband primary factors, which measure relatively specific behaviors, and a smaller number of higher-order factors, which are more abstract and general in nature.

RECENT HISTORY OF THE MULTIVARIATE PARADIGM

Raymond B. Cattell

Raymond B. Cattell (1905–1998), the founding father of the multivariate paradigm, received his PhD under Spearman at University College London in 1928. His intellectual development was clearly influenced by Spearman, Fisher, Cyril Burt, and others in the eugenic tradition that prevailed there at that time (Cattell, 1984). Thus his later advocacy of "multivariate experimental research" (Cattell, 1966) stemmed naturally from his association with both Spearman (factor analysis) and Fisher (analysis of variance), and he quite naturally developed interests in genetics, intelligence, and the eugenic issues raised by Galton (1884). Of much greater historical significance, however, was Cattell's (1933) prescient recognition that the methods employed in the study of human intelligence could be applied to the study of personality structure.

Cattell's Grand Plan

Cattell had a grand plan for the study of personality, which he and his associates implemented over a period of 65 years: (1) to determine the totality of behaviors encompassed by the term "personality" (the "personality sphere"), and to identify the basic and universal clusters of phenotypic "surface traits"; (2) to reduce these clusters of surface traits by factor analysis to their underlying "source traits"; and (3) to confirm, by multivariate analysis and experimentation, the generalizability of these source traits across the observational media of (a) life records ("L-data"), (b) self-report questionnaires ("Q-data"), and (c) behavioral responses to controlled test stimuli ("T-data"). These three aspects of the grand plan are now considered separately.

The Personality Sphere and the Lexical Tradition[2]

Cattell's first attempt to stake out the totality of human behavior in the personality sphere was done with reference to a dictionary of the English language. There was considerable precedent at the time for this approach, which is now called the lexical tradition in personality research (see Goldberg, 1981). Not surprisingly, this type of research was first reported by Galton (1884):

> I tried to gain an idea of the number of the more conspicuous aspects of the character by counting in an appropriate dictionary the words used to express them. Roget's Thesaurus was selected for that purpose, and I examined many pages of its index here and there as samples of the whole, and estimated that it contained fully one thousand words expressive of character, each of which has a separate shade of meaning, while each shares a large part of its meaning with some of the rest. (p. 181)

In 1926, Klages estimated that there were approximately 4,000 German words descriptive of the "inner states" of persons. The first systematic psychological study of trait-descriptive terms was conducted by Baumgarten (1933), who assembled 1,093 separate German trait terms from dictionaries and from the writings of psychologists. The following year, Thurstone (1934) described a study in which 1,300 raters were provided with a list of 60 trait-descriptive adjectives and asked to describe someone they knew well. Factor analysis of the intercorrelations among adjectives revealed that five factors were sufficient to account for most of their common variance, and Thurstone concluded that "the scientific description of personality might not be so hopelessly complex as it is sometimes thought to be" (1934, p. 14). He suggested that efforts be directed toward the identification of adjectives that formed "clusters" on the surface of the sphere formed by the five underlying factors.

Although the scientific description of personality may not be hope-

---

[2] Oliver John (1990) has provided a comprehensive historical overview of dimensions of personality in the natural language.

lessly complex, it is nonetheless complex when one considers that there were approximately 18,000 trait-descriptive adjectives in the English language available to Thurstone at that time, and that his only rationale for employing his particular set of 60 adjectives was that they were "in common use." What was needed was a lexicon of trait-descriptive adjectives that would permit investigators to select and sample terms on a systematic basis.

The task of identifying and organizing all of the trait-descriptive adjectives within a language can be overwhelming in its complexities. However, the benefits can be equally impressive. If something is of importance to people, they will develop a word for it. How important something is can also be suggested by the number of words within the language that are associated with that attribute (e.g., describing its variations, degrees, qualifications, expressions, and manifestations). That is, the most important domains of personality functioning are represented by the greatest number of trait terms within the language. A language is a sedimentary deposit of persons' observations over the thousands of years of the language's existence. Investigators can then mine this language to determine objectively and empirically what has been of most importance to persons as they have been developing and enriching the language.

Allport and Odbert (1936) were impressed by Thurstone's rating study: "Theoretically it would be possible to apply this ingenious method to a *complete* list of trait terms" (p. 33; emphasis added). And they took upon themselves the task of compiling an exhaustive list of 17,953 terms from the approximately 400,000 terms in the 1925 *Webster's New International Dictionary* that distinguished "the behavior of one human being from that of another" (p. 240). These terms were then classified alphabetically under the four broad categories shown in Table 4.4.

TABLE 4.4. Classification of Terms in Allport and Odbert's Lexicon

Category	Criteria	Examples
I	Neutral terms designating possible personal traits	Friendly, dutiful, curious
II	Terms primarily descriptive of temporary moods or activities	Delighted, repelled, dumbfounded
III	Weighted terms conveying social or characterical judgments of personal conduct, or designating influence on others	Abnormal, immoral, ignorant
IV	Miscellaneous: Designations of physique, capacities, and developmental conditions; metaphorical and doubtful terms	Bovine, full-grown, limpid

Note. Data from Allport and Odbert (1936).

The terms classified in the first category (I) were those that appeared to have the potential for capturing the most "objective" and "realistic" attributes describing lasting structures, as opposed to temporary states (II), censorial and evaluative terms (III), and metaphorical and doubtful terms (IV). In addition to providing a fertile source of items for subsequent scale and instrument development in other paradigms (e.g., Gough & Heilbrun, 1965), this lexicon served a critical role in the development of both the lexical and structural approaches within the multivariate paradigm.

Surface Traits

Surface traits are clusters of observable attributes that tend to be encoded in the ordinary language of personality and may be considered to constitute the "language personality sphere" (Cattell, 1946, p. 216). In this sense, surface traits constitute the *phenotypic* variables of personality that require, rather than provide, explanations of the behaviors they describe. Using cluster-analytic procedures, Cattell (1943) reduced the Allport–Odbert list of approximately 18,000 terms to 35 bipolar clusters of surface traits (see John, 1990, pp. 69–71).

Source Traits

Source traits are determined from a factor analysis of surface trait clusters and they represent, according to Cattell, the *genotypic* variables in personality research. In other words, source traits are assumed to be associated with environmental and genetic influences that are thought to cause characteristic surface behaviors (Cattell, 1957). Within Cattell's plan, source traits should be identified in three media of observation in order to establish their generalizability. As noted above, these are life record data (L-data), which are obtained from naturalistic observation of participants in everyday life situations (e.g., peer ratings); questionnaire data (Q-data), which are obtained from participants' responses to self-report personality inventories; and objective test data (T-data), which are obtained from the behavioral responses of participants to controlled stimulus situations (e.g., psychophysiological measures).

Cattell began his studies "through the *L*-medium because this domain of observed behavior was (and is) the most down-to-earth reality in human behavior (used as the 'criterion' in much predictive work)" (1979, p. 53; emphasis in original). The 35 surface trait clusters extracted from the Allport–Odbert taxonomy were administered in a series of peer rating studies. Initially, Cattell (1944) identified 12 source trait factors underlying the intercorrelations among the 35 peer rating scales. Over the ensuing years, Cattell and his colleagues conducted an unprecedented number of studies in the life record, questionnaire, and objective test media. They published,

among other tests, the widely used Sixteen Personality Factor Questionnaire (16 PF; Cattell, 1949), which is discussed later in this chapter.

Other Early Investigators

The Guilfords (Guilford & Guilford, 1936, 1939) were also pioneers in the
application of factor analysis to personality data, and they assembled evidence for four interpretable factors that would now be called Extraversion,
Conscientiousness, Neuroticism, and Intellect; these, together with Agreeableness, constitute the currently important five-factor model (FFM) of
personality (Digman, 1996). A few years later, Eysenck (1944) factored the
intercorrelations among presenting symptoms of psychiatric patients and
interpreted the first two factors as Neuroticism and Introversion. Cattell
(1945) rotated Eysenck's factor matrix a different way and offered a different interpretation.[3] Later, Eysenck (1947) argued for Extraversion and
Neuroticism on the basis of theoretical (Jung, 1923) and empirical (MacKinnon, 1944) precedents (see Eysenck, 1990). By the 1950s, the systems of
Eysenck (1953), Cattell (1957), and Guilford (1959) had become prominent alternative theories of personality structure.

As the method of factor analysis became a standard tool of investigation, both the number and nature of reported factors proliferated. In 1953,
John W. French and his associates at Educational Testing Service (ETS)
took on the Herculean task of identifying and categorizing the approximately 450 factors that had been reported in the literature. A wealth of detail was provided on the nature of the studies, the factors found, and their
replications by others. A factor was considered "established" if it was identified in at least three studies, at least two of which were from different lab-
oratories. Perusal of the alphabetical list of factors reveals the presence of
such factors as Gregariousness, Agreeableness, Dependability, Emotionality, and Intelligence, which were not accorded any special significance at
the time, but which would later (under slightly different names) be recognized as the "Big Five" factors of personality structure.

Comparison of one factorial study with another involves an element of
subjectivity unless there are common marker scales employed in the two
studies being compared. Based on an additional literature review by French
(1973) and on empirical confirmation studies (e.g., Derman, French, &
Harman, 1974), brief and internally consistent marker scales were constructed for 18 well-established factors in the literature, and published
marker scales were cited for an additional 10 (Derman, French, & Harman, 1978). Marker scales for Gregariousness, Agreeableness, Dependability, Emotional Stability, and Open-Mindedness survived this short list,

---

[3] These interchanges continued for the next 50 years.

although again without special emphasis. Despite the pioneering and illuminating contributions of the ETS group, the long-awaited consensus on the basic factors of personality was to come from quite another line of historical development.

THE EMERGENCE OF THE "BIG FIVE" FACTORS

As mentioned earlier, after Cattell reduced the Allport–Odbert taxonomy to 35 surface clusters, he constructed bipolar rating scales for the clusters and conducted a series of peer rating studies, which suggested that 12 source traits accounted for the personality sphere. Subsequent investigations in the line of research initiated by Cattell led to remarkable agreements concerning both the lexical basis of personality (i.e., surface traits) and the structural organization of personality (i.e., source traits). The four studies outlined in Table 4.5 have been selected as the most influential from a larger number of studies that have reported similar findings.

The Fiske Studies

Twenty-two of Cattell's bipolar peer rating scales were employed in the Michigan Veterans Administration Selection Research Project on the selection of graduate students in clinical psychology (Kelly & Fiske, 1951). These rating scales were used to obtain self-ratings, teammate ratings, and staff assessment ratings for all trainees in the study. In a now classic study, Fiske (1949) found that the factorial results from these different rating sources were highly consistent, and that 5 (not 12) factors were sufficient to

TABLE 4.5. Milestones in the "Big Five" Lexical Tradition

	Fiske (1949)	Tupes and Christal (1961)	Norman (1963)	Goldberg (1977)
Source	Cattell clusters	Cattell clusters	Cattell clusters	Norman clusters
I	Confident Self-Expression	Surgency	Surgency	Surgency
II	Social Adaptability	Agreeableness	Agreeableness	Agreeableness
III	Conformity	Dependability	Conscientiousness	Conscientiousness
IV	Emotional Control	Emotional Stability	Emotional Stability	Emotional Stability
V	Inquiring Intellect	Culture	Culture	Intellect

account for most of the variance among rating scales from different sources. Unfortunately, the results of this study were largely ignored until the 1970s (Goldberg, 1995).

The Tupes and Christal Studies

The suspicion that Cattell might have "overfactored" the personality language sphere in his original studies was later strongly confirmed in an equally classic series of studies by Tupes and Christal (1958, 1961), who demonstrated what they felt was the "universal" nature of a five-factor solution within Cattell's surface trait variables. Tupes and Christal named these factors (I) Surgency, (II) Agreeableness, (III) Dependability, (IV) Emotional Stability, and (V) Culture.

The Norman Studies

In a highly influential paper entitled "Toward an Adequate Taxonomy of Personality Attributes," Norman (1963) set forth in detail both the rationale and specific procedures for developing a "well-structured" taxonomy of personality attributes. Although clearly impressed by the robustness of the five recurrent factors of the personality language sphere reported by previous investigators, Norman felt that "it is time to return to the total pool of trait names in the natural language—there to search for additional personality indicators not easily subsumed under one or another of these five recurrent factors" (p. 582).

Using the unabridged 1961 *Webster's Third New International Dictionary*, Norman (1967) added new personality terms that had appeared in the language since the time of Allport and Odbert's search. Of greater importance were Norman's criteria for eliminating unsuitable terms from his master list of 18,125 terms. Terms were eliminated from the list that were (1) solely evaluative (e.g., "evil"); (2) ambiguous, vague, or metaphorical (e.g., "nebulous"); (3) difficult or obscure (e.g., "Icarian"); or (4) descriptive of anatomical or physical conditions (e.g., "hairy"). The reduced list of items was then sorted into the three major classes of terms illustrated in Table 4.6. Ratings of word familiarity by college students resulted in further reduction of the list to approximately 1,600 terms. Finally, Norman classified items as falling at either the positive or negative pole of the five factors identified in earlier studies (e.g., Tupes & Christal, 1961).

The Goldberg Studies

Norman's taxonomy of personality attributes and his preliminary classification of terms within five factors were subsequently employed by Goldberg (1977, 1980) as a starting point in an ongoing program of method-

TABLE 4.6. Classification of Terms in Norman's Lexicon

Category	Criteria	Examples
I. Stable Traits	Terms that designate typical, generalized, and personalized characteristics of a person or his or her behavior	Calm, daring, genial, lazy
II. Temporary States	Terms descriptive of activities or actions of a person that are typically brief or episodic in duration	Arguing, disagreeing, obeying
III. Social Roles	Terms connoting particular social roles, relationships, status, or position of a person vis-à-vis some other person, group, or social institution	Adversary, captive, employed, leader, scapegoat

Note. Data from Norman (1967).

ologically elegant research on the natural language of personality. This research firmly established the dimensions identified by earlier investigators, which Goldberg referred to as the "Big Five."[4] Goldberg (1981) described the theoretical foundation of his research program as follows:

> The most promising of the empirical approaches to systematizing personality differences have been based on one critical assumption: *Those individual differences that are of the most significance in the daily transactions of persons with each other will eventually become encoded in their language.* . . . Moreover, this fundamental axiom has a highly significant corollary: *The more important is an individual difference in human transactions, the more languages will have a term for it.* (pp. 141–142; emphasis in original)

Goldberg reduced Norman's taxonomy by deleting uncommon terms, structured his own taxonomy according to strict rules, generated a large number of categories that mapped onto higher-order dimensions, and evaluated the final taxonomy by several rigorous criteria. In light of his finding five, and only five, robust factors under different methods of extraction and

---

[4] In an earlier review of the literature of personality structure, I (Wiggins, 1968) referred to the dimensions of Extraversion and Neuroticism (Anxiety) as the "Big Two" because of their prominence in published studies of scales and inventories at that time. Subsequently, Saucier and Goldberg (1996a) suggested that the expression "Big Five" be restricted to taxonomic studies in the lexical tradition, as opposed to the "five-factor model" (FFM) tradition of questionnaire studies of personality traits. The two expressions are generally used interchangeably, as they are here, on the grounds that they are the same variables at two stages in Cattell's grand plan.

rotation in both self-ratings and peer ratings, Goldberg (1990) proposed an alternative "description of personality" to that originally proposed by Cattell (1943). Some representative trait-descriptive adjectives from this taxonomy are shown in Table 4.7. With respect to the generalizability of the structure of the Big Five across languages, as mentioned in the quote above, there have been substantial confirmations of this hypothesis in several languages by interlinguistic teams of investigators (e.g., Hofstee, Kiers, De Raad, Goldberg, & Ostendorf, 1997).

ASSESSMENT INSTRUMENTS

As discussed earlier, Cattell's original grand plan was to (1) define the totality of the personality sphere with reference to the language of personality; (2) reduce the basic clusters of phenotypic surface traits by factor analysis to their underlying source traits; and (3) confirm the generalizability of these source traits in various media, including especially the multivariate personality questionnaire. The FFM has had considerable influence on contemporary scales and inventories (Wiggins & Trapnell, 1997). The extent of this influence has been clearly stated by Ozer and Reise (1994):

> Personality psychologists who continue to employ their preferred measure without locating it within the five-factor model can only be likened to geographers who issue reports of new lands but refuse to locate them on a map for others to find. (p. 361)

With one exception, the six major personality inventories considered here can be easily "mapped" onto the FFM. Table 4.8 presents these locations.

TABLE 4.7. Goldberg's "Big Five" Taxonomy

Dimensions	Positive pole	Negative pole
I. Surgency	Extraverted, talkative, assertive, verbal	Introverted, shy, quiet, restrained
II. Agreeableness	Kind, cooperative, warm, sympathetic	Cold, unkind, distrustful, demanding
III. Conscientiousness	Organized, systematic, thorough, practical	Disorganized, careless, inefficient, undependable
IV. Emotional Stability	Relaxed, unemotional, unenvious, unexcitable	Anxious, moody, emotional, irritable
V. Intellect	Intellectual, creative, complex, imaginative	Simple, shallow, uncreative, imperceptive

Note. Data from Goldberg (1990).

Earlier Inventories

Sixteen Personality Factor Questionnaire

As the venerable Sixteen Personality Factor Questionnaire (16 PF; Cattell, Cattell, & Cattell, 1993) approached its 50th anniversary, a handsome new technical manual was issued (Conn & Rieke, 1994b) that emphasized continuity with the extensive empirical literature of the past, while ensuring a place in the future for this pioneering multivariate inventory. In the construction of the fifth edition of the 16 PF, revisions occurred at both the item level and the primary factor scale level, and these revisions have increased both the psychometric precision and interpretability of the 16 primary factor scales (H. E. P. Cattell, 1994).

Although Cattell himself was no fan of the "five big factors heresy" (R. B. Cattell, 1994, p. 9), the new manual places an increased emphasis on the interpretation of the five second-order factor scales that are now called global factor scales "to better reflect the broad personality domains that they represent" (H. E. P. Cattell, 1994, p. 13). The convergence of the five global factor scores with other questionnaire measures of the FFM of personality are presented in detail in the 16 PF test manual. These include correlations with the facet scores of the NEO Personality Inventory, the five global factor scores of the Personality Research Form, the California Psychological Inventory, and the Myers–Briggs Type Indicator (Conn & Rieke, 1994a). As shown in Table 4.8, the five global factor scales of the 16 PF are labeled Extraversion, Independence, Self-Control, Anxiety, and Tough Mindedness. Although the primary factors of the 16 PF are still the major foci of some "Cattellians" (e.g., Krug, 1994), others stress that "Cattell's second-order traits were a fundamental part of his theory from the beginning" and emphasize the historical priority of the 16 PF in this respect (H. E. P. Cattell, 1996, p. 5).

Eysenck Personality Questionnaire—Revised

The widespread use of the Eysenck Personality Questionnaire (EPQ-R; Eysenck & Eysenck, 1993) in its present and earlier forms has been due in no small part to the extraordinary research productivity of Eysenck and his colleagues in England (Eysenck, 1990). The three substantive scales of the EPQ-R provide measures of the factors of Psychoticism, Extraversion, and Neuroticism, which are referred to by the acronym of PEN. Few would contest the importance of Extraversion and Neuroticism in the assessment of personality, and Eysenck's pivotal role in establishing both the conceptual and empirical bases of these dimensions is universally recognized (e.g., Eysenck, 1960, 1970–1971). However, earlier versions of the Psychoticism scale have been criticized on psychometric grounds (e.g., Block, 1977b; Stricker, 1978), as well as for being unrelated to the clinical syndrome of

TABLE 4.8. The FFM in Personality Questionnaires

Author(s)	Test	I	II	III	IV	V
Cattell et al. (1993)	16 PF	Extraversion	Independence (–)	Self-Control	Anxiety	Tough-Mindedness (–)
Eysenck and Eysenck (1993)	EPQ	Extraversion	Psychoticism (–)		Neuroticism	
Jackson et al. (1996)	PRF	Extraversion	Agreeableness	Achievement/Methodicalness	Independence	Openness
Costa and McCrae (1992)	NEO-PI-R	Extraversion	Agreeableness	Conscientiousness	Neuroticism	Openness
Hogan and Hogan (1992)	HPI	Ambition/Sociability	Likeability	Prudence	Adjustment (–)	Intellectance/School Success
Goldberg (1999)	IPIP	Surgency	Agreeableness	Conscientiousness	Emotional Stability (–)	Intellect

Note. (–) indicates that a scale measures the opposite pole of the dimension from that normally emphasized (e.g., "Adjustment" and "Emotional Stability" may be seen as representing *low* Neuroticisim).

psychoticism (Block, 1977a; Bishop, 1977). Studies of the PEN dimensions with reference to the FFM (McCrae & Costa, 1985) and the Big Five lexical framework (Goldberg & Rosolack, 1994) have established the convergences of EPQ/EPQ-R Extraversion and Neuroticism with their factorial counterparts in these two traditions, and have also shown that the less reliable dimension of Psychoticism has moderate negative loadings on both Agreeableness and Conscientiousness.

Personality Research Form

The Personality Research Form (PRF; Jackson, 1984) was not initially constructed by factor-analytic procedures. Instead, the instrument was developed under a construct-oriented approach to Murray's (1938) need variables, which utilized a sophisticated sequential system for scale development designed to maximize convergent and discriminant content saturation (Jackson, 1970). The result was a multiscale inventory with impeccable psychometric properties (Wiggins, 1989) that has proven useful in a variety of contexts, including that of the personological paradigm (e.g., Nasby & Read, 1997a, 1997b). The PRF has been found to conform to the FFM by Costa and McCrae (1988) and by Jackson, Paunonen, Fraboni, and Goffin (1996). The latter authors found the most optimal fit to be a six-factor solution in which the Conscientiousness factor was split into Achievement and Methodicalness components. Neuroticism was renamed Independence to reflect its loadings by the Autonomy, Social Recognition (–), and Succorance (–) need scales of the PRF.

More Recent Inventories

Revised NEO Personality Inventory

The Revised NEO Personality Inventory (NEO PI R) was published by Costa and McCrae in 1992. The acronym "NEO" was applied to an earlier three-factor version of this inventory that had its origins in the Neuroticism (N) and Extraversion (E) dimensions identified by Eysenck and Cattell, and in the Openness to Experience (O) dimension suggested by Rogers (1961) and identified by Coan (1974). To these three dimensions were added the dimensions of Agreeableness (A) and Conscientiousness (C) identified by Goldberg (1980) in his lexical studies of the Big Five dimensions of natural language. In its present form, the NEO PI-R is considered a questionnaire measure of the major dimensions of personality traits that have been identified within the venerable multivariate-trait paradigm (McCrae & Costa, 1996), and that have come to be known as the FFM of personality characteristics.

The NEO PI-R provides global measures (i.e., domain scores) for each

TABLE 4.9. Domains and Facets of the Revised NEO
Personality Inventory (NEO PI-R)

Neuroticism	Agreeableness
N1. Anxiety	A1. Trust
N2. Angry Hostility	A2. Straightforwardness
N3. Depression	A3. Altruism
N4. Self-Consciousness	A4. Compliance
N5. Impulsiveness	A5. Modesty
N6. Vulnerability	A6. Tender-Mindedness

Extraversion	Conscientiousness
E1. Warmth	C1. Competence
E2. Gregariousness	C2. Order
E3. Assertiveness	C3. Dutifulness
E4. Activity	C4. Achievement Striving
E5. Excitement-Seeking	C5. Self-Discipline
E6. Positive Emotions	C6. Deliberation

Openness

O1. Fantasy
O2. Aesthetics
O3. Feelings
O4. Actions
O5. Ideas
O6. Values

of the five factors, and six more specific measures (i.e., facet scores) within each of the five domains of Neuroticism, Extraversion, Openness to Experience, Agreeableness, and Conscientiousness, as indicated in Table 4.9. Note that the facets can be represented by letter–number labels (e.g., "N1" for the "Anxiety" facet of Neuroticism). The "astonishingly fruitful research collaboration" (Block, 1995, p. 200) of Costa and McCrae has produced more than 100 publications that document the substantive, structural, and empirical validity of this instrument.

Hogan Personality Inventory

Historically, the FFM arose in the context of peer ratings (Wiggins, 1973b). Hogan and Hogan (1992), in their manual for the Hogan Personality Inventory (HPI), have provided an explicit rationale for interpreting the dimensions of the FFM in that context:

> The FFM concerns the structure of reputation . . . based on social consensus regarding trends in a person's behavior. . . . What is it that creates a person's reputation? Behavior during social interaction consists at least in part of actions designed to establish, defend or enhance that person's identity

... personality assessment measures self-presentational behavior. (p. 3; emphasis added)

This perspective led the Hogans to formulate an alternative seven-factor representation of the FFM—one more directly focused on those aspects of a person's reputation that have implications for his or her potential contributions to a social group or organization (see Hogan, 1983). Each factor contains from four to eight Homogeneous Item Composites (HICs), which identify specific subthemes within each domain. With reference to the original roman numeral ordering assigned to them (Tupes & Christal, 1961), the factors (and their highest-loading HICs) are as follows:

Ia. Ambition (competitive; competent).
Ib. Sociability (likes parties; likes crowds).
II.   Likeability (easy to live with; sensitive and caring).
III. Prudence (moralistic; virtuous).
IV. Adjustment (empathy; not anxious).
Va. Intellectance (science ability; curiosity).
Vb. School Success (education; math ability).

Within the traditional first factor, the impulsivity and need for interaction of Sociability are distinguished from the desire for status, power, and recognition of Ambition. Within the traditional fifth factor, the interest in culture and ideas of Intellectance are distinguished from the academic performance of School Success. The HPI is very much intended to be an "applied" instrument, and the range and number of personnel selection problems to which it has been successfully applied are most impressive (Wiggins & Trapnell, 1997).

International Personality Item Pool

In introducing his International Personality Item Pool (IPIP), Goldberg (1999) wrote:

> I envisage an international effort to develop and continually refine a broad-bandwidth personality inventory, whose items are in the public domain, and whose scales can be used for both scientific and commercial purposes. No one investigator alone has access to many diverse criterion settings; but the international scientific community has such access, and by pooling our findings we should be able to devise instruments over the next decade that make our present ones seem like ancient relics. (p. 8)

Goldberg's dissatisfaction with the commercial test-publishing industry is based in part on his concern that copyright regulations may restrict the free use of tests by investigators who might further develop, refine, or revise such instruments—procedures that have not been high among the priorities of many commerical publishing firms. As a consequence, he has taken his mission to the World Wide Web (http://www. ipip.ori.org) with an open invitation for international collaboration among those interested in accelerating the development of the multivariate paradigm.

In 2002, the IPIP included 1,956 items, measuring 280 personality scales. Approximately 750 of those items were originally developed by a Dutch team (Hendriks, 1997), and about 1,200 new English items were later added to that set. This pool was developed by Goldberg for the purposes of (1) taxonomy refinement, (2) scale construction, and (3) scale validation. Most importantly, the total pool of items was administered to a large adult community sample; test forms were mailed to a sample of approximately 800 individuals who agreed to participate in the IPIP study for a period of 5–10 years, and who were compensated for their participation. Over time, these same participants completed a number of standard personality inventories, including the 16 PF, California Personality Inventory, NEO PI-R, and HPI. IPIP equivalents of these standard personality inventories were created from the IPIP item pool with remarkable success (Goldberg, in press).

The IPIP items are presented as succinct behavioral statements preceded by active verbs (e.g., "Make friends easily"). The self-applicability of each statement is rated on a 5-point Likert scale ranging from "very inaccurate" (1) to "very accurate" (5). Table 4.10 presents representative IPIP items and their NEO PI-R counterparts for each of the five factors.

TABLE 4.10. Representative IPIP Items and Their NEO PI-R Counterparts

Factor	IPIP	NEO PI-R
Surgency	Make friends easily.	I really like most people I meet.
Agreeableness	Trust others.	I tend to be cynical and skeptical of others' intentions.[a]
Conscientiousness	Complete tasks successfully.	I am efficient and effective at my work.
Emotional Stability	Worry about things.	I am not a worrier.[a]
Intellect	Have a vivid imagination.	I have a very active imagination.

[a] Reversed scoring.

Hierarchies in Multivariate Inventories

Orthogonal and Oblique Factor Rotations

When factors are extracted from an intercorrelation matrix, it is up to the investigator to decide whether the factors will be correlated with each other (i.e., oblique) or uncorrelated with each other (i.e., orthogonal). Although the orthogonal varimax rotational procedure employed in our earlier numerical example has much to recommend it, there is considerable historical precedent for oblique factors. For example, Cattell (1957) argued that relations in the natural world are oblique rather than orthogonal, and Thurstone (1934) suggested that although height and weight are correlated, they have nevertheless proved to be useful categories in the study of physique. To the extent that factors are correlated with each other, it is possible to factor the intercorrelations among these factors to obtain second-order factors. The relation between the lower-order and higher-order factors is conceived of as hierarchical; the first orders are thought to reflect specific facets closer to behavior, and the higher-order factors are thought to represent broader and more abstract categories.

Big Five Hierarchies

It should be clear from the earlier summaries of different instruments that the current multivariate paradigm represents personality as a *hierarchical structure* (Goldberg, 1993; Hampson, John, & Goldberg, 1986; John, Hampson, & Goldberg, 1991). Cattell's (1949) 16 primary factors were correlated with each other, and factor analysis of the intercorrelations among these primaries revealed four clear second-order factors. A fifth second-order factor was later recognized (Cattell, Eber, & Tatsuoka, 1970), and these global factor scales are now routinely interpreted within the Big Five tradition (H. E. P. Cattell, 1994). A similar relationship between first- and second-order factors is reflected in the lower- and higher-order scales of the PRF, the facets and domains of the NEO PI-R, and the HICs and factor scales of the HPI. Although Eysenck (1992, 1994) examined a number of first-order factors, he mainly preferred to interpret the second-order "Giant Three" of the EPQ (see Cattell, 1973).

Bandwidth and Fidelity

Shannon and Weaver's (1949) information theory was developed in the context of electronic communication systems in which the concepts of "bandwidth" and "fidelity" were first introduced. "Bandwidth" refers to the amount or complexity of information obtained in a given space or time. "Fidelity" refers to the clarity with which that information is transmitted.

The evolution of the modern compact disc from the original gramophone record is a history of attempts to optimize these two parameters. Cronbach and Gleser (1957) applied these two concepts to psychological tests and personnel decisions. For example, administration of the Strong Vocational Interest Blank (Strong, 1959), followed by career counseling, is a strategy that has both high bandwidth and high fidelity. An inexpensive paper-and-pencil test provides an excellent mapping of the field of vocational interests; the more focused interview determines the implications of these scores for a particular client (Cronbach, 1960).

From the standpoint of prediction of specific criteria, it may be the case that appropriate first-order primaries, facets, and HICs of the 16 PF, NEO PI-R, and HPI (being more concrete in nature) would be able to predict specific behaviors with greater precision than would the broader, more abstract, second-order Big Five factors. Recent findings tend to substantiate this possibility (e.g., Ashton, Jackson, Paunonen, Helmes, & Rothstein, 1995; Mershon & Gorsuch, 1988). The higher-order factors of the Big Five may be broader in bandwidth and lower in fidelity, whereas the lower-order factors may be narrower in bandwidth and higher in fidelity.

COMPARATIVE VALIDITY OF MULTIVARIATE INVENTORIES

Although each of the major instruments considered in this chapter has distinctive and desirable features, the "proof of the pudding" of any assessment instrument resides in its ability to forecast socially relevant criteria (Wiggins, 1973b). A number of studies have compared the extent to which different instruments are correlated with one another or appear to have similar structures, but prior to the study of Goldberg (in press) reported in this section, there were virtually no studies reporting how inventories differ in the variety of different outcomes they can predict (their bandwidth) and in the extent to which they can predict each outcome (their fidelity).

Goldberg's Comparative Validity Study

Predictor Variables

Goldberg's (in press) study was based on the protocols of 423 participants in his community sample for whom complete data on all measures were available. The predictor variables included 16 PF, HPI, and NEO PI-R first- and second-order scales and their equivalent IPIP versions, making possible a comparison of the predictive validity of the two versions of each instrument. The predictors developed from the IPIP also included Big Five marker scales and the bipolar adjective clusters identified in a previous large-scale study (Hofstee, De Raad, & Goldberg, 1992). In sum, instruments included the following: the 16 PF (16 primaries, 5 global factors); the HPI (44 homogeneous item clusters, 7 factors); the NEO PI-R (30 facets, 5 domains); and IPIP equivalents of each of the foregoing scales, as well as 45 IPIP-derived bipolar facet scales and Big Five markers. It was thus possible to compare the relative predictive efficiency of lower-order and higher-order scales across a variety of instruments.

Criterion Variables

Participants were also asked to complete a substantially modified version of the Objective Behavior Inventory (Loehlin & Nichols, 1976). With this item pool, respondents estimated the frequency with which they have performed a variety of specific acts on a 5-point scale ranging from (1) "Never in my life" to (5) "More than fifteen times in the past year." For purposes of the present study, the 400 acts in this inventory were empirically reduced to six reliable clusters: (1) Drug Use (14 acts) (e.g.,"Smoked marijuana"); (2) Undependability (7 acts) (e.g., "Did not return a phone call"); (3) Friendship (8 acts) (e.g., "Did a favor for a friend"); (4) Creative Achievements (11 acts) (e.g., "Played a piano or other instrument"); (5) Reading (6 acts) (e.g., "Bought a book"); and (6) Writing (8 acts) (e.g., "Wrote a postcard").

Comparative Validity of Multivariate Inventories

For each commercial inventory and its IPIP counterpart, lower-order scales were multiply regressed on each of six criterion composites. Table 4.11 displays these comparative correlations. From this table it can be seen, for example, that the 16 primaries of the 16 PF were correlated .42 with Drug Use, and that the 16 corresponding IPIP scales were correlated .55 with the same criterion. The final column shows that the average correlation of the 16 PF across criteria was .46, and that the average cross-criteria correlation of the IPIP counterpart was .51.

What is immediately apparent from this table is that all inventories were reasonably predictive of a variety of criteria. If one were to pick a winner among the commercial inventories, it would be the 16 PF by a nose. (This venerable instrument is clearly not ready to be put out to pasture.) However, the overall winner appeared to be the IPIP version of the 16 PF, although it should be noted that the IPIP equivalent scales were constructed within this sample, which might be associated with higher internal consistencies (and therefore more predictive power) for the IPIP scales compared to their commercial counterparts. Nonetheless, the IPIP equivalent scales appeared to be representative of their original counterparts, with the IPIP versions correlating between .60 and .75 with their commercial counter-

TABLE 4.11. Cross-Validity Scale Correlations of Regression Analyses with Act Criteria

Test	Drug Use Orig.	IPIP	Friendship Orig.	IPIP	Dependable Orig.	IPIP	Reading Orig.	IPIP	Writing Orig.	IPIP	Creative Orig.	IPIP	Mean Orig.	IPIP
16 PF	.42	.55	.48	.47	.34	.49	.56	.56	.45	.45	.48	.52	.46	.51
HPI	.43	.48	.34	.47	.43	.46	.57	.57	.38	.42	.48	.48	.44	.48
NEO PI-R	.49	.54	.45	.48	.35	.43	.37	.44	.43	.46	.46	.53	.43	.48
Mean	.45	.53	.42	.47	.37	.46	.48	.50	.42	.44	.47	.51	.44	.49

Note. Data from Goldberg (in press).

parts. As Goldberg (in press) noted, these correlations were between .85 and .95 when corrected for the unreliabilities of the scales involved.

Comparative Validity of Lower-Order and Higher-Order Scales

It is generally believed that lower-order scales tend to predict specific behaviors with greater precision than do broader, more abstract second-order factors. Cattell emphasized this point consistently, and this in part explains his resistance to the FFM (see Wiggins & Trapnell, 1997). The findings in Table 4.12 indicate that, with the exception of the possibly less reliable HICs of the HPI, lower-order scales consistently tended to outpredict their higher-order representations. However, the magnitude by which they did so was considerably less than has previously been suggested. This and other features of the present comparative validity study raise questions concerning the generalizability of these findings to other criteria and to other populations. But that, of course, is the question that Goldberg (1999) would like others to consider in the context of his invitation for all to participate in his plan to devise instruments over the next decade that make "our present ones seem like ancient relics" (p. 8).

Johnson's Comparative Validity Study

An Alternative Criterion for Comparative Validity Studies

Johnson (2000) has made a convincing case for the importance of observer ratings as criteria against which self-report inventories should be validated. The way that one is viewed by significant others, and one's social reputation in general, define the limitations and opportunities of one's social life (e.g., Gough, 1987; Hogan & Hogan, 1992). With this in mind, Johnson assessed the comparative validity of higher-order and facet scales of the NEO PI-R (Costa & McCrae, 1992), the HPI (Hogan & Hogan, 1992), and the California Psychological Inventory (CPI; Gough, 1987) in predicting acquaintance ratings on four sets of Big Five scales. Undergraduate students (n = 148) were asked to complete the aforementioned personality inventories and to obtain Big Five ratings from two acquaintances who knew them well. The four different sets of Big Five rating scales represented variants in scoring procedures suggested by Hogan and Johnson (1981), McCrae and Costa (1987), Norman (1963), and Goldberg (1992).

Johnson explored a number of important methodological issues in addition to the main effects of comparative validity. The comparative validity findings were quite clear:

> In 25 of the 27 possible comparisons of the three self-report inventories, the NEO-PI-R scales equaled or surpassed the abilities of the other self-report scales to predict the acquaintance ratings. In the other two cases, the NEO-PI-R-based correlation was within r = .02 of the strongest predictor. Overall, the average validity coefficient for the NEO-PI-R primary scales was r = .42; for the CPI, r = .28, and for the HPI, r = .30. (Johnson, 2000, p. 12)

Secondary Loadings of the Big Five Factors

Johnson's (2000) comparative validity study was also designed to explore what he considered to be an equally important methodological issue that has been neglected by other investigators of the comparative validity of Big

TABLE 4.12. Comparisons between Higher-Order and Lower-Order Scales in Predicting Act Criteria

Test	Drug Use Orig.	IPIP	Friendship Orig.	IPIP	Dependable Orig.	IPIP	Reading Orig.	IPIP	Writing Orig.	IPIP	Creative Orig.	IPIP	Mean Orig.	IPIP
16 PF														
Globals	.36	.31	.39	.39	.28	.43	.47	.43	.43	.33	.43	.49	.39	.40
Primaries	.42	.55	.48	.47	.34	.49	.56	.56	.45	.45	.48	.52	.46	.51
HPI														
Factor scales	.46	.50	.35	.39	.26	.37	.42	.44	.23	.25	.35	.43	.34	.40
HICs	.43	.48	.34	.47	.43	.46	.57	.57	.38	.42	.48	.48	.44	.48
NEO PI-R														
Domains	.40	.39	.33	.35	.32	.38	.35	.39	.33	.35	.40	.52	.36	.40
Facets	.49	.54	.45	.48	.35	.43	.37	.44	.43	.46	.46	.53	.43	.48
Means														
Higher-order	.41	.40	.36	.38	.29	.39	.41	.42	.33	.31	.39	.48	.36	.40
Lower-order	.45	.52	.42	.47	.37	.46	.50	.52	.42	.44	.47	.51	.44	.44
Big Five markers														
Domains	—	.38	—	.43	—	.39	—	.43	—	.34	—	.46	—	.41
AB5C facets	—	.44	—	.42	—	.40	—	.41	—	.49	—	.54	—	.45

Note. Data from Goldberg (in press).

Five instruments. As indicated in Chapter 2, advocates of both multivariate and circumplex models initially viewed their respective models as complementary rather than competitive (e.g., McCrae & Costa, 1989; Trapnell & Wiggins, 1990). A further step toward coordination of the two models may be found in the Abridged Big Five Dimensional Circumplex (AB5C; Hofstee et al., 1992). As Hofstee and colleagues (1992) note, trait names tend to represent *blends* of factors, rather than loading univocally on only one factor. Circumplex models provide the precise location of items within the 360 degrees of a circle whose coordinates are two orthogonal factors. As such, "[they] provide much more opportunity for identifying clusters of traits that are semantically cohesive" (Hofstee et al., 1992, p. 146).

The AB5C model locates items within the 10 two-dimensional circumplexes formed by considering all possible pairings of the Big Five factors of (I) Surgency, (II) Agreeableness, (III) Conscientiousness, (IV) Emotional Stability, and (V) Intellect. Only the first two highest loadings of an item are considered. For example, if an item has its *primary* loading on Surgency (e.g., .65), and its second highest loading is insignificant (e.g., .09), the item is classified as I+I+ to indicate that it is primarily defined by a positive loading on Surgency (e.g., "talkative"). If an item loads primarily on Surgency and has a significant secondary loading on Emotional Stability, the item is classified as I+IV+ to reflect this pattern (e.g., "courageous").

Johnson (2000) explored the possibility that in comparative validity studies, the AB5C locations of the criterion variables and the AB5C locations of the predictor variables might affect the validity correlations between the two. For example, a given correlation between self-reports and acquaintance ratings might be highest if both predictor and criterion were measured with V+III– variables, lower if predictor and criterion variables differed in their secondary loadings (e.g., V+III– vs. V+II+), and still lower if predictor and criterion variables differed in *sign* on their secondary loadings (e.g., V+III– vs. V+III+). And this was exactly what Johnson found in his own comparative validity study. For all the domain scales in his study, the predictor–criterion correlations averaged .36 when predictors and criteria shared the same AB5C locations; .28 when predictors and criteria had the same primary, but different secondary, AB5C locations; and .15 when predictors and criteria had the same primary location and opposite signs on secondary locations. The same pattern was found for the NEO PI-R facet scales and the HPI HICs.

The predictive superiority of the NEO PI-R domain and facet scales to those of the CPI and HPI was, in Johnson's view, due mainly to the superior internal consistency (homogeneity) of the NEO PI-R scales. The AB5C criterion scales themselves were all quite homogeneous and were located very near to their appropriate vectors. Whereas the variance of each CPI and HPI scale tended to be relatively spread out over the five-factor space, each NEO PI-R scale was located more closely and more precisely to an AB5C vector. Johnson (2000) concluded that "as future researchers respond to Goldberg's (1999) request for comparative validity studies, they might be well advised to consider both the primary and secondary loadings of predictors and criteria." (p. 13).

CLINICAL APPLICATIONS AND CURRENT STATUS

Personality Disorders and the FFM

The third edition of the American Psychiatric Association's (APA's) *Diagnostic and Statistical Manual of Mental Disorders* (DSM-III; APA, 1980) was a landmark in the history of clinical assessment within the multivariate paradigm. A group of disorders were identified on the basis of *"personality traits* [that when] inflexible and maladaptive and cause either significant impairment in social or occupational functioning or subjective distress . . . constitute *Personality Disorders"* (APA, 1980, p. 305; emphasis in original). The definition of these disorders in terms of dysfunctional personality traits stimulated an unprecedented collaborative effort to find common grounds for characterizing these disorders among psychiatrists, psychologists, and psychometricians (e.g., Widiger & Frances, 1985). The fourth edition of the manual (DSM-IV; APA, 1994) reported the results of field trials and other research (coordinated by clinical psychologist Thomas A. Widiger), and this enterprise involved the cooperation of more than 1,000 individuals and numerous professional organizations (APA, 1994, p. xiii).

Morey, Waugh, and Blashfield (1985) developed Minnesota Multiphasic Personality Inventory (MMPI) Personality Disorder Scales (MMPI-PD) under a combined rational–empirical strategy that yielded self-report measures for the 11 personality disorders described in DSM-III. Strack's (1987) Personality Adjective Check List (PACL) provided scales for eight personality disorders, based on 8 of the 11 personality styles described in Millon's (1969, 1981) theory of psychopathology. A colleague and I (Wiggins & Pincus, 1989) evaluated the differing conceptions of personality inherent in the MMPI-PD and PACL personality disorder scales with reference to the five domains and the 18 facets available in an earlier version of the NEO PI (Costa & McCrae, 1985). In a university sample, we found that conceptions of personality disorders were strongly and clearly related to dimensions of normal personality traits. We concluded that:

> although the two conceptions of personality used were operationalized *independently* of the five-factor model of personality, the canonical analysis indicated that these conceptions in fact share five dimensions with the personality trait domain that are readily interpretable as the "Big Five" factors of personality. (Wiggins & Pincus, 1989, p. 314; emphasis in original)

Costa and McCrae (1990) attempted to generalize these findings across populations, observers, and instruments. In a community sample, self-report, spouse, and peer ratings were obtained for the original NEO PI, as were self-reports on the Millon Clinical Multiaxial Inventory (MCMI; Millon, 1987), which provided measures of DSM personality disorders. Their results were sufficiently congruent with the earlier study for Costa and McCrae to observe:

> A few years ago, the notion that new personality disorders might be discovered by looking at normal dimensions of personality would probably have been ignored by psychiatrists and personality psychologists alike. The results of recent research show that psychiatric conceptions of disorder are not worlds apart; in fact, they share five basic dimensions. With shared measures, shared constructs, and a shared vocabulary, the fruitful integration of personality research and psychiatric nosology seems much more likely today. (1990, pp. 370–371)

An example of such an integration was the demonstration that both the APA (1987) DSM-III-R diagnostic criteria for personality disorders and the associated clinical literature on these disorders were compatible with descriptions of each disorder generated by the facets of the NEO PI-R (Widiger, Trull, Clarkin, Sanderson, & Costa, 1994). Table 4.13 presents the results of this collaborative enterprise. (Widiger, Trull, Clarkin, Sanderson, & Costa, 2002, have since revised and updated this table for the APA [1994] DSM-IV diagnostic criteria.) In this table, the personality disorders appear as columns: paranoid (PAR), schizoid (SZD), schizotypal (SZT), antisocial (ATS), borderline (BDL), histrionic (HST), narcissistic (NAR), avoidant (AVD), dependent (DEP), obsessive–compulsive (OBC), and passive–aggressive (PAG). The rows of this table are the 30 facets of the NEO PI-R, which are arranged under their corresponding domains of Neuroticism, Extraversion, Openness, Agreeableness, and Conscientiousness. In the body of the table, the DSM-III-R diagnostic criteria for the disorders appear in upper-case H (high) and L (low). Features that are not in themselves diagnostic, but are sometimes associated with the disorder appear in lower-case h (high) and l (low). Features that have been reported in the literature but are not presently part of the diagnosis appear in bold type.

From the paranoid personality disorder (PAR) column, it is clear that the defining features of this disorder are hostility, lack of trust, lack of straightforwardness (crafty, deceptive), and lack of compliance (competitive). Features associated with this disorder also include a decided lack of warmth, gregariousness, and positive emotions; a lack of openness to aesthetics (art/beauty) and inner feelings; and a lack of modesty and tender-mindedness. In the research literature, it has been reported that individuals

TABLE 4.13. DSM-III-R Personality Disorders and the FFM

Criteria	PAR	SZD	SZT	ATS	BDL	HST	NAR	AVD	DEP	OBC	PAG
Neuroticism											
N1. Anxiety	h		h	h/L	H			H	H		
N2. Hostility	H	L		H	H	H	H			h	h
N3. Depression			h	h	H		h/L	h	H	h	
N4. Self-Consciousness		L	H	L	H	H	H	H	h	h	
N5. Impulsiveness				H	H						
N6. Vulnerability			h		H	h	H	H	H		
Extraversion											
E1. Warmth	l	L	L	l		H		L/H	h	L	
E2. Gregariousness	l	L	L		h	h		L			
E3. Assertiveness					h		H	L	L	H	
E4. Activity-Seeking						h		L			
E5. Excitement-Seeking		L			H	h		L		l	
E6. Positive Emotions	l	L			h	H					
Openness											
O1. Fantasy			H			h	H				
O2. Aesthetics	l										
O3. Feelings	l	L	L			H				L	
O4. Actions	L					h		L			
O5. Ideas			H			l					
O6. Values			h							L	
Agreeableness											
A1. Trust	L		L			h					
A2. Straightforwardness	L			L	L	l	l				L
A3. Altruism				L		L	L		H	L	
A4. Compliance	L	h		L	L				H	L	L
A5. Modesty	l			L			L		H		
A6. Tender-mindedness	l			L			L		h		
Conscientiousness											
C1. Competence	h				l		h				L
C2. Order										H	
C3. Dutifulness				L						H	L
C4. Achievement Striving		l			L		h		L	H	
C5. Self-Discipline				L		L					L
C6. Deliberation				L						H	

Note. Adapted from Widiger, Trull, Clarkin, Sanderson, and Costa (1994, p. 42). Copyright 1994 by the American Psychological Association. Adapted by permission.

with paranoid personality disorder are not open to alternative actions, such as trying different activities or going to new places.

Empirical Confirmation

That the five higher-order factors of the FFM may be useful in distinguishing among the DSM personality disorders has been demonstrated in both normal and clinical samples, with a variety of assessment procedures (e.g., Costa & McCrae, 1990; Duijsens & Diekstra, 1996; Soldz, Budman, Demby, & Merry, 1993; Wiggins & Pincus, 1989). Nevertheless, there are limitations on the fidelity with which these global factors can measure the heterogeneous personality disorder categories (e.g., Clark, 1993; Coolidge et al., 1994; Schmidt, Wagner, & Kiesler, 1993).

As illustrated in Table 4.13, and as discussed with reference to the paranoid personality disorder example, the 30 facets of the NEO PI-R provide finer-grained predictions than do the factor scales. As a consequence, the accuracy of the predicted relationships in Table 4.13 should be given high priority as a research topic in future empirical investigations. Dyce and O'Connor (1998) have reported preliminary evidence in this respect. They administered the NEO PI-R, along with a revised version of the MCMI (MCMI-III; Millon, 1994), to a university sample. The MCMI-III provides measures of DSM-IV personality disorders, and the correlations between the NEO PI-R facets and each of the personality disorders listed in Table 4.13 were used to evaluate the predictions made in that table. Dyce and O'Connor concluded that

> (a) 63% of the predicted facet relationships were significant, although many unpredicted relationships also emerged; (b) facet-level analyses did not yield substantially stronger effect sizes than domain-level analyses; but (c) facet-level analysis provided much better discrimination between personality disorders than domain-level analyses. (p. 31)

Domain- versus Facet-Level Classification of Personality Disorders

More recent research by Morey, Gunderson, Quigley, and Lyons (2000) has called into question Dyce and O'Connor's (1998) conclusion that facet-level analysis provides better diagnostic discrimination than domain-level analysis. Morey and his collaborators compared the utility of the Widiger and colleagues (1994) diagnostic classification scheme based on NEO PI *facets* with predictions generated from NEO *domain* scores. In effect, they were assessing the relative merits of "categorical" (combinations of facets) and "dimensional" (broad domains) predictions. Their sample was a carefully selected research sample of 144 psychiatric patients in which there was a high prevalence of personality disorders (diagnosed via structured interviews)[5]. For comparative purposes, the facet-level predictions of Widiger and colleagues (Table 4.13) were aggregated into domain-level predictions (e.g., paranoid personality disorder = low Extraversion + low Openness + Low Agreeableness).

The results were generally supportive of the hypothesis that additive regression models based on domain-level NEO PI scores are more predictive of DSM diagnoses; 9 of the 11 additive models achieved significance (models for schizotypal and borderline personality disorders did not). However, although predictive validity was encouraging, discriminative validity was poor. The profiles of personality disorder groups were in general quite different from those found in community norms, but the configurations for the 11 personality disorders were all *highly* similar to one another in having "above average Neuroticism, below average Extraversion, Conscientiousness, and Agreeableness; and few distinguishing features on Openness" (p. 212). This was especially evident when the results were viewed from the perspective of the DSM-III-R personality disorder clusters: (A) odd–eccentric (schizoid, schizotypal, paranoid); (B) dramatic–emotional (antisocial, borderline, histrionic, narcissistic); and (C) anxious–fearful (avoidant, dependent, obsessive–compulsive, passive–aggressive) (APA, 1994, pp. 629–630, 634). Not only were patterns within these clusters highly similar to each other, but the overall patterns across these clusters were also highly similar. In fact, the median configural correlation among profiles of all 11 disorders in this study was found to be .983! And no evidence for interaction effects within disorders was found.

> For the nine disorders where more than one personality dimension had been hypothesized to be salient, hierarchical regressions were performed to determine the increment achieved by a consideration of the interaction among personality features. In none of these analyses did the interaction provide a significant increment in description above the simple additive combination of features. These results indicate that, in those instances where these personality dimensions are useful in describing Axis II disorders, the utility of these dimensions is largely independent rather than in combination with other features. (p. 212)

Morey and his collaborators attributed their rather surprising findings to, at least in part, the extensive comorbidity that has been found among the personality disorders. They also suggested that the classifications of

---

[5] As has been found in most other samples, there was a high degree of "comorbidity" (meeting DSM criteria for more than one personality disorder) in this sample as well. Some 64.5% of the Morey and colleagues (2000) sample met criteria for at least two specific personality disorders.

Widiger and colleagues (Table 4.13) may be viewed as pure *prototypes* that are nevertheless "a rare exception to the general rule of Axis II diagnostic overlap" (p. 212).

ADDITIONAL ISSUES IN THE APPLICATION OF THE FFM TO THE PERSONALITY DISORDERS

Internal and External Correspondence

Shopshire and Craik (1994) made a distinction between internal and external correspondence of the DSM personality disorders to the dimensions of personality within the FFM. Thus the Wiggins and Pincus (1989) and Costa and McCrae (1990) findings were considered to be based on an *external* conceptual analysis in which both personality disorders and dimensions of normal personality (FFM) were measured within the same medium (Q-data) and in which "the personality disorder concepts are translated into a set of inventory items (i.e., MMPI-PD) that may or may not correspond directly or precisely to the DSM-III-R diagnostic categories" (Shopshire & Craik, 1994, p. 42).

In contrast, Shopshire and Craik's (1994) own analysis of the relation between personality disorders and the FFM was based on an *internal* conceptual analysis in which the behavioral diagnostic criteria of DSM-III-R were rephrased into a common format of behavioral descriptors. Thus the avoidant personality disorder criterion "is easily hurt by criticism" was rephrased as the behavioral descriptor "He (or she) is easily hurt by criticism." A total of 110 such behavioral descriptors were constructed. From previous work on trait constructs thought to be relevant to personality disorders (e.g., Buss & Craik, 1987), 43 trait constructs were assembled (e.g., "shallow," "mistrustful," "oversensitive"). A panel of 260 undergraduates was asked to rate the extent to which each behavioral descriptor was a "good example" of each trait on a 7-point scale. These prototypicality judgments (Broughton, 1990) were used to evaluate the internal correspondence of traits and personality disorder criteria. The results of this study led the authors to conclude:

> Correspondence between the FFM dimensions of personality structure and the DSM-III-R categories of personality disorder reported by Wiggins and Pincus (1989) and by Costa and McCrae (1990) is largely replicated in this analysis. . . . This convergence between studies using the methodologically different internal and external forms of analysis is impressive. (p. 49)

Dimensional versus Categorical Assessment

Psychiatric diagnosis has a long history of employing a categorical "disease entity" model (see Chapter 5), and the most recent editions of DSM (DSM-

III-R and DSM-IV) are no exception to this tradition. The various personality disorder categories are conceived of as discrete, discontinuous, and either present or absent, in accord with current conceptions of other psychiatric disorders (Carson, 1991). That the multivariate paradigm in general, and the FFM in particular, are dimensional in nature is obvious. That judgments regarding the presence or absence of psychopathology are dimensional in nature is less obvious. Dimensions of personality are quantified continua, along which the *extent* to which a person may be characterized as, for example, "distrustful" is assessed. Dimensions of psychopathology are also continua, although in this instance "distrustful" is but one of several characteristics that is taken into account in determining the *extent* to which a person may be characterized as having "paranoid personality disorder."

The mounting empirical evidence that the personality disorder categories of DSM-III-R and DSM-IV are not categorical in nature has led to repeated suggestions that this subgroup of disorders be diagnosed by dimensional rather than categorical procedures (e.g., Clark & Watson, 1999; Livesley, Schroeder, Jackson, & Jang, 1994; Widiger & Frances, 1985, 1994). Widiger's (1991) earlier suggestions to (1) retain the categorical approach but provide a conversion table; (2) revise criteria for severity rating; or (3) include a dimensional model in an appendix to DSM-IV have not been implemented to date.

The "Atheoretical" Nature of the FFM

Although the well-documented occurrence of five-factor solutions of personality variables does not in itself constitute a theory of personality (McAdams, 1992), it would be inaccurate to suggest that the model is without theoretical import (cf. Eysenck, 1994). The FFM has been interpreted from a variety of theoretical perspectives that have guided conceptually driven research. And it has provided unprecedented opportunities for "communication and the sharing of ideas among some of the major figures in contemporary personality research, investigators whose subdisciplinary 'boundaries' might otherwise have proven less permeable to such exchanges" (Wiggins, 1996c, p. viii).

Although the lexical perspective on the FFM is primarily concerned with phenotypic variables, it has nonetheless provided a firm psycholinguistic basis for trait measurement (Saucier & Goldberg, 1996b). The trait perspective on the FFM attempts to combine the conceptual insights of classic theories of personality and contemporary research within a meta-theoretical framework for "a new generation of personality theories" (McCrae & Costa, 1996). The dyadic–interactional perspective on the FFM combines the insights of interpersonal and social-psychological theorists in assigning conceptual priority to the first two factors of the model, and in emphasizing the manifestations of agency and communion within the remaining three factors (Wiggins & Trapnell, 1996). The socioanalytic perspective on the FFM combines the insights of psychoanalytic and socio-logical theorists in describing the manner in which the FFM provides the societal standards by which individuals are evaluated (Hogan, 1996). And, finally, the evolutionary perspective on the FFM illuminates the manner in which problems of social adaptation, such as the forming of strategic alli-ances and the avoidance of strategic interference, may be represented in di-mensional terms (Buss, 1996). Given the variety and potential fruitfulness of these perspectives, it is clearly not accurate to suggest that the FFM is "atheoretical" in nature.

APPLICATION OF THE FFM TO CLINICAL PRACTICE

An Alternative Perspective on Psychodiagnosis

We might conclude that normal and abnormal personality are not merely related phenomena but are in fact equivalent and that the personality disorders of the DSM-III-R are not qualitatively new forms of personality but are merely descriptions of individual differences in personality as they are seen in psychiatric patients. . . . [This] more radical approach is justified by serious problems with the DSM-III-R system, which has been criticized as being arbitrary, overlapping, and without a clear empirical basis.

—MCCRAE (1994a, p. 27)

In effect, McCrae is suggesting that instead of assuming the validity of the DSM diagnostic categories of personality disorders and seeking the personality correlates of such classifications, we might reaffirm the valid-ity of established dimensions of personality and investigate the difficulties in living associated with being comparatively either very high or very low on these dimensions (see also Horowitz, 1979). Table 4.14 is adapted from a table in another chapter by McCrae (1994b) and is meant to be illustrative of this alternative approach. Here it is important to note that "the FFM is not itself a theory of psychopathology, and many different theories of psychopathology would be compatible with it" (McCrae, 1994a, p. 28).

Treatment Characteristics Associated with Standing on the FFM

Miller (1991) reported that the dimensions of the original NEO PI were helpful in anticipating and understanding clients' private experience, antici-pating problems presented in treatment, formulating treatment plans, and anticipating "opportunities and pitfalls for treatment" (p. 417). On the

TABLE 4.14. Problems Associated with High and Low Standing on FFM Personality Dimensions

Dimension	High	Low
Neuroticism	Chronic negative affects; difficulty in inhibiting impulses; irrational beliefs; unfounded somatic concerns; helplessness and dependence.	Lack of appropriate concern for potential problems in health or social adjustment; emotional blandness.
Extraversion	Excessive talking, inappropriate self-disclosure and social friction; inability to spend time alone; attention seeking; reckless excitement seeking.	Social isolation, interpersonal detachment, and lack of support networks; flattened affect; lack of joy and zest for life; social inhibition and shyness.
Openness	Preoccupation with fantasy and daydreaming; lack of practicality; eccentric thinking (e.g., belief in ghosts, reincarnation, UFOs); diffuse identity.	Difficulty adapting to social or personal change; low tolerance or understanding of different points of view or lifestyles; excessive conformity to authority.
Agreeableness	Gullibility; indiscriminate trust of others; excessive candor and generosity, to detriment of self-interest; inability to stand up to others and fight back.	Cynicism and paranoid thinking; inability to trust even friends or family; quarrelsomeness; readiness to pick fights; exploitation and manipulation.
Conscientiousness	Overachievement; workaholic absorption in job or cause, to the exclusion of family, social, and personal interests; compulsiveness.	Underachievement; not fulfilling intellectual or artistic potential; poor academic performance relative to ability; inability to discipline self.

Note. Adapted from McCrae (1994b, p. 306). Copyright 1994 by the American Psychological Association. Adapted by permission.

basis of his experiences with 119 patients in private-practice, outpatient psychotherapy and their family members over a period of 2 years, he concluded:

> Neuroticism (N) influences the intensity and duration of the patient's distress, Extraversion (E) influences the patient's enthusiasm for treatment, Openness (O) influences the patient's reactions to the therapist's interventions, Agreeableness (A) influences the patient's reaction to the person of the psychotherapist, and Conscientiousness (C) influences the patient's willingness to do the work of psychotherapy. (Miller, 1991, p. 415)

Although data are not presented to substantiate these impressions, the author's rationale for his conclusions is highly convincing.

Clinical Interpretation of the NEO PI-R

Piedmont (1998) has provided a comprehensive, integrative, and highly readable introduction to the rationale, research literature, and clinical interpretation of the NEO PI-R. He emphasizes that the FFM is *not* a measure of psychopathology, but rather a measure of "the larger internal forces that have brought the individual to his or her current situation" (p. 60), and the "potential psychological risks a person may face" (p. 61). As a consequence, "the traits of the five-factor model of personality provide a strong paradigm for organizing personality dysfunctioning" (p. 63), in which "a dimensional model does better represent the qualities underlying the personality disorders than does a categorical model" (p. 63).

That the FFM is equally applicable to interpreting normal and abnormal behavior is evident in the seamless nature of interpretations made by Piedmont (1998) of NEO PI-R profiles of both highly effective persons and those with severe problems of living. Piedmont's interpretations of profiles of relatively normal individuals provide some further confirmation of the usefulness of the FFM in personnel work (e.g., Barrick & Mount, 1991). His interpretation of the following case of a 42-year-old white married female is more relevant to the clinical interpretation of the FFM:

> She presents with many problems, including suicidal ideations. She has repeatedly injured herself in a number of ways, including cutting and burning herself. She has been on drugs for 10 years and abused alcohol for at least 5 years. She is also a compulsive spender, having spent her husband's credit card to their limits several times. Even when everything is confiscated, she continually opens new credit card accounts and proceeds to "max them out." She reports being a victim of child abuse. (Piedmont, 1998, p. 131)

Not surprisingly, this patient was diagnosed as having borderline personality disorder, and her NEO PI-R profile (presented in Figure 4.1) is highly consistent with this diagnosis. One is immediately impressed with the *variability* of this profile, both within and between domains. In light of the "off-the-chart" Neuroticism domain score, Piedmont immediately considers the "control" dimension of Conscientiousness, which reflects a person's ability to function despite emotional distress. The equally "off-the-chart" competence facet (C1) and the remaining "very low" Conscientiousness facets give little evidence of the client's ability to deal with her anxiety (N1), anger (N2), depression (N3), insecurity (N4), impulsiveness (N5), and feelings of vulnerability (N6). "When she is in pain, she seeks *any* outlet for relief, whether it is spending money, attempting to kill herself, or

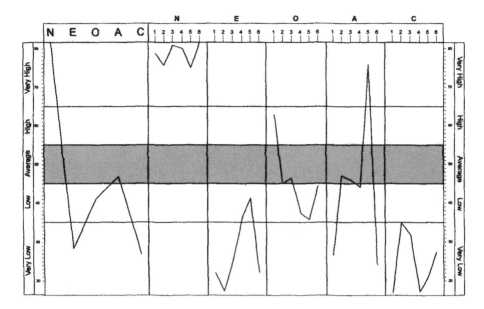

FIGURE 4.1. NEO PI-R profile of a 42-year-old white married female. From Piedmont (1998). Copyright 1998 by Plenum Publications, Inc. Reprinted by permission.

abusing controlled substances" (Piedmont, 1998, p. 131; emphasis in original).

The low levels of Extraversion facets suggest an isolated, detached individual with few social attachments. Although her generally low levels of Openness to Experience suggest rigidity and a need for structure, the peak on fantasy (O1) may suggest an active inner world to which she may retreat from her emotional suffering. The generally low scores on Agreeableness characterize a person who is distrustful (A1), devious (A2), selfish (A3), stubborn (A4), and cold (A6) in interpersonal transactions. The peak on the modesty facet (A5) of Agreeableness suggests that "Her modesty may help to keep others from looking critically at her and protect her from any additional psychological insults" (Piedmont, 1998, p. 133). In Piedmont's view, the basic personality structure of this unfortunate individual has brought her to this current situation with all of its potential psychological risks.

HEREDITY REVISITED

The multivariate paradigm arose in the context of statistical methods for the study of the inheritance of mental abilities, which were thought to be stable characteristics of individuals over their life span. The founder of the paradigm, Raymond B. Cattell, considered temperamental characteristics to also be stable and heritable, and he developed methods for assessing the relative contributions of nature and nurture to these characteristics (Cattell, 1953). Some 40 years later, Costa and McCrae (1994) provided extensive evidence for the longitudinal stability of the Big Five personality traits. After the age of 30, these traits, as William James put it, appeared to be "set like plaster." Costa and McCrae reported retest correlations ranging from .60 to .80, even after an interval of 30 years.

Recent advances in the methodologies of twin, family, and adoption studies have made it possible to establish the substantial heritability of the Big Five dimensions of personality (e.g., Bergeman et al., 1993; Heath, Neale, Kessler, Eaves, & Kendler, 1992; Jang, Livesley, & Vernon, 1996; Loehlin, 1992; Riemann, Angleitner, & Strelau, 1997). Although much work remains to be done in sorting out the precise contributions of heredity and environment in this area (Rose, 1995), the findings to date lend considerable credence to McCrae and Costa's (1996) view of the five factors as "basic tendencies" in human behavior. And the implications of this view continue to be explored widely (e.g., Costa & McCrae, 2000).

OVERVIEW

It should be apparent that the factor-analytic model that evolved at University College London at the turn of the 20th century has been the cornerstone of the multivariate paradigm—from the early days when this procedure was labor-intensive and restricted to a small number of variables, to the present computer era of apparently unbounded potential. However, as computational procedures expanded, so did the number of factors identified; the paradigm became fractionated with disagreements over the number and nature of personality factors, as well as over procedures for extracting, rotating, and interpreting such factors.

In this chapter, I have traced the gradual consolidation of the multivariate paradigm with respect to an evolving consensus on the importance of the Big Five factors in personality assessment. This is not to say that the consolidation has occurred in the absence of strong and often well-reasoned resistance to the FFM. In fact, this resistance was most widespread in the decade in which consolidation occurred (e.g., Block, 1995; Eysenck, 1992; Hough, 1992; McAdams, 1992; Pervin, 1994). Perhaps this is the karma of our "preparadigms" of personality assessment (see the Introduction).

Although the FFM appears to be a "new look" within the multivariate paradigm, it should be apparent from the present chapter that its origins are far from recent. As Digman (1994) has observed,

> Now, after many years of lying on the closet shelf of personality theory, the model has been dusted off, "as good as new," and appears to be for many researchers . . . a very meaningful theoretical structure for organizing the myriad specifics implied by the term *personality*. (p. 13; emphasis in original)

5

The Empirical Paradigm

A response to a personality inventory is an interesting and significant bit of verbal behavior, the non-test correlates of which must be discovered by empirical means.
—MEEHL (1945, p. 297)

THE DISEASE MODEL OF MENTAL ILLNESS

Emil Kraepelin (1856–1926) was a student of Wilhelm Wundt, the founder of experimental psychology. After receiving a medical degree, Kraepelin accepted the position of medical director at an insane asylum in East Prussia. His subsequent influence on descriptive psychiatry is legendary:

> Emil Kraepelin fell upon a psychiatric world exhausted with arranging and reordering symptoms along psychological lines largely without medical significance. He sought in psychological phenomena the key to *disease* states. Although an experimental psychologist and student of Wundt, and a lifetime investigator of what is today called psychopharmacology, he had little interest in psychological facts for themselves. . . . His overriding interest was disease and disease processes in the pathological tradition of Virchow; it was to the discovery and elucidation of diseases that the greatest part of his work was directed. He brought to the task enormous energy, a long life, and the gift of marshaling large numbers of facts about a few, powerful ideas. (Havens, 1965, p. 16; emphasis in original)

Kraepelin's (1896) taxonomy of mental and nervous diseases emphasized organic states, toxic psychoses, endogenous psychoses, and deviant personalities. With the eventual addition of a category of neurotic disorders, this system is basically the one now adhered to by the American Psychiatric Association (1994). Over the years, there has been a broad spectrum of criticism, from a variety of disciplines, concerning what is now called the "medical model" of psychiatric disorders (e.g., Goffman, 1961; Lacan, 1977; Rosenhan, 1973; Sarbin, 1997; Szasz, 1961; Zubin, 1967). Despite these criticisms, the so-called "neo-Kraepelinians" (e.g., Klerman, 1978) have prevailed (see Blashfield, 1998, for an excellent historical overview).

Quite aside from the etiological and treatment issues raised by the medical model is the question of choosing an appropriate measurement model for the assessment of psychopathology. In her discussion of trait-structural models, Loevinger (1957) discussed "class models," which describe "a class of people rather than a trait present to a greater or lesser degree in all of us" (p. 666). She noted that such models postulate a syndrome as either present or absent, with no degrees in between: "To take an example from medicine, fever and cough may indicate several diseases, fever and rash may also indicate several diseases, but fever, cough, and rash strongly suggest a diagnosis of measles" (p. 666).

A disease is a syndrome that comprises a unique combination of symptoms. Thus it is not possible for a psychiatric patient to be a little bit schizophrenic, a little bit manic–depressive, or the like. For these and other reasons, Widiger and Frances (1994) have argued for a "dimensional," as opposed to a class-based or "categorical," approach to the assessment of psychopathology. The Minnesota Multiphasic Personality Inventory (MMPI; Hathaway & McKinley, 1943), which has been the principal focus of the empirical paradigm, was originally developed to provide differential diagnoses among Kraepelinian categories. The reasons why an instrument that was constructed on such shaky foundations became the most widely used inventory in the world is one of the more intriguing stories in the history of personality assessment.

ORIGINS OF THE MMPI

Robert S. Woodworth is generally credited with constructing the first personality inventory. His Personal Data Sheet (Woodworth, 1917) was developed as a screening device for identifying neurotic symptoms among recruits for military service during World War I. Designed as a substitute for psychiatric interviews, it consisted of 116 questions of the form "Do you usually feel well and strong?", to which respondents answered "yes" or "no." Respondents who answered a large number of items in the "neurotic" direction were referred to a psychiatrist. This approach to test construction was later called a "rational approach," because item construction or selection was based largely on a test author's (rational) judgments or beliefs concerning the likely validity of the item's assessment. Items selected in this manner would often consist of rather straightforward, direct questions concerning the presence or absence of the construct or criterion being assessed, and therefore relied heavily on honesty or accuracy in self-description. For example, Woodworth perhaps naively assumed, among other things, that a respondent who claimed *not* to feel "well and strong" was neurotic, rather than possibly not interested in risking his life in combat. Another version of a rationally derived test was Pressey's (1921) Cross Out Test. This test provided respondents with sets of words (e.g., "disgust, fear, sex, suspicion, aunt") with instructions to cross out those words that were unpleasant and to circle the most unpleasant word. More importantly, Pressey developed a scoring system for measuring emotional maladjustment that was based on *norms* for infrequent (deviant) word choices.

Strong's (1927) Vocational Interest Blank was the first instrument to employ the test construction strategy of "contrasted groups," in which the item responses of a criterion group (e.g., architects) were statistically compared with those of a control group (e.g., men in general) in the construction of a scale (e.g., an "empirical" architects' scale). In the following decade, a number of papers criticized the older "rational" approach to test construction and called for a more empirical approach (e.g., Landis & Katz, 1934; Landis, Zubin, & Katz, 1935).

The Humm–Wadsworth Temperament Scale (HWTS; Humm & Wadsworth, 1935) was the first inventory of psychopathology that was based on the strategy of contrasted groups. The item responses of groups of psychiatric patients (e.g., patients with hysteroid, manic, or paranoid diagnoses) were statistically compared with those of normal respondents, to determine the keying direction of empirically significant items for scales measuring hysteroid, manic, and other dispositions. "The [HWTS] reports the temperamental constitution of an individual by means of what was called a Profile or psychograph" (Humm & Humm, 1944, p. 55). A measure of "response bias" was employed, which corrected scale scores for the number of items denied ("no-count"). The validity of the inventory and that of the response bias measure were investigated by comparing HWTS profiles with independently obtained case histories (Humm & Humm, 1944). As will become apparent, all of these innovations, and many of the HWTS items (Meehl, 1989), were incorporated into the development of the MMPI.

The epigraph to this chapter is from Meehl's classic critique of rational approaches to test construction, which has been referred to as the "empirical manifesto." In that paper, Meehl (1945) defined the meaning of a response to an objective test item as "an intrinsically interesting and significant bit of verbal behavior, *the nontest correlates of which must be discovered by empirical means*" (p. 297; emphasis added). The empirical paradigm (which has come to be associated with the MMPI) subsequently explored this line of inquiry with a vengeance.

DESCRIPTION OF THE MMPI

Universe of Content

In assembling self-reference statements that reflected "behavior of significance to the psychiatrist," Hathaway and McKinley (1940, p. 249) consulted psychiatric examination forms, psychiatry textbooks, previously published attitude and personality scales, clinical reports and case summaries, and their own clinical experience. "As a matter of convenience in handling and in avoiding duplication" (p. 250), these statements were classified into 25 "content categories" (e.g., general health, gastrointestinal system, political attitudes, obsessive and compulsive states). Because of their empirical inclinations and distrust of rational inventories, the authors of the MMPI deemphasized the apparent "content" of the items that entered into their empirically derived scales (Wiggins & Vollmar, 1959).

Validity Scales

One of the most important failings of almost all structured personality tests is their susceptibility to "faking" or "lying" in one way or another, as well as their even greater susceptibility to unconscious self-deception and role-playing on the part of individuals who may be consciously quite honest and sincere in their responses.
—MEEHL AND HATHAWAY (1946, p. 525)

From the beginning, the authors of the MMPI were seriously concerned with both measuring and correcting for respondents' tendencies to deceive themselves or others in answering items of potential pathological significance. The so-called "validity indicators"—the L, F, and K scales—were developed with this in mind. The Lie (L) scale consists of 15 items, modeled on an earlier scale of Hartshorne and May (1928), which express common human foibles (e g , "Once in a while I laugh at a dirty joke") that are denied by very few respondents. Answering too many of these items in the "saintly" direction ("false") raises questions concerning the truthfulness of the respondent.

The Infrequency (F) scale consists of 64 items for which less than 10% of the Minnesota normative sample answered in the keyed direction (e.g., a "true" response to "My soul sometimes leaves my body"). There are a variety of reasons why F may be elevated in a given profile, including carelessness in responding, poor reading comprehension, poor visual acuity, and acute psychotic reactions. MMPI profiles with highly elevated F scores are therefore interpreted with caution, if at all.

The Correction (K) scale consists of 30 items that were developed by an elaborate set of procedures, which included a contrasted-groups analysis of items differentiating clinically abnormal respondents with normal MMPI profiles from clinically normal respondents with normal MMPI profiles (Meehl & Hathaway, 1946). The items in the K scale are quite heterogeneous in nature, and their relation to defensiveness is not always evident (e.g., a "false" response to "I have periods in which I feel unusually cheerful without any special reason"). One of the primary purposes for developing the K scale was the possibility of adding corrective weights of K to the clinical scales to compensate for a patient's "defensiveness" in responding to items on some of the clinical scales (Meehl & Hathaway, 1946). Opinion has been divided on the usefulness of this "K-correction" (e.g., Greene, 1980), but the K scale itself has proven to be a useful member of the triad of validity scales.

Construction of the Clinical Scales

Strategy of Contrasted Groups

Items in the initial MMPI item pool were administered to visitors to the University of Minnesota Hospitals, who served as a control group in the development of the MMPI clinical scales. The same items were also administered to groups of psychiatric inpatients who had been diagnosed in a number of different Kraepelinian diagnostic categories; these served as "criterion groups" in scale development. The manner in which the strategy of contrasted groups was applied to selection of items for the Hypochondriasis (Hs) scale is illustrated in Table 5.1. "The group of cases for scale construction was selected with meticulous care to exclude those with manifestations of the major psychoses; as far as it was possible for us to determine, only pure, uncomplicated hypochondriasis was included" (McKinley & Hathaway, 1940, pp. 255–256).

In Table 5.1, hypothetical percentages of response are provided for 3 of the 504 items that were originally contrasted between the control and criterion groups. On the first item, the control group was evenly divided— half of the group answering "true," the remainder answering "false." The slight difference in percentage between the endorsement of this item in the control and criterion groups (50% vs. 51%) was clearly not significant, and therefore this item was not included in the Hs scale (zero weights for "true" and "false" responses). Significant differences were obtained on the next two items, and they were scored (weighted) in the appropriate directions on the final Hs scale.

Table 5.2 on page 171 presents the scale labels, criterion groups, and typical interpretations of elevated scores for the validity scales, eight clinical scales (Hypochondriasis [Hs], Depression [D], Hysteria [Hy], Psychopathic Deviate [Pd], Paranoia [Pa], Psychasthenia [Pt], Schizophrenia [Sc], and Hypomania [Ma]), a scale of Masculinity/Femininity (Mf), and a Social Introversion (Si) scale. These scales constitute the final MMPI profile that

TABLE 5.1. Strategy of Contrasted Groups Applied to the Measurement of Hypochondriasis

	Control group (n = 527 normal individuals)		Criterion group (n = 50 patients with hypochondriasis)		Difference in percentage between two groups		Scoring weights for Hs scale	
Items	T	F	T	F	T	F	T	F
I like mechanics magazines	50	50	51	49	+1	−1	0	0
I feel weak all over much of the time	5	95	35	65	+30	−30	+1	0
I seldom worry about my health	80	20	50	50	−30	+30	0	+1

was normed and standardized on the original sample of normal control subjects.

MMPI Profile

The manner in which the standard MMPI profile is displayed may be seen in Figure 5.1. Each of the validity and clinical scales has been standardized with respect to a population of normal subjects, the so-called "Minnesota normative group." Raw scores on the scales are expressed as standardized *T*-scores with a mean of 50 and a standard deviation of 10. The dark horizontal lines indicate the mean of the normative population (50) and two standard deviations above (70) and below (30) that mean value. The 3-variable configuration of validity scales and the 10-variable configuration of clinical scales are indicated by dark lines. Of particular interpretive interest here are the general *shapes* of these two configurations.

Although the MMPI clinical scales were derived by the method of contrasted groups, it soon became evident that they were subsequently rather unsuccessful in discriminating pathological groups from normal control groups (Benton, 1949). For example, Morris (1947) found that the MMPI profiles of patients diagnosed as having psychoneurosis, constitutional psychopathic state, and schizoid personality were "markedly similar" to one another and concluded that "the Minnesota Inventory cannot be regarded as a practical clinical tool the results of which can be accepted as valuable diagnostic aids to the psychiatric member of the clinical team" (p. 374). It has been suggested that many of the "subtle items" on these scales (i.e., items with no obvious substantive relation to the diagnostic categories) may have been selected by chance and not subjected to appropriate cross-

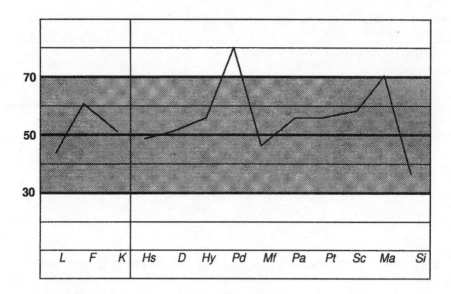

FIGURE 5.1. MMPI profile of standard clinical and validity scales.

validation (Jackson, 1971).[1] As a consequence of these findings, the original emphasis within the paradigm on properties of single scales shifted to an emphasis on the correlates of diagnostic patterns (Gough, 1946) and on clinical scale configurations (Meehl, 1950). In keeping with the empirical philosophy, there was also a shift of emphasis from the scale labels in Table 5.2 (e.g., *Sc* for Schizophrenia) to the more neutral characterization of scale numbers in the same table (e.g., "Scale 8" for Schizophrenia).

Code Types

The first major MMPI book was *An Atlas for the Clinical Use of the MMPI* (Hathaway & Meehl, 1951a), in which a large number of MMPI case records were classified with respect to a coding system that employed the numbers of each of the clinical scales. An alternative coding system was devised by Welsh (1948), and it has become more or less standard. The latter system is described in Table 5.3. There is no need to master the details of this coding system, except to note that scale numbers are presented in descending order of magnitude and grouped according to standard deviations above and below that of the normative population, as indicated by sym-

---

[1] Ben-Porath and Graham (1995) state that "Hathaway and McKinley did not have sufficient resources to cross-validate item selections using large samples" (p. 7).

TABLE 5.2. Standard Validity and Clinical Scales of the MMPI

Scale label	Scale name	Criterion group	No. of items	Interpretation of elevated scores
L	Lie	—	15	Denial of common frailties; saintliness
F	Infrequency	—	64	Validity of profile is doubtful
K	Correction	50 psychiatric patients with low MMPI profiles	30	Defensive; minimizes social and emotional complaints
(1) Hs	Hypochondriasis	50 patients with hypochondriasis	33	Numerous physical complaints
(2) D	Depression	50 patients with depression	60	Severely depressed
(3) Hy	Hysteria	50 patients with hysteria	60	Immature, suggestible, egocentric, demanding
(4) Pd	Psychopathic Deviate	Unspecified number of patients with psychopathy	50	Rebellious and nonconformist
(5) Mf	Masculinity–Femininity	13 homosexual men	60	Artistic interests; effeminate
(6) Pa	Paranoia	Unspecified number of patients with paranoia	40	Resentful and suspicious of others
(7) Pt	Psychasthenia	20 patients with psychasthenia	48	Fearful, ruminative, agitated
(8) Sc	Schizophrenia	50 patients with schizophrenia	78	Withdrawn, reclusive; bizarre thinking
(9) Ma	Hypomania	24 patients with mania	46	Impulsive, expansive, distractible
(0) Si	Social Introversion	50 high and 50 low scorers on social introversion test	70	Introverted, shy, self-effacing

bols. Scales within 1 *T*-score point of each other are underlined, and the configuration of validity scales (indicated by letter) appears at the end. Virtually all the significant information about the profile in Figure 5.1 is contained in the code: 4″9′8<u>36</u>-721/50:F-K/L (except for the additional information that this profile was obtained from a 22-year-old female who was in serious trouble with the law).

In practice, most coding systems emphasize "high-point codes"—that is, the two or three scales on which a profile is most highly elevated. In the actuarial prediction system developed by Marks, Seeman, and Haller

TABLE 5.3. The Welsh (1948) Coding System Applied to the Profile in Figure 5.1

Welsh (1948) coding system	
T-score values	All followed by
90 and above	*
80–89	"
70–79	'
60–69	-
50–59	/
40–49	:
30–39	#
29 or below	Recorded to right of #

Profile in Figure 5.1			
Scale	T-scores	Scale	T-score
L	47	5	49
F	64	6	60
K	53	7	59
1	51	8	62
2	55	9	75
3	60	0	40
4	84		

Welsh code: 4"9'836-721/50:F-K/L

Note. Scales within 1 T-score point of each other are underlined.

(1974), a given profile was compared with previously established code types of patient samples for whom extensive criterion data were available (e.g., Q-sort ratings of personality descriptors by professional staff). Within the Marks and colleagues system, the profile shown in Figure 5.1 would be classified as a "4-9" profile to emphasize the "double spikes" on 4 (Psychopathic Deviate) and 9 (Hypomania). In Marks and colleagues' normative sample of psychiatric patients with a close fit to this configuration, 80% were diagnosed as having "Personality disorder: sociopathic/emotionally unstable" (p. 118). Actuarially derived Q-sort ratings of "4-9" patients described them as "incapable of controlling impulses and acts with insufficient deliberation and poor judgment . . . histrionic, self-dramatizing, egocentric, self-centered, selfish, narcissistic, and self-indulgent" (p. 119). Unfortunately,

> The 4-9 type is distinctive in that it is the only one which maintains its code under all instructional sets (admission, projected discharge, and discharge). It is as though they are announcing: "I am a 4-9; I plan to remain a 4-9." And, in fact, they do! No other code type behaves in this way. (Marks et al., 1974, p. 119)

Variants of the Standard Clinical Scales

Over the years, the scoring of the original clinical and validity scales has been modified in a number of ways to serve a variety of research and interpretive purposes. For example, Wiener and Harmon (1946) found that five of the clinical scales could be divided into "subtle" and "obvious" subscales for scoring purposes. Thus, in the Hysteria (Hy) scale, items with an obvious relation to the criterion (e.g., a "true" response to "I am troubled by attacks of nausea and vomiting") are scored on the Hy-O subscale, and items that bear a subtle relation, if any, to the criterion (e.g., a "false" response to "I enjoy detective or mystery stories") are scored on the Hy-S subscale. Although the use of subtle items might in principle circumvent problems of defensiveness in MMPI self-report, the evidence for this to date is not impressive (e.g., Duff, 1965).

Harris and Lingoes (1955) were among the first to express an interest in the distinguishably different "content" that exists *within* six of the standard clinical scales. Within the Hy scale, for example, they developed subscales such as Hy_1 (Denial of Social Anxiety) and Hy_4 (Somatic Complaints). An earlier count of the number of such variants of the standard clinical and validity scales found 89 of them (Dahlstrom, Welsh, & Dahlstrom, 1972). Interest in item content (as opposed to item discriminative capacity) eventually resulted in sets of content scales for the entire item pools of the MMPI (Wiggins, 1966) and the MMPI-2 (Butcher, Graham, Williams, & Ben-Porath, 1990).

MMPI Supplementary Scales

One of the virtues of the contrasted-groups strategy is its *generality*. Given criterion groups that differ from control groups only in their status on the criterion variable of interest (demographic and other characteristics being equal), it should in principle be possible to construct almost any kind of scale with this methodology. Thus, if one is interested in predicting response to psychotherapy, one might contrast the MMPI item responses of a criterion group of patients who clearly improved after 6 months with a comparable control group of patients who appeared to differ only in their failure to improve. This is precisely what Barron (1953a, 1953b) did in developing a supplementary MMPI scale to measure improvement in psychotherapy. Examination of a wide range of correlates of this empirically derived scale led Barron to consider it a measure of Ego Strength (Es).

The appeal of this empirical approach to scale construction, and the relative ease with which scales of this type may be developed, have produced an embarrassment of riches. It has been estimated that more than 700 of these scales had been developed by the end of the 1980s (Friedman,

Webb, & Lewak, 1989), and the number of MMPI supplementary scales now clearly exceeds the number of items in the MMPI. The variety of criteria employed in the development of these scales is suggested by the labels of a more or less random assortment: Success in Baseball (*Ba*; La Place, 1954); Graduate School Potential (*Gr*; Gough, 1957); Pharisaic Virtue (*Pv*; Cook & Medley, 1954); Homosexuality (*Hsx*; Panton, 1960); Choice of Nursing (*Nc*; Beaver, 1953); Promiscuity (Finney, 1965); Tired Housewife (Pearson, Swenson, & Rome, 1965); Neurodermatitis (Allerhand, Gough, & Grais, 1950); and Brain Lesions (Hovey, 1964).

CONTRASTING VIEWS ON THE MEANING OF TEST RESPONSES

The rationales underlying five distinguishable views of the *meaning* of responses to objective tests have guided both scale construction and interpretation over the 80+-year history of the objective testing enterprise (Wiggins, 1973b).

1. The "rational" (correspondence) view assumes a one-to-one correspondence between a patient's report ("I am anxious") and a palpable internal state of the subject (e.g., the experience of anxiety) (Buchwald, 1961). This assumption was the cornerstone of introspectionism in early experimental psychology, and it was the principal rationale underlying the earliest personality inventories (e.g., Woodworth, 1917).

2. The "empirical" (instrumental) view regards a patient's utterance as "an intrinsically interesting and significant bit of verbal behavior, the nontest correlates of which must be discovered by empirical means" (Meehl, 1945, p. 297). If it were established empirically that a "false" response to the item "I am anxious" was more characteristic of hospitalized patients with hysteria than of a normal control group, that particular bit of verbal behavior would become meaningful and would illustrate the instrumental value of verbal behavior as a "tool" in psychodiagnostics. As Buchwald (1961) put it, the tester "has his attention focused on what *he* can conclude about the subject on the basis of the subject's verbal utterances rather than on what the subject can tell him" (p. 464; emphasis in original). This philosophy was evident in the early behaviorist critique of introspectionism in experimental psychology and in later critiques of existing rational personality inventories of the 1930s. The empirical viewpoint is, of course, the one most closely associated with the empirical paradigm.

3. The "construct" view interprets a patient's response as a "postulated attribute of people assumed to be reflected in test performance" (Cronbach & Meehl, 1955, p. 283). Such a construct must be embedded in an interlocking system of laws that relate constructs to one another and to

observable properties of the environment. The *meaning* of a construct is given by the empirical laws into which it enters, and the *significance* of a construct is given by the number of such lawful relations discovered. The construct validity of a personality scale is estimated from "the proportion of test score variance that is attributable to the construct variable" (Cronbach & Meehl, 1955, p. 289).

4. The "interpersonal" (self-presentational) view regards a patient's response as an interpersonal *communication* between the patient and the clinician (or the institution that the clinician represents) (Carson, 1969b; Leary, 1957). The meaningfulness of such a communication is dependent upon both the patient's and the clinician's views of the meaning of test responses in a particular testing situation (e.g., hospital admission, vocational guidance). For example, the patient may mean to communicate a complaint ("I am anxious"), and the clinician (or the scoring system employed by the institution) may encode this as "neuroticism." The patient may view the testing situation as an opportunity for self-disclosure (Jourard, 1964), and the clinician may view it as an opportunity for impression management (Goffman, 1959). In Leary's (1957) formulation of the interpersonal paradigm, responses to the MMPI are considered on two levels: (a) the impact or interpersonal pressure exerted on the *clinician* by the patient's symptoms; and (b) the way the *patient* experiences and communicates his or her phenomenal world. The former might be said to involve "diagnosability" and the latter "communicability."

5. The "extended construct" (substantive) view was expressed in Loevinger's (1957) extension of Cronbach and Meehl's (1955) formulations. Loevinger proposed a "more radical reformulation of the validity problem" (p. 637). In particular, she argued that items employed in scale construction should be sampled from a conceptually specified *universe of content*, in such a way as to correspond to "traits which have real existence in some sense" (p. 640). As such, Loevinger assigned equal importance to the (a) substantive (content), (b) structural (dimensional), and (c) empirical (external correlates) components of construct validity.

EVOLUTION AND DEVELOPMENT OF THE PARADIGM

Impact and Influence of the MMPI

The MMPI is, and has been for many years, the most widely used inventory of personality and psychopathology; it has been estimated that over 10,000 articles, chapters, and books related to this instrument have been published (Archer, 1989). But perhaps of greater interest is the manner in which the scientific community associated with the empirical paradigm has functioned—a manner that would seem to fit the Kuhnian account more closely than any other paradigm we have considered.

To understand the 60+-year history of this instrument is to understand the history of objective personality assessment for the same time period. As Craik (1986) put it in his historical survey of personality research methods, "the MMPI came to serve as the centerpiece of this period's [post-World War II] predominant or mainstream agenda" (p. 21). Within that agenda, one can discern the operation of two separate dialectical processes over time: (1) ongoing disputes *between* the developers of the MMPI and their critics, and (2) bipolar shifts in conceptualization that have occurred *within* the evolving conceptual and interpretive frameworks of the developers of the MMPI. The ongoing disputes reflect the fact that, because of its prominence, the MMPI came to be associated with such contentious issues as clinical versus statistical prediction (Meehl, 1954) and response styles (Wiggins, 1962). These shifts in conceptualization reflect the virtuosity and intellectual flexibility of members of the empirical paradigm, who were able to shift from typological categories to continuous trait dimensions; from discriminative validity of differential diagnoses to the construct validity of scales and profiles; and from denigration of self-reports to the canonization of item content (Ben-Porath, 1994).

Conceptual Contributions of Paul E. Meehl

Although the empirical paradigm was originally characterized as "dust-bowl empiricism," the specific directions that the paradigm has assumed over the years have been determined as much by conceptual as by empirical considerations. These conceptual directions were strongly influenced by the writings of Paul E. Meehl; Table 5.4 lists a selection of Meehl's writings to illustrate this point.[2] As mentioned earlier, Meehl's (1945) "empirical manifesto" proclaimed that the meaning of responses to objective test items must be discovered by empirical means. Meehl (1989) later observed: "Although I now think the pure 'dustbowl empiricism' keying doctrine too strong as I presented it 44 years ago, the paper made several points important at the time and is still being cited" (p. 350). Meehl and Hathaway's (1946) suggestions for measuring test-taking attitudes that might compromise scale validity were years ahead of their time, and they initiated considerable research on "response styles" that were uniquely associated with the empirical paradigm (Wiggins, 1962). Similarly, Meehl's (1950) paper on configural scoring and the interpretation of patterns of scale scores, so essential to MMPI interpretation, was influential both inside and outside the empirical paradigm. And, of course, Meehl's (1954) well-known argument

---

[2] A more extensive collection of Meehl's early writings may be found in his selected papers (Meehl, 1973). An extensive collection of papers *on* Meehl may be found in the two-volume work edited by Cicchetti and Grove (1991) and by Grove and Cicchetti (1991).

TABLE 5.4. Conceptual Contributions of Paul E. Meehl

Title	Reference
"The Dynamics of 'Structured' Personality Tests"	Meehl (1945)
"The *K* Factor as a Suppressor Variable in the MMPI"	Meehl and Hathaway (1946)
"Configural Scoring"	Meehl (1950)
Clinical versus Statistical Prediction	Meehl (1954)
"Construct Validity in Psychological Tests"	Cronbach and Meehl (1955)
"Wanted—A Good Cookbook"	Meehl (1956)
"Schizotaxia, Schizotypy, Schizophrenia"	Meehl (1962)
Multivariate Taxonomic Procedures: Distinguishing Types from Continua	Waller and Meehl (1998)

that empirical methods of data combination will equal or exceed "intuitive" data combination in the forecasting of outcomes was highly influential within the empirical paradigm—although, unfortunately, it was generally ignored outside that paradigm (Grove & Meehl, 1996).

Cronbach and Meehl's (1955) classic paper on construct validity had a major influence on almost all paradigms of personality assessment, but was particularly influential in the paradigm shift to construct-oriented interpretation within the empirical paradigm itself. As Hathaway (1960) noted, "the MMPI began with validity based upon the usefulness of the various diagnostic groups from which its scales were derived. Now the burden of its use rests upon construct validity" (p. vii). Cronbach and Meehl viewed constructs as "open-ended" rather than operationally defined. The meaning of a construct becomes apparent in the nature and number of correlates that enter into the empirical network that has been established for that construct. Thus, for example, the *Pd* scale was derived by contrasting item responses of individuals diagnosed as "psychopathic deviates" with normal Minnesota residents, but this operation did not define the construct. To illustrate this point, Cronbach and Meehl (1955, pp. 20–21) cited the following empirical findings regarding the *Pd* scale of the MMPI:

1. *Pd* was found to be reasonably predictive of "delinquency" (Hathaway & Monachesi, 1953).
2. A survey of hunting accidents in Minnesota showed that hunters who "carelessly" shot someone had elevated *Pd* scores (*Minnesota Casualty Study*, 1954).
3. High school students judged by their peers to be least "responsible" were elevated on *Pd* (Gough, McClosky, & Meehl, 1952).
4. Professional actors were found to have elevated *Pd* scores (Chayatte, 1949).

5. Nurses rated by their supervisors as "not shy" and "unafraid of mental patients" were high on *Pd* (Hovey, 1953).
6. High *Pd* predicted dropping out of high school (Roessel, 1954).
7. Low *Pd* was associated with ratings of being "good-natured" (Gough, McKee, & Yandell, 1953).

Cronbach and Meehl (1955) concluded:

> The point is that all seven of these "criterion" dispositions would be readily guessed by any clinician having even superficial familiarity with MMPI interpretation; but to mediate these inferences explicitly requires quite a few hypotheses about dynamics, constituting an admittedly sketchy (but far from vacuous) network defining the genotype *psychopathic deviate.* (p. 21)

In his presidential address to the Midwestern Psychological Association, Meehl (1956) reported encouraging Q-sort personality correlations of MMPI code types found in a doctoral dissertation (Halbower, 1955), and he urged clinicians to develop more "cookbooks" of this sort. Clinicians within the empirical paradigm took up this challenge and developed actuarial prediction systems of the type long employed within the insurance industry (e.g., Gilberstadt & Duker, 1965; Marks & Seeman, 1963; Sines, 1966).

In his presidential address to the American Psychological Association, Meehl (1962) used the occasion to share his long-standing interest in genetic interpretations of schizophrenia. Briefly, Meehl assumed that four core behavioral traits ("cognitive slippage," "interpersonal aversiveness," "anhedonia," and "ambivalence") are inherited and together constitute the predisposition of "schizotaxia." The social learning histories of such individuals may result in the personality organization of the "schizotype." A minority of such schizotypic individuals may be disadvantaged by a variety of factors (e.g., what were then called "schizophrenogenic mothers," who would probably be referred to as "high in expressed emotion" today) and thus may develop schizophrenia.

In accord with his interests in the etiology of schizophrenia, Meehl (1995) was for many years interested in solving the basic classification problem involved in developing multivariate taxonomic procedures that can distinguish discontinuous personality "types" (e.g., the schizotype) from the continuously distributed individual differences that have come to be the subject matter of most contemporary personality psychology. In a sense, this may be thought of as a renewed emphasis on the disease model of mental illness, with reference to which the original MMPI was constructed:

> But I want to argue that we can do considerably better than we have been, by adopting the unpopular medical model (with suitable adaptations to

psychodiagnosis) and asking ourselves what would be the nearest equivalent to a pathologist's report. (Meehl, 1973, p. 288)

The term "taxon" has been used more or less interchangeably with such terms as "syndrome," "type," "disease entity," and "latent class." Although taxonicity is sometimes distinguished from "dimensional" measurement, Waller and Meehl (1998) emphasized that taxonicity does not imply the absence of a dimension. The defining characteristic of a taxon is the *discontinuity* that exists among categories within a taxonomy. The taxonomic procedures developed by Meehl and his colleagues have permitted the estimation of "latent parameters," such as base rate and indicator validity, in the absence of a criterion variable (e.g., Golden & Meehl, 1979; Meehl & Yonce, 1994, 1996). The availability of computer programs for taxonomic analysis (Waller & Meehl, 1998) has stimulated considerable research of this kind. These procedures have been used to investigate the latent structure of schizotypy (Korfine & Lenzenweger, 1995; Lenzenweger & Korfine, 1992); children at risk for schizophenia (Erlenmeyer-Kimling, Golden, & Cornblatt, 1989); borderline personality disorder (Trull, Widiger, & Guthrie, 1990); psychopathy (Harris, Rice, & Quinsey, 1994); and dissociative identity disorder (Waller, Putnam, & Carlson, 1996). It should be borne in mind that these procedures are not limited to the identification of pathological syndromes, and that they have had more general psychometric applications (e.g., Strong, Green, & Schinka, 2000).

My selection of eight from among the many papers of Paul Meehl to illustrate the influence of conceptual considerations upon the evolution of the empirical paradigm hardly does justice to the breadth and depth of his *oeuvre*. Meehl's (1973) own selection of his papers is perhaps more representative in this respect, and clinicians who have not yet read "Why I Do Not Attend Case Conferences" are strongly encouraged to consult the 1973 volume as well.

SOURCE BOOKS IN THE EARLY HISTORICAL DEVELOPMENT OF THE PARADIGM

From the beginning, the empirical paradigm has been "empirical" in several meanings of that word. The meaning and significance of MMPI profiles were established by their nontest correlates, which were discovered in a series of empirical investigations that continues today. As a consequence, competent users of the test must have some familiarity with what has now become the largest empirical literature associated with any existing personality test. Although a number of single articles have represented clear achievements and have tended to solidify the paradigm, the evolution of the paradigm itself is perhaps best understood with reference to certain canonical books and manuals that have appeared over the last 50 years.

There is substantial agreement within the empirical community that the works listed in Table 5.5 are among the most important that appeared during the first 40 years of paradigm development. Similarly, there is general agreement that the works listed later in Table 5.6 (see the next section) are representative of more contemporary developments and refinements within the empirical paradigm. Note, however, that the division of the history of the evolution of the empirical paradigm into two tables is meant to illustrate a radical change in the basis of that paradigm—a change that occurred over time. As will become evident later, this change does not qualify as a Kuhnian "paradigm shift," but it does provide an example of the manner in which a paradigm "crisis" was resolved.

The 799-page *An Atlas for the Clinical Use of the MMPI* (Hathaway & Meehl, 1951a) is a collection of 968 short case histories with associated MMPI scale codes "that might serve to recall similar cases with MMPI patterns similar to the one being considered" (p. iii). Diagnoses and demographics were presented for individual cases, which themselves were ordered in the atlas by MMPI scale codes to facilitate "matching." Also available at that time was an Army and Air Force technical manual, *Military Clinical Psychology* (Departments of the Army and the Air Force, 1951), which served a similar function for postwar military clinical psychologists to that of Rapaport's (1944–1946) wartime manual. The postwar Army and Air Force manual provided bottom-line summaries of the Wechsler–Bellevue Scale (by David Wechsler), the Rorschach technique (by Bruno Klopfer), the Thematic Apperception Test (by Henry Murray), and the MMPI (by Starke Hathaway and Paul Meehl). The suggestions for MMPI interpretation offered by Hathaway and Meehl (1951b) were generally conservative in nature (e.g., "the MMPI profile does not directly provide a diagnosis with the majority of patients" [p. 72]), and they also reflected an early shift of emphasis from the original Kraepelinian nosological

TABLE 5.5. Source Books in the Historical Development of the Empirical Paradigm

Author(s)	Description
Hathaway and Meehl (1951a)	Atlas for clinical use
Hathaway and Meehl (1951b)	Chapter in military assessment manual
Welsh and Dahlstrom (1956)	Basic readings
Dahlstrom and Welsh (1960)	Interpretive and research handbook
Butcher (1972)	Changing perspectives
Dahlstrom, Welsh, and Dahlstrom (1972)	Expanded interpretive handbook
Dahlstrom, Welsh, and Dahlstrom (1975)	Expanded research handbook
Dahlstrom and Dahlstrom (1980)	Revised basic readings

categories to "code combinations" (profile types) and their empirical correlates (e.g., as found in adjective checklists).

The seminal *Basic Readings on the MMPI in Psychology and Medicine* (Welsh & Dahlstrom, 1956) was meant to represent "the major research and clinical developments in the use of the MMPI during the last fifteen years" (p. v). From an MMPI bibliography of 689 entries, 66 were selected on the grounds of "historical priority, completeness of analysis, representativeness of the sample, or imaginative design" (p. v). These carefully selected and well-annotated articles served to introduce the scope, depth, and applicability of the empirical paradigm to at least several generations of clinicians and researchers, and their historical importance cannot be overestimated.

As discussed in the Introduction, the accomplishments of earlier workers in the field are often emphasized as "paradigmatic" in the training of students. Such accomplishments provide the basis for current and future practice, and also illustrate the rules and standards of the paradigm. The *Basic Readings* served this function well, and Harrison Gough's (1956) chapter on "Some Common Misconceptions about Neuroticism" provides an excellent illustration of this principle. Members of a criterion group of clinicians were asked to answer all items in the MMPI as they would be answered by a patient "experiencing a psychoneurotic reaction" (Gough, 1956, p. 52). A control group consisted of patients diagnosed with neuroses who had taken the MMPI. A contrasted-groups analysis of the items that distinguished the former group ("dissimulators") from the latter group (bona fide patients with neuroses) yielded a 74-item dissimulation scale, which (1) illustrated the misconceptions clinicians had about neuroticism (e.g., overemphasizing physical complaints) and (2) discriminated subsequent groups of instructed fakers from genuine patients with neuroses (e.g., 93% of instructed dissimulators were correctly identified). Graduate students of that era (including myself) rarely failed to be impressed by the ingenuity, elegance, and promise of this paradigmatic tour de force.

The first edition of *An MMPI Handbook* (Dahlstrom & Welsh, 1960) was meant to introduce novice clinicians to "current MMPI usage in clinical practice together with the findings to date on its various validities" (p. xiii). It provided a wealth of detail on MMPI administration, interpretation, and clinical applications, plus a series of useful appendices, such as one providing scoring keys for the 213 MMPI "supplementary scales" that were available at that time.

In a sense, the foregoing scholarly texts described the halcyon days of the empirical paradigm, with little awareness of the dark days that awaited personality assessment in the 1960s. The MMPI developed in the 1940s was, by more contemporary standards, based on inadequate and outdated norms, replete with offensive and anachronistic items, and unsuited in many ways to the diagnostic task for which it was devised. Pressures to

(1) restandardize, (2) revise, or (3) replace this relic had existed almost from its inception, culminating in a historically important summit meeting in which the third option was seriously considered (Wiggins, 1973a). Butcher's (1972) *Objective Personality Assessment: Changing Perspectives* contained invited addresses to the Fifth Annual Symposium on Recent Developments in the Use of the MMPI. The general question addressed by the participants was "whether the MMPI was in need of revision and what problems would surround such an enterprise" (p. x). Many of the answers to these questions reflected the "paradigm crisis" alluded to earlier:

> From a strictly diagnostic viewpoint, the Multiphasic is a mess! Its original clinical criteria are anachronistic; its basic clinical scales are inefficient, redundant, and largely irrelevant for their present purposes; its administrative format and the repertoire of responses elicited are, respectively, inflexible and impoverished; and its methods for combining scale scores and for profile interpretation are unconscionably cumbersome and obtuse. (Norman, 1972, p. 64)

Somewhat ironically, the first volume of Dahlstrom, Welsh, and Dahlstrom's (1972) meticulously revised *An MMPI Handbook* (on clinical interpretation) appeared in the same year as the Butcher volume, and was followed 3 years later by an equally thorough revision of a second volume (on research applications; Dahlstrom, Welsh, & Dahlstrom, 1975). Together, these volumes constitute a milestone in the history of personality assessment that might well serve as exemplars for other paradigms. To revise the original MMPI and thus threaten the continuity of accumulated clinical and research knowledge appeared unthinkable, to some at least.

Dahlstrom and Dahlstrom's (1980) revision of the *Basic Readings on the MMPI*, when compared with the original (Welsh & Dahlstrom, 1956), provides both a more complete account of the development of the MMPI clinical scales and an indication of some of the challenges to the validity of the paradigm that occurred over a period of 24 years. The latter included issues pertaining to the effects of "response styles," on the MMPI (e.g., Block, 1980; Edwards, 1980; Jackson & Messick, 1980); the possibility of "content scales" for the MMPI (Wiggins, 1980b); and the possibility of removing "offensive" items from the MMPI pool (Butcher & Tellegen, 1980; Walker, 1980).

SOURCE BOOKS IN THE CONTEMPORARY DEVELOPMENT OF THE PARADIGM: THE MMPI-2 AND MMPI-A

Ten years after the historic summit conference in Minneapolis, the University of Minnesota Press appointed the MMPI Restandardization Committee to supervise the long-awaited revision of the MMPI.[3] The following were the overall goals of this committee: (1) to replace obsolete items (e.g., "I used to like drop-the-handkerchief"), potentially offensive items (e.g., "I have never had any black, tarry-looking bowel movements"), and items that might be difficult to process (e.g., "I have often wished that I were a girl. [Or if you are a girl] I have never been sorry that I am a girl"); (2) to restandardize the normative base of the MMPI with a more recent and more representative sample of respondents; and (3) to maintain continuity with the original clinical and validity scales, "so as to allow test-interpreters to continue to rely on decades of accumulated research and clinical experience with these scales" (Ben-Porath, 1994, p. 380).

Table 5.6 lists the canonical works regarding the MMPI-2 that have already appeared in the brief period of time that has elapsed since the original MMPI was officially put to rest. It is evident from both editions of the manual for administering and scoring the MMPI-2 (Butcher, Dahlstrom, Graham, Tellegen, & Kaemmer, 1989; Butcher et al., 2001) that the original clinical and validity scales of the MMPI have been preserved more or less intact. However, newer and more sophisticated procedures for *norming* these scales (e.g., the "uniform *T*-scores" developed by Tellegen & Ben-Porath, 1992) have raised questions regarding the applicability of previously established interpretations of MMPI scale configurations to MMPI-2 scale configurations. Nevertheless, empirical comparison of code types using both linear and uniform *T*-score transformations has established that these differences are negligible (Graham, Tinbrook, Ben-Porath, & Butcher, 1991).

A question has also been raised concerning the comparability of MMPI and MMPI-2 profile configurations—a topic that is most relevant to the validity of MMPI-2 interpretations based on the extensive literature of the original MMPI. The answer to this question is detailed (see Graham, 2000, pp. 205–211), but the bottom line is that "MMPI-2 code types can be interpreted similarly to their MMPI counterparts" (Graham, 2000, p. 211). As Nichols (1992) observed in his review of MMPI-2 for the *Eleventh Mental Measurements Yearbook*, "what was broke was fixed, what was not broke was left alone" (p. 567).

Publication of the first edition of the manual for the MMPI-2 (Butcher et al., 1989) was followed closely by a series of publications that extended the paradigm to include item "content," enlarged the scope of the paradigm to specifically include adolescent populations, and made available new interpretive systems for clinical use.

---

[3] This committee was coordinated by Beverly Kaemmer, test manager for the University of Minnesota Press, and consisted of James N. Butcher, W. Grant Dahlstrom, John R. Graham, and Auke Tellegen.

TABLE 5.6. Source Books in the Contemporary Development
of the Empirical Paradigm

Author(s)	Description
Butcher et al. (1989)	MMPI-2 manual
Butcher et al. (1990)	MMPI-2 content scales
Butcher et al. (1992)	MMPI-A (adolescent version)
Williams et al. (1992)	MMPI-A content scales
Butcher (1993)	MMPI-2 Minnesota Report
Ben-Porath (1994)	Historical overview of paradigm
Nichols and Greene (1995)	MMPI-2 Structural Summary
Graham (2000)	MMPI-2 interpretation
Butcher et al. (2001)	MMPI-2 revised manual

Validity Scales for the MMPI-2

From its inception, developers of the empirical paradigm have maintained a somewhat skeptical view of self-report data. The "meaning" of a test response was held to reside in the empirically demonstrated correlates of that response. And the validity scales (L, F, K) provided a means of identifying respondents' tendencies to present an unrealistically favorable or unfavorable portrait of themselves. The development of rational content scales for the MMPI-2 and the new adolescent version of the MMPI (MMPI-A) does not in itself represent a retreat from the earlier skeptical view of self-report data. On the one hand, it should be noted that my earlier MMPI content scales (Wiggins, 1966) were encouraged from their inception by most of the major figures in MMPI research (Wiggins, 1990). On the other hand, the published MMPI-2 content scales were accompanied by no fewer than five new validity scales!

As can be seen from Figure 5.2, the validity scale portion of the MMPI-2 profile sheet now lists eight scales. The original scales of F, L, and K retain their interpretive significance. The Variable Response Inconsistency ($VRIN$) scale consists of 67 pairs of items for which a particular pattern of responding is semantically inconsistent (e.g., answering "true" to both "My sleep is fitful and disturbed" *and* "I wake up fresh and rested most mornings"). Whereas the $VRIN$ measures more or less random inconsistency, the True Response Inconsistency ($TRIN$) scale measures fixed patterns of inconsistency: answering all true to pairs of inconsistent items (acquiescent response style) or answering all false to pairs of inconsistent items (counteracquiescent response style).

The F scale still measures the tendency to endorse items that have a very low probability of endorsement in normal populations, and it is still used to raise questions of "faking bad" or random responding. However,

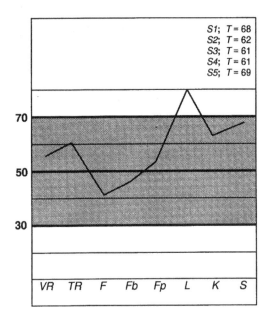

S1; T = 68
S2; T = 62
S3; T = 61
S4; T = 61
S5; T = 69

FIGURE 5.2. Profile of MMPI-2 validity scales. Adapted from Butcher (1999, p. 33). Copyright 1999 by the American Psychological Association. Adapted by permission.

because all of the original *F* items appeared within the first 370 items on the test form, additional *F* items were developed for the remaining part of the test form. The *Fb* scale consists of items toward the later part of the test ("back") that have a low probability of endorsement in normal populations. Thus it measures (among other things) random responding due to loss of interest, or to becoming bored and fatigued toward the end of this very long test (Berry, Baer, Rinaldo, & Wetter, 2002). In addition, *Fp* (Infrequency Psychopathology) was developed to examine the in frequency of responses in psychiatric inpatients. It is "the most sensitive and specific measure of overreporting on the MMPI-2" (Nichols, 2001, p. 49).

The Superlative Self-Presentation *(S)* scale was developed by Butcher and Han (1995) to provide a more differentiated assessment of defensiveness than is found in the *K* scale. In a contrasted-groups analysis, a highly defensive group of job applicants served as a criterion group, and the new normative MMPI-2 sample served as a control group. There are five subscales of *S* whose items reflect different components of superlative self-presentation: *S1*, Beliefs in Human Goodness; *S2*, Serenity; *S3*, Contentment with Life; *S4*, Patience and Denial of Irritability and Anger; and *S5*, Denial of Moral Flaws.

Content Scales for the MMPI-2 and MMPI-A

Adults (MMPI-2)

The development of "official" content scales for the MMPI-2 signaled a final shift in conceptual perspective—from the original "dustbowl empiricism," to a construct-oriented perspective, to the even more substantive view of construct validity first proposed by Loevinger (1957). This extended view of construct validity has been discussed earlier in this chapter (see "Contrasting Views on the Meaning of Test Responses"). Interest in the content of patients' communication of complaints via the MMPI remained minimal until the appearance of the Wiggins (1966) MMPI content scales. In terms of Loevinger's (1957) distinctions, these content scales appeared to provide (1) representative coverage of the *universe of content* of the MMPI item pool (see Johnson, Butcher, Null, & Johnson, 1984); (2) psychometrically sound measures of 13 self-report dimensions that were interpreted with reference to previous studies of the *factorial structure* of the MMPI (Welsh, 1956); and (3) *empirical evidence* of convergent and discriminant validity with reference to psychiatric diagnostic categories (Wiggins, 1966; Payne & Wiggins, 1972). Perhaps of greater interest to the MMPI community was the potential usefulness of these content scales in individual psychodiagnostic appraisal (e.g., Nichols, 1987).

In the course of revising the MMPI item pool, a number of the original items were dropped, including some that had been included in the Wiggins (1966) content scales. As a consequence, a new set of 15 content scales was developed for use with the MMPI-2. The development of these new scales was based on a "deductive approach, including theoretical, rational, and construct-oriented methods" (Butcher, Graham, Williams, & Ben-Porath, 1990, p. 3). In the spirit of "The Prototypical Wiggins Content Scales" (Butcher et al., 1990, p. 9), a heavy emphasis was placed on *communicability* between patient and tester. New items were prepared to cover content areas of contemporary interest, such as substance abuse, Type A behaviors, and treatment compliance.

The 15 MMPI-2 content scales are listed in Table 5.7. Although some of these scales resemble the original Wiggins content scales, many of them represent more recent concepts in descriptive psychiatry.[4] In addition, although the original MMPI content scales were each constructed to represent a single homogeneous dimension, some of the new content scales represent more than one dimension. The third column of the table indicates the number of distinguishable content components that were found for each content scale (Ben-Porath & Sherwood, 1993). For instance, all the

---

[4] The Wiggins content scales were based on Hathaway and McKinley's (1940, p. 249) original survey of "behavior of significance to the psychiatrist."

TABLE 5.7. The MMPI-2 Content Scales

MMPI-2 content scale	No. of items	No. of component scales
Anxiety (ANX)	23	—
Fears (FRS)	23	2
Obsessiveness (OBS)	16	—
Depression (DEP)	33	4
Health Concerns (HEA)	36	3
Bizarre Mentation (BIZ)	24	2
Anger (ANG)	16	2
Cynicism (CYN)	23	2
Antisocial Practices (ASP)	22	2
Type A (TPA)	19	2
Low Self-Esteem (LSE)	24	2
Social Discomfort (SOD)	24	2
Family Problems (FAM)	25	2
Work Interference (WRK)	33	—
Negative Treatment Indicators (TRT)	26	2

Note. Data from Butcher et al. (1990).

items in the Anxiety content scale measure a single component of anxiety (ANX). However, the Fears content scale includes the two separate components of Generalized Fearfulness (FRS1) and Multiple Fears (FRS2). The Depression content scale includes the four components of Lack of Drive (DEP1), Dysphoria (DEP2), Self-Deprecation (DEP3), and Suicidal Ideation (DEP4).

In terms of test–retest reliability, the Wiggins content scales and the MMPI-2 content scales were found to be generally comparable (Butcher et al., 1990). On average, the MMPI-2 content scales tended to be more internally consistent than the Wiggins scales. Most importantly, it soon became apparent that the new content scales provided *incremental validity* in the differential diagnosis of psychopathology; that is, they contributed unique predictive variance over and above that provided by the standard clinical scales (e.g., Archer, Aiduk, Griffin, & Elkins, 1996; Ben-Porath, Butcher, & Graham, 1991).

Adolescents (MMPI-A)

From the beginning, the MMPI has been used in adolescent populations, particularly in the prediction of juvenile delinquency (e.g., Capwell, 1945; Hathaway & Monachesi, 1953). The applicability to an adolescent population of a test designed for adults "has not provided a consistent or comprehensive way to use and interpret the test" (Kazdin, 1992, p. xiv). The MMPI-A was specifically designed for an adolescent population (Butcher et al., 1992). New items were written to reflect adolescent concerns in such areas as peer group influence, family relations, school, and teachers, and the overall length of the test was reduced. In accord with the now standard view that "Content scales, in effect, provide a means of psychometrically appraising direct communications between patient and clinician" (Butcher et al., 1992, p. 135), 15 content scales were constructed for the MMPI-A (Williams, Butcher, Ben-Porath, & Graham, 1992). These content scales reflect areas of concern that are specific to this age group (e.g., Adolescent Alienation, Adolescent Low Self-Esteem, Adolescent School Problems).

Supplemental Scales for the MMPI-2

In the revision of the MMPI, items in the traditional clinical scales were retained (often in edited form) to ensure continuity of these scales with their counterparts in the MMPI-2. Rather than attempting to choose which of the literally hundreds of special scales of the MMPI should be left intact, the authors focused instead on the development of new supplemental scales that focused on clinical problems not directly addressed in the original MMPI. Table 5.8 lists the supplemental scales of the MMPI-2, which were designed to appraise currently important clinical problems.

Among these current social problems are problems of substance abuse (i.e., the psychiatric sequelae of overindulgence in alcohol and in a wide range of mind-altering drugs). Notwithstanding its history of occasional misapplication (Gottesman & Prescott, 1989), the MacAndrew Alcoholism scale has proven useful in the detection of potential substance abuse problems, as has the newly constructed MMPI-2 Addiction Potential scale (Weed, Butcher, McKenna, & Ben-Porath, 1992). The Addiction Acknowl-

TABLE 5.8. Supplemental Scales for the MMPI-2

Label	Scale	Author(s)	Application
MAC-R	MacAndrew Alcoholism—Revised	MacAndrew (1965)	Potential substance abuse problems
APS	Addiction Potential	Weed et al. (1992)	Potential substance abuse problems
AAS	Addiction Acknowledgment	Weed et al. (1992)	Substance abuse acknowledged
MDS	Marital Distress	Hjemboe et al. (1992)	Marital problems or relationship difficulties
Ho	Hostility	Cook & Medley (1954); Han et al. (1995)	Cynicism and hostility; associated with coronary disease

edgment scale, developed by the same authors, assesses a patient's willing-ness (or unwillingness) to acknowledge problems of abuse.

Marital distress is another social problem of current concern, and re-search employing the MMPI-2 has demonstrated that the *Pd* clinical scale and the Family Problems (*FAM*) content scale are significantly related to marital distress (Hjemboe & Butcher, 1991). Hjemboe, Almagor, and Butcher (1992) developed an MMPI-2 supplemental scale for measuring marital distress, which was found to be even more strongly related to mari-tal problems. Cook and Medley's (1954) Hostility (*Ho*) scale has long been identified as a critical component of the "Type A" personality that is asso-ciated with coronary disease. During the revision of the MMPI, the *Ho* scale (with slightly reworded items) was found to be significantly related to MMPI-2 scale measures of cynicism and hostility.

The MMPI-2 Structural Summary

Advances in more conceptually oriented scale construction have been ac-companied by advances in more conceptually oriented *interpretation* of the MMPI scales. This is perhaps most clearly illustrated by the MMPI-2 Struc-tural Summary approach. Nichols and Greene (1995), the authors of the manual explaining the Structural Summary, state:

> The history of the interpretation of the MMPI/MMPI-2 may be seen as an ever expanding set of perspectives for viewing the respondent's perfor-mance . . . Thus, the contemporary approach to the interpretation of MMPI/MMPI-2 encourages an integration of these combined perspectives. (pp. 1–2)

The unique feature of this system is that it incorporates previous advances made under the empirical, construct, interpersonal, and extended construct viewpoints within a comprehensive interpretive system that places full em-phasis on the (1) substantive (content), (2) structural (dimensional), and (3) empirical (external correlates) components of construct validity.

The Structural Summary is organized into six major sections. These are meant to represent the kinds of clinical interpretations that may be made with varying degrees of confidence from 108 scales and indices, which include standard validity and clinical scales (e.g., *Hy*, Hysteria); variants of standard clinical scales (e.g., *Hy-S*, Subtle Hysteria); supplemen-tary scales (e.g., *Es*, Ego Strength); MMPI-2 content scales (e.g., *HEA*, Health Concerns); and special scoring indices (e.g., False %, Percentage of False Responses). An overview of the six major sections is provided in Table 5.9, in which only two illustrative subcategories are listed for each section. (The actual number of subcategories within each section varies from 2 to 12, with some subsections containing further divisions.) In contrast to previous computer-generated reports, which organized MMPI scales into types or origins, the Structural Summary organizes scales with respect to their *interpretive meanings*:

> The composition of the Structural Summary emphasizes face or content validity, supported through studies of item overlap; examination of scale internal consistencies; and confirmation of patterns of covariation among measures using correlation and factor analysis. These operations were, however, embedded within a rational and intuitive process that focused on the concepts a new organization of MMPI-2 scores might address and on how measures could be arranged to best address those concepts selected. (Nichols & Greene, 1995, p. 3)

Although not yet subjected to extensive empirical confirmation, the Structural Summary, along with other new interpretive materials for MMPI-2 (e.g., Butcher & Williams, 2000; Graham, 2000), has facilitated clinical applications of this promising new instrument. Butcher (1999) has also written the remarkable *A Beginner's Guide to the MMPI-2*, which employs his "quick immersion" technique of presenting didactic material in the context of clinical case studies. This book has obviously benefited from Butcher's 35 years of experience in teaching the MMPI to graduate students and professionals. It is highly recommended to the beginner as an introduction to the MMPI, the MMPI-2, or both.

John R. Graham is also a highly experienced teacher of the MMPI who was extensively involved in the restandardization project. His textbook (Graham, 2000) is in the classic empirical tradition of the MMPI, because it presents an exceptionally well-integrated and up-to-date summary of the MMPI and MMPI-2 research literature—a literature that provides the basis for Graham's interpretation of MMPI-2 protocols. In addition to being the best available summary of recent literature for the researcher, this book provides sound and unambiguous advice to clinicians. For example, Gra-

TABLE 5.9. The MMPI-2 Structural Summary

Test-taking Attitudes	*Cognitions*
Self-Favorable	Paranoid Thought Processes
Self-Unfavorable	Defense Mechanisms
Factor Scales	*Interpersonal Relations*
First Factor Scales (distress)	Social Alienation
Second Factor Scales (overcontrol)	Authority Conflict
Moods	*Other Problem Areas*
Depression	Substance Abuse
Anxiety	Suicidal Ideation

Note. Data from Nichols and Greene (1995).

ham notes that in a forensic setting, "Clinicians are advised to limit their interpretations to issues for which the MMPI/MMPI-2 has been adequately validated and to avoid making interpretations that cannot be supported by reference to empirical research" (2000, p. 362). Regarding computer administration of MMPI-2, he states: "The computer time required to complete the test on-line is so great that in most settings this form of administration is not appropriate" (p. 293).

Around the World with the MMPI-2

Over 150 translations of the MMPI-2 have been developed, and the test has been employed in at least 46 countries (Butcher et al., 1998, p. 279). An international handbook on MMPI-2 translation and clinical use contains 56 contributions from psychologists and psychiatrists from around the world (Butcher, 1996). The focus of this international enterprise has been upon the validity of MMPI-2 computer-based test reports. The "official" MMPI-2 computer-based interpretive system is now the MMPI-2 Minnesota Report (Butcher, 1993). In tandem with efforts to establish the validity of the report in its country of origin, studies of the validity of the report in other parts of the world have been conducted.

In one such study, computer-based MMPI-2 reports were evaluated in Australia, France, Norway, and the United States (Butcher et al., 1998). A broad range of clients were administered the MMPI-2 in each country. Clinicians who were seeing their clients for psychological evaluation or therapy were instructed to rate the accuracy and appropriateness of their clients' MMPI-2 computer-based reports, with reference to such areas as accuracy of self-report, symptomatic pattern, interpersonal relations, diagnosis, and treatment recommendations. Overall, the various indices of "consumer satisfaction" were promising:

> Relatively few of the practitioners in any of the four countries found the reports inappropriate or inaccurate. The sections for which most of the reports were considered as valuable and to provide in-depth information were the validity considerations, the symptomatic patterns, and the interpersonal relations sections and, to a lesser degree, the diagnostic and the treatment considerations. (Butcher et al., 1998, p. 289)

OVERVIEW

Ben-Porath (1994) has provided an excellent historical summary of the "reinvention of the MMPI" following the failure of the empirical strategy and its subsequent evolution into an omnibus measure of personality within a construct-oriented perspective. The highlights of this shift over a 50-

year period of unprecedented research and clinical work include emphases upon (1) MMPI profile configurations, rather than on single scales; (2) normal correlates of profile types; (3) additional empirically and substantively derived scales that have broadened the nomological network of MMPI investigation (e.g., Morey, Waugh, & Blashfield, 1985); and (4) actuarial prediction systems based on configural profile types.

One cannot help noting the contrast between Hathaway's (1972) earlier pessimistic assessment of the future of the paradigm—"So, in summary, we are stuck, I think, with the MMPI . . . for a dreary while longer" (p. 40)—and Ben-Porath's (1994) optimistic challenge to those who would develop instruments intended to augment or replace the MMPI-2:

> . . . tests that are intended to replace the MMPI-2 are faced with the daunting challenge of matching its empirical and experiential data base, whereas instruments designed to augment the MMPI-2 must be shown to possess incremental clinical validity in the assessment of clinically relevant phenomena. (p. 389)

These contrasting opinions were expressed by individuals representing widely separated generations within the highly "inbred" empirical paradigm.[5] As an obvious heir apparent to a guiding role in the future development of the empirical paradigm, Ben-Porath has a gratifyingly deep appreciation of the history and significance of that remarkable endeavor.

---

[5] Starke Hathaway was the founding father of the empirical paradigm, and his student, Grant Dahlstrom, was the mentor of James Butcher, who in turn was the mentor of Yossef Ben-Porath.

6

Convergences among Paradigms
The Individual and Society

METAPSYCHOLOGICAL CONSIDERATIONS

Metaconcepts are "concepts about concepts," which may be employed to illuminate, on an abstract level, the root metaphors that underlie the world views of philosophical or scientific models (Pepper, 1942). In this context, David Bakan's (1966) metaconcepts of "agency" and "communion" may be thought of as social constructions that serve to identify the common metaphors and philosophical–political assumptions underlying a variety of disciplines in the humanities and social sciences. "Agency" refers to the condition of being a differentiated *individual*, and it is manifested in the strivings for mastery and power that enhance this differentiation. "Communion" refers to the condition of being part of a larger *social or spiritual entity*, and it is manifested in strivings for intimacy, union, and solidarity within that larger entity.

Bakan's (1966) wide-ranging essay related these metaconcepts to such diverse topics as religion, science, myth, death, and disease. Subsequently, I (Wiggins, 1991) illustrated the centrality of these concepts to the worldviews of philosophers from Confucius to Bakan, and of personality theorists from Freud to McAdams; to psycholinguistic and historical-developmental studies of the language of personality; and to the conceptions of men and women from a variety of disciplines. In Chapter 2 of this book, I have considered the manner in which conceptions of agency and communion in the social and behavioral sciences provided a conceptual foundation for the interpersonal paradigm. In the present chapter, I consider the possibility that agency and communion are central metaconcepts within all paradigms of personality assessment.

Although there is some disagreement concerning Bakan's interpretation of the *relation* between these two fundamental modalities of human experience (e.g., Leonard, 1997), agency and communion are viewed by most as being independent of, or orthogonal to, each other (Wiggins, 1991, 1997). Thus it is possible to be both a strongly differentiated person and a nurturantly engaged person, to be one and not the other, and so forth.

The variety of guises that the metaconcepts of agency and communion have assumed within the five paradigms of personality assessment is suggested by Table 6.1. Within the psychodynamic, interpersonal, and personological paradigms, agency and communion may be thought of as conceptual assumptions concerning the nature of human nature; they underlie not only differences among these paradigms, but differing assumptions that have been made within paradigms as they have developed over time. Within the multivariate and empirical paradigms, for example, agency and communion may be thought of as interpretations that emerged from empirical findings in the later stages of paradigm development.

AGENCY AND COMMUNION WITHIN THE PARADIGMS OF PERSONALITY ASSESSMENT

Man is an essentially individual animal; man is an essentially social animal. The history of Western social and political philosophy has revolved around the tension between these two views of the nature of human experience.
—GREENBERG AND MITCHELL (1983, p. 400)

In what is unquestionably one of the more sophisticated and enlightening conceptual introductions to the psychodynamic paradigm, Greenberg and Mitchell (1983) have called attention to a fundamental paradox in the hu-

TABLE 6.1. Bakan's (1966) Metaconcepts of Agency and Communion within the Five Paradigms of Personality Assessment

Paradigm	Agency	Communion	Author(s)
Psychodynamic	Drive/structure model (Freud)	Relations/structure model (Sullivan)	Greenberg and Mitchell (1983)
Interpersonal	Self-esteem (Sullivan)	Security (Sullivan)	Wiggins (1991)
Personological	Power (Winter)	Intimacy (McAdams)	McAdams et al. (1996)
Multivariate	Factor Beta	Factor Alpha	Digman (1997)
Empirical	Egoistic bias	Moralistic bias	Paulhus and John (1998)

man condition. On the one hand, we are all individuals who live in our own subjective world with our own desires and dreams, and our existence in this world is but temporary. On the other hand, we cannot survive without living in a human community and a culture that give meaning to our lives, and that will survive us. Greenberg and Mitchell have provided a succinct summary of opposing agentic and communal views of the human condition throughout the recent history of Western philosophy.[1]

Agency in Western Political Philosophy

The English philosophers Thomas Hobbes (1588–1679) and John Locke (1632–1704) both believed that the natural state of persons was to pursue and fulfill their own pleasures and satisfactions. But the totally unchecked pursuit of individual desires can, as they both experienced, lead to war (i.e., the English Civil War of 1642–1646). In order to prevent the subversion of individual fulfillment, some form of intervention by the state is required— either by the power of royalty (Hobbes's view) or by the power of Parliament (Locke's view). As Greenberg and Mitchell pointed out, Sir Isaiah Berlin (1958) referred to this concept as "negative liberty"; that is, the society prevents something negative from happening to individual fulfillment.

Communion in Western Political Philosophy

Greenberg and Mitchell have identified an alternative school of political philosophy that originated in the works of Jean-Jacques Rousseau (1712–1778) and G. W. F. Hegel (1770–1831), and that culminated dramatically in the writings of Karl Marx (1818–1883), who stated: "But the human essence is no abstraction inherent in each single individual. In its reality it is the ensemble of the social relations" (Marx, 1845, p. 244). In this ultracommunal view, human nature is intrinsically social and can only be fulfilled through interactions with others. Berlin (1958) referred to this concept as "positive liberty"; that is, the state serves a positive function by providing an entity for the fulfillment of the communal needs of individual citizens.

THE PSYCHODYNAMIC PARADIGM

> The persistence and tenacity of the drive model and the relational
> model derive from the fact that they draw on two of the most

---

[1] Although Greenberg and Mitchell's (1983) formulation of this issue appears to have been developed independently of Bakan's (1966) earlier work, I use Bakan's terms of "agency" and "communion" to designate their distinctions.

fundamental and compelling approaches to human experience,
approaches which have dominated our civilization and entered into the
thinking of each of us.
—GREENBERG AND MITCHELL (1983, p. 403)

As discussed in Chapter 1, Greenberg and Mitchell have made a fundamental conceptual distinction between the agentic drive/structure model of Freud and the communal relations/structure model of Sullivan. As indicated in the quote above, they attributed the persistence of these models over time to their lucid representations of the two universal aspects of human experience.

The Drive/Structural Model

The bit of truth behind all of this—one so eagerly denied—is that men are not
gentle, friendly creatures wishing for love, who simply defend themselves if they
are attacked, but that a powerful measure of desire for aggression has to be
reckoned as part of their instinctual endowment. The result is that their neighbor
is to them not only a potential helper or sexual object, but also a temptation to
them to gratify their aggressiveness on him, to exploit his capacity for work
without recompense, to use him sexually without his consent, to seize his
possessions, to humiliate him, to cause him pain, to torture and to kill him.
Homo homini lupus.[2]
—FREUD (1930, p. 85)

In his annotations to Freud's writings, Peter Gay (1989) says of the wolf metaphor: "This harsh saying evokes the tough-minded, realistic political thought of Thomas Hobbes, with which Freud's ideas are often contingent" (p. 749). Certainly no one would mistake this saying as representative of the communal tradition in Western political philosophy, and Greenberg and Mitchell (1983) have also depicted that Freud's drive/structural model as a prototype of agentic philosophy. In that model, the *individual* psychic apparatus is the basic unit of study, and the dynamics are provided by primitive sexual and aggressive instincts striving for expression against the constraints of society. Negative liberty protects individuals from their neighbors, but prevents them from expressing their most basic desires in other than disguised or symptomatic forms.

The Relations/Structural Model

No great progress in this field of study can be made until it is realized that the
field of observation is what people do with each other, what they can
communicate to each other about what they do with each other. When that is
done, no such thing as the durable, unique, individual personality is ever clearly
justified. For all I know every human being has as many personalities as he has

---

[2] "Man is a wolf to man."

interpersonal relations; and as a great many of our relations are actual
operations with imaginary people—that is, in-no-sense-materially-embodied
people—and as they may have the same or greater validity and importance in
life as have our operations with materially-embodied people like the clerks in the
corner store, you can see that even though "the illusion of personal
individuality" sounds quite lunatic when first heard, there is at least food for
thought in it.

—SULLIVAN (1950, pp. 220–221)

Sullivan's exclusive emphasis upon interpersonal relations posed a radical
alternative to the drive/structural model. He subscribed to the biological
principle of communal existence (Eldridge, 1925), according to which "the
living cannot live when separated from what might be described as their
necessary environment" (Sullivan, 1953b, p. 31)—and, for Sullivan, the
necessary environment for humans must include *culture*. The positive liberty provided by culture permits the satisfaction of communal needs that
cannot be fulfilled in isolation from others.

Incommensurability of the Two Models

Like the differing agentic and communal assumptions in Western political
philosophies, the drive/structure and relations/structure models are, in
Greenberg and Mitchell's view, based on fundamentally incompatible
claims. As a consequence, mixed models within the psychodynamic paradigm (e.g., Kohut, 1977; Sandler, 1981) are "unstable, at times contrived"
(Greenberg & Mitchell, 1983, p. 380). It is at this point that Greenberg and
Mitchell's view appears to diverge from Bakan's (1966) interpretation of
the paradox of agency and communion. As indicated earlier, the most fruitful interpretation of the structure of agency and communion has been that
of two orthogonal dimensions (i.e., dimensions that can appear in all possible combinations). That the metaconcepts of both agency and communion
can be consistently incorporated within the psychodynamic paradigm is evident in the more recent theorizing of Sidney Blatt, whose concepts of "interpersonal relatedness" (communion) and "self-definition" (agency) have
clear implications for personality development, psychopathology, psychotherapy, and the dynamics of depression (Blatt, 1990; Blatt & Blass, 1992;
Blatt & Zuroff, 1992). Furthermore, by incorporating Sullivan's (1953b)
neglected "chumship" stage of development within Erikson's (1950) psychosocial theory, Blatt and Blass (1996) have illuminated the developmental origins of attachment, as well as those of self-identity.

THE INTERPERSONAL PARADIGM

In Chapter 2, I have outlined the argument that Bakan's (1966) metaconcepts of agency and communion should serve as the conceptual coordi-

nates for the understanding and measurement of interpersonal behavior (see also Wiggins, 1991). In so doing, I have stressed the centrality of these metaconcepts to closely allied disciplines within the social and behavioral sciences, as well as the manner in which Sullivan's (1953b) concepts of self-esteem (agency) and security (communion) provided the basis for their subsequent representation as orthogonal dimensions of the interpersonal circumplex. This argument is to some extent at variance with Greenberg and Mitchell's (1983) dichotomous distinction between the drive/structure model of Freud and the relations/structure model of Sullivan. Although it is certainly true that this dichotomy reflects the differing *emphases* of the two models in their original forms, it is a less than accurate representation of subsequent developments within the two paradigms. Within the later psychodynamic paradigm, Blatt's (1990) communal concept of interpersonal relatedness is granted equal status with the agentic concept of self-definition. And within the original interpersonal paradigm itself, agentic concepts can be discerned.

In his brilliant although occasionally opaque writing style, Sullivan was inclined to exaggerate his own position in order to emphasize the lack of a communal perspective in the psychoanalytic thought of his time. A case in point is Sullivan's notion of "the illusion of personal individuality," for which he was widely criticized.

> This criticism, we believe, is based on a misreading of Sullivan's statements regarding "individuality" and a failure to differentiate between his concept of the self, which is explicitly narcissistic and conformistic, and his characterization of the rest of the personality, which contains many constructive, unique, and authentic features. (Greenberg & Mitchell, 1983, p. 113)

In fact, Sullivan's view of differentiated individuality (agency) is not dissimilar to Allport's (1937) later view; Sullivan (1936) described "the real unique individuality of each psychobiological organism—an individuality that must always escape the methods of science" (p. 16).

THE PERSONOLOGICAL PARADIGM

A review of milestones in the historical development of case studies and psychobiographies in Chapter 3 makes it clear that various theoretical orientations have been applied to the study of lives. These include the psychodynamic (Erikson, 1969; Freud, 1905, 1910; Jones, 1910), the personological (Allport, 1965; McClelland, 1951; Murray, 1938), and the interpersonal (Alexander, 1990). There are of course no limits to the theoretical orientations that may be brought to bear on the study of a life (Runyan, 1982), and some psychobiographers prefer to select the theory that best fits the facts of the subject of their psychobiography (e.g., Elms, 1994). In more recent times, however, there is evidence for a convergence—not upon a single theory, but upon the metaconcepts of agency and communion as an organizing framework for the study of lives.

The most significant advances in Murray's (1938) personology occurred on both empirical and conceptual fronts. Murray's concept of the need for achievement was elaborated and operationalized in an extraordinary series of studies by McClelland and Atkinson (e.g., Atkinson, 1958; McClelland, 1961; McClelland, Atkinson, Clark, & Lowell, 1953). In an innovative application of Murray's Thematic Apperception Test (TAT), McClelland and colleagues (1953) devised reliable scoring categories for achievement motivation. Subsequently, Winter (1973) developed TAT scoring categories for power motivation, and McAdams (1980, 1989) developed a thematic coding system for intimacy motivation.

The concepts of power (agency) and intimacy (communion) are central to McAdams's (1985a, 1985b, 1989, 1993) approach to the study of lives. As suggested in Chapter 3, McAdams is perhaps the most influential theorist within the personological paradigm today. His explicit operationalization of the metaconcepts of Bakan may be taken as evidence of the increased recognition of their importance to this paradigm. Moreover, McAdams (1985a) is particularly clear on the metatheoretical nature of these concepts:

> This is not to say, however, that intimacy motivation *is* communion or that power motivation *is* agency. Bakan's constructs are much broader, encompassing a host of personality variables at a number of different levels of analysis. Thus, communion and agency are highly general thematic clusterings in lives which may be mirrored in conscious values, specific attitudes, particular interests, stylistic traits, characteristic self-schemata and social motives such as intimacy and power. (p. 89; emphasis in original)

The generalizability of coded themes of agency and communion in life stories to other conceptually appropriate measures was demonstrated in a study employing more than 300 community adults and college students (McAdams, Hoffman, Mansfield, & Day, 1996). In this study, the four agentic themes of self-mastery, status, achievement/responsibility, and empowerment in life stories were found to be positively associated with TAT measures of achievement and power motivation, self-report scales of dominance and achievement, and personal strivings concerning being successful and feeling strong. The four communal themes of love/friendship, dialogue, care/help, and community were positively associated with intimacy motivation, needs for affiliation and nurturance, and personal strivings concerned with warm and close relationships.

I have also emphasized in Chapter 3 that Nasby and Read's (1997a,

1997b) case study of Dodge Morgan is a recent milestone in the historical development of the personological paradigm, and that it is likely to have a solidifying effect on that paradigm. In this study, McAdams's life story model (with its conceptual underpinnings of agency and communion) was contrasted with the five-factor model (FFM) of personality from the multivariate tradition, in order to evaluate the relative utilities of these two conceptual frameworks. As will become evident in the next section, these two paradigms may be thought of as sharing common metatheoretical coordinates.

THE MULTIVARIATE PARADIGM

Conceptual convergences between the FFM of the multivariate paradigm and the circumplex model of the interpersonal paradigm have been increasingly noted in recent times. That the first two factors of the FFM (Surgency/Extraversion and Agreeableness) are rotational variants of the two coordinates of the interpersonal circumplex (dominance and nurturance) is generally agreed upon (e.g., McCrae & Costa, 1989; Trapnell & Wiggins, 1990). We (Wiggins & Trapnell, 1996) have taken a more radical position on this convergence, granting conceptual priority to the first two factors of the FFM on the grounds of their relative purity as lower-order indicants of the metaconcepts of agency and communion. In our view, the remaining three dimensions of the FFM (Conscientiousness, Emotional Stability, and Openness/Intellect) are dimensions that facilitate the development and maintenance of agentic and communal enterprises within a social group. It was not our intention to minimize the importance of the remaining three factors of the FFM; instead, we proposed that these factors be interpreted within the broader context of the two basic dimensions of social experience. A similar line of reasoning was presented by Digman (1997):

> Are these factors "basic," as Costa and McCrae (1992) have contended? That is, are they *the* fundamental trait dimensions, with nothing beyond them other than evaluation (Goldberg, 1993)? One might also ask, where in this system is there a place for the grand theories of the past—for example, the theories of personal growth, social interest, attachment, and the struggles between instinctual impulse and conscience? (p. 1246; emphasis in original)

Digman proposed that the five orthogonal factors of the FFM be subjected to higher-order factor analysis, on the grounds that it is "at this abstract level of conceptual organization that links with theoretical accounts of the 'why' of personality may be found" (p. 1246). For Digman, higher-order factor analysis of the FFM involved factoring the intercorrelations among the five factors, using multivariate procedures for which there is considerable historical precedence (e.g., Cattell, 1945; Thurstone, 1934). Digman factored the correlations among the five factors of the FFM in 14 diverse samples, which included teacher's ratings of children and early adolecents, self-ratings by adults, and peer ratings of adults. A consistent *two-factor* solution was found in all samples.

The first factor was consistently loaded by Agreeableness, Emotional Stability, and Conscientiousness; it was interpreted as being related to theories of *socialization*, in which impulse restraint and conscientiousness, and the reduction of hostility, aggression, and neurotic defense, facilitate the development of a sense of community. The second factor was consistently loaded by Extraversion and Openness/Intellect; it was interpreted as being related to theories of *personal growth*, in which, as Rogers (1961) put it, "the organism has one basic tendency and striving—to actualize, maintain, and enhance the experiencing organism" (p. 487). Most important, Digman (1997) recognized that theories of *both* agency and communion (such as those proposed by Bakan, 1966; McAdams, 1985b; and Wiggins, 1991) "appear to have addressed both of these abstractions" (p. 1250).

Digman's findings do not suggest that the dimensions of the FFM can be "reduced" to the dominance and nurturance dimensions of the interpersonal circumplex. Nor do they suggest that the two circumplex dimensions capture the full spectrum of important individual differences that characterize human transactions. What they do suggest, however, is that the metaconcepts of agency and communion are manifested in both the circumplex and the FFM, and that they may serve to clarify the nature of the conceptual convergences between these two models.

THE EMPIRICAL PARADIGM

As discussed in Chapter 5, the empirical paradigm, which has been primarily focused on the MMPI, has shifted over time from typological categories to continuous trait dimensions; from discriminative validity of differential diagnoses to the construct validity of scales and profiles; and from denigration of self-reports to the canonization of item content (Ben-Porath, 1994). It was also noted that because of its durability and prominence, the MMPI came to be associated with various contentious issues of the times, such as the question of "response styles" (Jackson & Messick, 1958; Wiggins, 1962). This prolonged controversy focused attention on the "content" of the MMPI clinical scales, and particularly on the manner in which clients *respond* to such content—topics that had heretofore not been of great interest to those working within the empirical paradigm. Ironically, it was just such considerations that, after 40 years, suggested the roles of agency and communion within the empirical paradigm.

Within the psychodynamic paradigm, ego defenses have come to be viewed as "styles" representing fundamental components of character (e.g., Shapiro, 1965). In contrast, workers within the empirical paradigm have generally relegated the notion of defense to the status of an "error" in the self-reporting of symptoms. But efforts to measure and "correct" for defensiveness within the empirical paradigm have, after many years, eventuated in alternative theories of defensiveness that have suggested substantive parallels between these two (and the other) paradigms.

Social Desirability, Acquiescence, and the Factor Structure of the MMPI

Factor-analytic studies of the MMPI clinical scales have consistently revealed two large factors, which have been given a variety of interpretive labels. For example, Wheeler, Little, and Lehner (1951) interpreted the first factor as Psychotic (highest loadings on *Sc* and *Pt*, negative loading on *K*) and the second factor as Neurotic (highest loadings on *Hy*, *Hs*, and *D*). Welsh (1956) subsequently developed a set of marker scales for these factors, which he labeled *A* (Anxiety) and *R* (Repression), and these scales have been useful in identifying the original MMPI factors when additional scales are included in a factor analysis.

To the extent that the items in a given MMPI scale are rated by groups of judges as being clearly very high or very low in social desirability, respondents are likely to answer these items in such a manner as to create a favorable (or unfavorable) impression, rather than responding to the "content" of the items (Edwards, 1957). To the extent that the majority of items in a given scale are keyed in the same direction (e.g., "true"), respondents with tendencies to "acquiesce" or agree with most items will achieve high scores on that scale (Jackson & Messick, 1961). A number of scales have been developed that purport to measure respondents' tendencies to respond in a socially desirable direction, to acquiesce in their responses, or to exhibit a variety of other "response styles" (Wiggins, 1962). In general, the response style of social desirability has been associated with the first factor of the MMPI (Edwards & Heathers, 1962), and the response style of acquiescence has been associated with the second factor (e.g., Jackson & Messick, 1961).

Ego Resiliency and Ego Control

In a classic critique of response style formulations, Block (1965) presented a series of both logical and empirical arguments that cast serious doubt on the validity of both social desirability and acquiescence interpretations of the first two factors of the MMPI. His logical arguments were psychometric in nature and were based on manipulations of the item characteristics of social desirability and acquiescence. His empirical arguments were based on the results of five previous assessment studies, in which staff Q-sort behavior ratings were available for participants who had been administered the MMPI. The striking results of these investigations led Block to reject the social desirability and acquiescence interpretations of the first two factors of the MMPI, and to propose instead a substantive interpretation based on the constructs of "ego resiliency" and "ego control" (Block, 1971; Block & Block, 1979).

Ego Resiliency

"The word, resilient, implies the resourcefulness, adaptability, and engagement with his world that characterizes the individual placed high on this continuum. . . . [It] is intended to denote the individual's characteristic adaptation capability when under the strain set by new environmental demands" (Block, 1965, p. 112). In addition to a measure of Ego Resiliency, the other special scales that loaded on the first factor of the MMPI in Block's study were Ego Strength (*Es*; Barron, 1953a), Intellectual Efficiency (*Ie*; Gough, 1957), Leadership (*Lp*; Oettel, 1953), and Dominance (*Do*; Gough, McClosky, & Meehl, 1951).

Ego Control

"The construct of ego-control relates to the individual's characteristic mode of monitoring impulse. . . . [The individual] delays gratification even when pleasure is a sensible course of action, not threatening of long range intents" (Block, 1965, p. 115). In addition to a measure of Ego Control, the other special scales that loaded on the second factor of the MMPI were Social Participation (*Sp;* Gough, 1952) and Social Status (*St*; Gough, 1948).

Despite Block's impressive defense of a substantive basis for interpreting the first two factors of the MMPI, it should be emphasized that the other MMPI scales involved, as well as Block's Ego Resiliency and Ego Control measures themselves, "are susceptible to deliberate feigning attempts or to tendencies to deny—for reasons of which the responding individual may be unaware—actually existing personal frailties" (Block, 1965, p. 112). In other words, Block's analyses were not meant to discredit the general idea of defensiveness in self-report; they were meant to demonstrate that there is much more to the two major factors of the MMPI than "merely" defensiveness.

Measuring Social Desirability Response Style

Edwards's (1957) Social Desirability (*SD*) scale was the first of a number of scales developed from the MMPI item pool to measure respondents' tendencies to give socially desirable responses to statements in personality inventories. This scale consisted of a set of MMPI items that were presumably heterogeneous in content and for which judges were in complete agreement regarding the socially desirable response to each item (e.g., a "true" response to "I am liked by most people I know"). The *SD* scale has been shown to be highly correlated with the first factor of the MMPI and with the clinical scales that load on this factor (e.g., Edwards & Heathers, 1962).

In an early paper, I (Wiggins, 1959) took issue with the implication that the *SD* scale provided a means of detecting respondents who were attempting to foster a good impression. In keeping with the empirical tradition, I developed an alternative measure of Social Desirability Responding (*Sd*) by contrasting the item responses of college students who were explicitly instructed to indicate the desirable response for each item of the MMPI with the item responses of students who took the MMPI under standard instructions. On replication, the *Sd* scale was found to be considerably more effective than Edwards's *SD* scale in discriminating "socially desirable" respondents given instructions to make a favorable impression from respondents given standard instructions (e.g., Skrzypek & Wiggins, 1966). And, in fact, the *Sd* scale is still considered by some to be useful for identifying socially desirable self-presentation in clinical populations (e.g., Baer, Wetter, & Berry, 1992; Caldwell, 1997).

Alpha and Gamma Factors in Self-Deception

Early Studies

In an attempt to establish the contribution of response style measures to the structure of the MMPI, I (Wiggins, 1964) factor-analyzed the intercorrelations among 30 measures of stylistic response tendencies from a variety of instruments, along with Welsh's factor markers for the MMPI (*A* and *R*). Three of the six factors obtained had previously been identified within the MMPI. Using the neutral designations suggested by Block (1962), I labeled the three MMPI factors Alpha, Beta, and Gamma. Factor Alpha was marked by Welsh's *A* and Edwards's *SD* scales, and was loaded by additional measures of social desirability. Factor Beta was marked by Welsh's *R* scale, and was loaded by measures of both acquiescence and desirability. The heretofore unidentified Factor Gamma was loaded by the Wiggins *Sd* scale; an earlier Malingering (*Mp*) scale developed by the method of contrasted groups (Cofer, Chance, & Judson, 1949); the MMPI *L* scale; and a stylistic measure of "approval motivation" (*MC-SDS*; Crowne & Marlowe, 1960). This finding was later replicated by Nichols and Greene (1988) in 11 noncollege samples where the full MMPI was administered: Factor Alpha was best marked by Edwards's *SD* scale, with loadings averaging .91

across samples; and Factor Gamma was best marked by the Wiggins *Sd* and the Cofer and colleagues *Mp* scale, with average loadings of *.92* and *.85*, respectively.

The Paulhus Studies

In an elegant series of interlocking experimental and psychometric studies conducted over almost 20 years, Delroy Paulhus has brought conceptual clarity to the roles of Alpha and Gamma as components of socially desirable responding within the MMPI (see Paulhus, 2002); he has shown how each component is a combination of stylistic and content variance. In line with Sackheim and Gur's (1978) distinction between conscious and unconscious defenses, Paulhus (1984) developed a Self-Deceptive Enhancement scale (Alpha) and an Impression Management scale (Gamma), which were refined in several revisions (Paulhus, 1988, 1998b). The Self-Deceptive Enhancement scale was found to be associated with unconsciously motivated distortion (e.g., Hoorens, 1995; Paulhus, 1998b) and to involve agentic content (e.g., Bonanno, Siddique, Keltner, & Horowitz, 1997; Paulhus, 1998a). In contrast, the Impression Management scale was found to be more sensitive to situational demands (e.g., public vs. anonymous administration) and to involve communal content (e.g., Paulhus, 1988). Furthermore, the Self-Deceptive Enhancement scale was found be related to the Extraversion and Openness dimensions of the FFM, while the Impression Management scale was related to Agreeableness and Conscientiousness (Meston, Heiman, Trapnell, & Paulhus, 1998). Of even greater significance was the finding that the Self-Deceptive Enhancement and Impression Management scales were related to Block's measures of Ego Resiliency and Ego Control, respectively.

Alpha as Agency, and Gamma as Communion

The literature on personality traits and defense mechanisms suggests individual differences in two self-favoring tendencies, we label *egoistic bias* and *moralistic bias*. The two biases are self-deceptive in nature and can be traced to two fundamental values, agency and communion, that impel two corresponding motives, [need for power and need for approval]. The two sequences of values, motives, and biases form two personality constellations, *Alpha* and *Gamma*.
—PAULHUS AND JOHN (1998, p. 1025; emphasis in original)

In an exceptionally integrative conceptual formulation, Paulhus and John (1998) have consolidated evidence from all five paradigms of personality assessment to underscore their argument that agency and communion are the two sets of cultural values promoting "the socialization of two sets of value consistent traits" (p. 1039). As can be seen from Table 6.2, they identified the self-deceptive mechanisms which had their origin in the psychody-

TABLE 6.2. Constellations of Alpha and Gamma

	Value	Motive	Self-deceptive mechanisms	Self-favoring bias on
Alpha	Agency	Need for power	Egoistic bias	Extraversion/Openness
Gamma	Communion	Need for approval	Moralistic bias	Agreeableness/Conscientiousness

Note. Adapted from Paulhus and John (1998, p. 1041). Copyright 1998 by Blackwell Publishers. Adapted by permission.

namic paradigm (egoistic and moralistic); emphasized the two corresponding motives of the personological paradigm (need for power and need for approval); made reference to the metaconceptual basis of the interpersonal paradigm (agency and communion); and identified their manifestations in the multivariate paradigm (Extraversion/Openness and Agreeableness/Conscientiousness). All of this was accomplished with Alpha and Gamma scales from the empirical paradigm (Ego Resiliency and Ego Control).

INFLUENCE OF A SINGLE THEORIST ACROSS PARADIGMS

Although the historical taxonomy provided in Table Int.3 in the Introduction may have served as a useful basis for comparison of the development of different traditions within personality assessment, an emphasis upon the columns of the table does not do justice to the mutual influences and overlaps among the traditions that have occurred over time. As mentioned earlier, study of the literatures represented by rows would facilitate the kind of "historical perspective taking" advocated by Craik (1986). Moreover, the columns of Table Int.3 would add a more explicit conceptual framework to Craik's classic taxonomy of personality research methods. A concomitant emphasis upon *theorists* would reveal the influence of certain individuals upon several personality assessment paradigms, the most outstanding of whom was unquestionably Henry A. Murray.

Murray was an outspoken advocate of psychodynamic psychology at Harvard during a time when that perspective "had virtually no impact on academic psychology" (Anderson, 1988, p. 151). As such, he must be counted among the earliest contributors to the psychodynamic paradigm in personality assessment, in addition to being the founder of the closely related personological paradigm. His most obvious link to the psychodynamic tradition was through the development of the TAT (C. D. Morgan & Murray, 1935), in collaboration with others and apparently with some input from Robert Holt and David Rapaport (W. G. Morgan, 1995).

Murray's "multiform organismic system of assessment" (Office of Strategic Services [OSS] Assessment Staff, 1948, p. 28) included a broad array of assessment techniques that were interpreted by an extraordinarily diverse and talented group of assessors. In the Harvard study (Murray, 1938), for example, one finds the Rorschach test interpreted by Samuel J. Beck (pp. 687–689) and psychoanalytic interpretations of a dramatic productions test presented by Erik Homberger Erikson (pp. 522–582). The Institute of Personality Assessment and Research was founded after World War II by former OSS psychologists in order to continue Murray's multiform assessment tradition within a framework that placed heavy emphasis upon the empirical paradigm of personality assessment (Wiggins, 1973b, pp. 539–553).

The influence of Murray's taxonomy of human needs upon the multivariate paradigm cannot be overstated. Although Murray (1938) himself was less than sanguine about the prospects of personality questionnaires (p. 439), he provided 10–20 questionnaire items for each of his need variables (pp. 153–226) and established clusters or "syndromes" of the variables by correlational analysis. Unfortunately, "the chapter on the intercorrelations of variables and syndromes had to be omitted from this volume" (p. 30), and 15 years elapsed before the Murray needs entered the multivariate tradition through the work of Edwards (1953). From Goldberg's (1971) historical survey of personality scales and inventories, it is evident that the subsequent impact of the Murray need variables upon the multivariate tradition was considerable—both directly (e.g., Gough & Heilbrun, 1965; Jackson, 1967; Stern, 1970) and indirectly (e.g., Guilford, Christensen, & Bond, 1954). In more recent times, the structure of the Murray need scales from Jackson's (1974) Personality Research Form has been related to the FFM of the multivariate tradition (Costa & McCrae, 1988).

Murray's taxonomy of needs also influenced the development of the interpersonal paradigm (LaForge, 1985). A colleague and I (Wiggins & Broughton, 1985) have observed that on a conceptual level, "it is not difficult to find the seeds of an interpersonal, social exchange formulation in Murray's (1938) writings" (p. 5). Moreover, the variables of most interpersonal circumplex systems may be related directly to corresponding Murray needs. For example, the variables of the Wiggins (1979) circumplex correspond to Murray's needs for dominance (PA), aggression (BC), autonomy (DE), rejection (FG), infavoidance (HI), deference (JK), nurturance (LM), and affiliation (NO). With slight modifications, we (Wiggins & Broughton, 1985) were able to construct circumplex structures for selected Murray need scales from Stern's (1958) Activities Index, Campbell's Need Scales, Edwards's (1953) Personal Preference Schedule, Gough and Heilbrun's (1965) Adjective Check List, and Jackson's (1967) Personality Research Form.

For an individual who had no formal training in psychology and whose theory of personality was (as noted earlier), decidedly lacking in explicitness, it is difficult to understand why Henry Murray had a greater influence on *all* paradigms of personality assessment than did any other individual (including Freud). Perhaps the answer lies somewhere within Robinson's (1992) detailed psychobiography of one of our great psychobiographers.

PART II

A COLLABORATIVE CASE STUDY

ORGANIZATION AND DESIGN OF THE STUDY

The idea for this study arose in the course of innumerable conversations I have had with Krista Trobst in the course of writing this book. As should be evident in the book, I am a great fan of each of the five paradigms, and I believe that each of them can make unique contributions to the study of lives. To demonstrate this in a concrete way, however, required an extensive case study of a single individual who was assessed by procedures that are truly representative of each of the five paradigms. Our subject, whom we will call "Madeline G," is seen by her associates as quite a "character" and as having a great deal of "personality." More technically, Madeline is highly outgoing, a bit narcissistic, and open to all kinds of experiences. She saw this research as a highly interesting adventure and a potential learning experience. As such, she appeared to be an excellent subject for a collaborative case study, and indeed she was.

It should also be noted at the outset that some identifying details (which would not affect the interpretations) have been changed, including the name of the subject. Madeline was given an opportunity to select the name to be used here, and her first response was "Pussy Galore." Needless to say, she was asked to select another name. Her eventual choice was "Madeline G," with "G" retaining her earlier reference to "Galore."

209

THE ASSESSORS

To ensure that assessment procedures would be truly representative of each of the paradigms, I simply contacted the individuals whom I knew and whom I considered to be among the best in the business for each paradigm. Gratifyingly, no one turned me down. I explained the ground rules of the project to potential assessors in very clear, albeit slightly vulgar, terms: "This is not a pissing contest." I firmly believed that each of the five paradigms would make valuable and unique contributions to our understanding of the subject, and in that context, it is inappropriate to argue that one paradigm is "better" than another. Sidney Blatt has described my approach to assessment as "ecumenical," and I think that some of the other assessors would concur with this description. In any event, my success in enlisting an extraordinarily talented group of assessors for this study can be seen in Table II.1.

PROCEDURES

Testing within the psychodynamic paradigm (the Rorschach, the Wechsler Adult Intelligence Scale—Third Edition [WAIS-III], and the Thematic Apperception Test [TAT]) and the personological paradigm (the Life Story Interview) required face-to-face contact with the subject. Krista Trobst handled the daunting task of coordinating the travel schedule for our subject, which took her from Albuquerque, New Mexico, to New Haven, Connecticut; then to Evanston, Illinois; and back to Albuquerque—all during the height of the holiday air travel season in December 1999. This was a busy time of year for both the assessors and the subject, and the net result was a schedule involving long hours in airports, delayed flights, and lost luggage—all of which were taken in stride by our resilient subject. The first indication that this project might be a successful one came in an e-mail from Dan McAdams on December 22, 1999. In response to my suggestion that I thought the project a good idea, he replied: "Well, I do think it is a great idea. Part of the greatness of the idea is in the choice of subject. Madeline is amazing . . . I could write a book on this woman. (Maybe I will!)"

That kind of response from the "dean of life stories" was most encouraging, as was the report from our distinguished assessors in New Haven that our subject's projective test protocols were "highly interesting." And, later, an unsolicited message from Yossef Ben-Porath on March 7, 2000, relieved my concerns that the Minnesota Multiphasic Personality Inventory—2 (MMPI-2) might be at a disadvantage in characterizing a "normal" subject rather than a patient: "A very interesting mult, with lots to chew on!" ("Mult" is "MMPI slang" for Minnesota *Mult*iphasic Personality Inventory.)

Informed consent forms were signed by Madeline and her common-

TABLE II.1. Overview of the Collaborative Case Study

Paradigm	Instruments	Assessors	Affiliations
Psychodynamic	Rorschach; Wechsler Adult Intelligence Scale— Third Edition (WAIS-III); Thematic Apperception Test (TAT); Object Relations Inventory (ORI)	Rebecca S. Behrends Sidney J. Blatt	Yale University Yale University
Interpersonal	Interpersonal Adjective Scales (IAS); Inventory of Interpersonal Problems— Circumplex (IIP-C)	Aaron L. Pincus Michael B. Gurtman	Penn State University University of Wisconsin–Parkside
Personological	Life Story Interview; Big Five Inventory (BFI); Loyola Generativity Scale (LGS); Personal Strivings; Satisfaction with Life Scale; research version of TAT	Dan P. McAdams	Northwestern University
Multivariate	Revised NEO Personality Inventory (NEO PI-R)	Paul T. Costa, Jr. Ralph L. Piedmont	National Institute on Aging Loyola College, Maryland
Empirical	Minnesota Multiphasic Personality Inventory—2 (MMPI-2)	Yossef S. Ben-Porath	Kent State University

law husband. I mailed copies of the Interpersonal Adjective Scales, the Inventory of Interpersonal Problems—Circumplex, the Revised NEO Personality Inventory, and the MMPI 2 to our subject, who had arranged for specific times to take these tests in a quiet office. All of these tests (with the exception of the MMPI-2) were also mailed to the office of the subject's partner, who filled them out independently. The completed test forms were returned to me, and I, in turn, mailed them to the appropriate assessors. With one pair of exceptions, each assessor was provided with a copy of McAdams's report on the subject (see Chapter 7).[1] McAdams's report provided both a context and a general format of reporting that was employed by most of the assessors.

---

[1] Rebecca Behrends and Sidney Blatt preferred to do a "blind analysis" of our subject's Rorschach and TAT test results. Blatt believes that the best way to demonstrate the unique potential of the Rorschach is to present the results of a "blind analysis." Hence their analysis was done in the absence of McAdams's report.

7

Personological Assessment
The Life Story of Madeline G

DAN P. MCADAMS

ASSESSMENT METHODS AND RATIONALE

On December 21, 1999, I interviewed "Madeline G" for a project developed by Jerry Wiggins and Krista Trobst, wherein different experts in personality assessment would interpret the same person's life and personality. Madeline agreed to be the subject for this project. I met with her for a little over 3 hours. She read and signed a standard research consent form, which explained that her participation in the project was voluntary and that the data she provided would be confidential. She also completed a short demographic form; the 44-item Big Five Inventory (BFI; John & Srivastava, 1999); the 20-item Loyola Generativity Scale (LGS; McAdams & de St. Aubin, 1992); a shortened (10-item) version of Emmons's (1986) assessment of personal strivings; the 5-item Satisfaction with Life Scale (Diener, Emmons, Larson, & Griffin, 1985); and a research version of the Thematic Apperception Test (TAT), in which she told imaginative stories in response to five picture cues. I then interviewed Madeline according to the Life Story Interview protocol that I have used in past research (e.g., McAdams, 1993). The interview asks the subject to provide an outline of the main "chapters" in his or her life story; to describe in detail at least eight key scenes in the story (such as a high point, low point, turning point, and earliest memory); to explain what the subject sees as the central life challenge in the story; to identify the best and worst characters in the story; to imagine what the

213

future chapters of the story will bring; to describe some basic values and beliefs exemplified in the story (especially in the realm of religion and politics); and finally to identify the story's central theme or message. The interview typically requires about 2 hours to complete. In the current case, the interview lasted about 2 hours and 15 minutes.

The purpose of the Life Story Interview is to obtain an account of how the subject makes narrative sense of his or her life in the overall. According to my life story model of identity, the significance of this account is that it gives some indication of the contours of a person's identity. Both others and I have argued that adults provide their lives with a sense of unity and purpose—what Erik Erikson (1963) called an "identity"—by constructing internalized and evolving life narratives, complete with settings, scenes, characters, plots, and themes. Identity, then, is an internalized and dynamic narrative of the self that contains reconstructions of the past and imaginative anticipations of the future. The story is not a purely objective account of what has happened. But it is not a purely fictionalized fantasy, either. Containing elements of both fact and fancy, life stories are psychosocial constructions that serve to integrate a person's understandings of self— often by reflecting particular narrative forms and themes prevalent in the culture, wherein the person's life is made and made sense of. Consequently, the main purpose of the Life Story Interview is not to determine exactly what has happened in a person's life (as might be the central aim in, say, a "life history" approach). In the life story approach, the focus is less on what really happened in the past than on how the subject today conceives of the past and imagines the future. Nonetheless, my colleagues and I assume that the subject is not making it all up out of thin air. In that our research procedures aim to win our subjects' trust and to encourage candor, we make the assumption that subjects believe their stories to be true in some sense, and that the general outlines of what they select and describe for us correspond roughly to real events and people that have been or continue to be part of the subjects' lives.

Consequently, the interview can be used in different ways by different investigators. For me, the value lies in analyzing recurrent themes and images that reflect an underlying and implicit narrative of the self—a narrative that serves as a person's identity. Therefore, I would typically develop a psycholiterary interpretation of the case, tying it to what we have learned about people's life stories in past research and connecting it to dominant narrative themes in culture. But investigators can also use the interview in a more straightforward manner, as in getting a sense of what a subject thinks are some of the most important events and people in his or her life. In what follows, I use the interview in both of these ways. First, I provide a more or less objective description of the main events and people that Madeline presents in her interview. In essence, I summarize the manifest content of the interview. In the second part of this chapter, I provide my own interpretation of the interview in terms of life story theory, incorporating as well the data obtained from the TAT and the self-report measures.

DESCRIPTIVE SUMMARY

Madeline G is a 35-year-old woman who is employed in Albuquerque, New Mexico, as a defense attorney. She earns over $70,000 annually. She is legally single, but she has been intimately involved with the same man for about 6 years, in what she describes as a "common-law" marriage. Her partner is a college professor. The couple has no children. Madeline is a Native American (a member of the Navaho Indian tribe in North America).

In the interview, Madeline divides her life into three large chapters, which she entitles "Childhood," "Jail," and "The Present." In her account, she begins with "The Present," goes back to her years in jail as an adolescent, describes aspects of childhood, and then flashes forward again to the present. In what follows, however, I will follow a simple chronology.

Madeline describes a harrowing childhood, growing up in a small town in New Mexico. She was one of three children born to a Native American couple—two girls and a boy. But "there were no babies" in this family. "We were born, and they put boots on you and you went to work." The children were never indulged, never allowed to act as children. From a very early age, the children had to work hard around the house, doing cleaning, cooking, and gardening, and assuming many other adult responsibilities. But this is not what she remembers with most bitterness. More pervasive were the lack of any human warmth from the parents, the violence, and the neglect. As Madeline remembers it, both of her parents had serious drinking problems, but her father seems to have been worse. When drunk, he was often violent. He beat all the children regularly; he beat his wife. In one scene, a teacher at school would not let Madeline put on shorts and a T-shirt for gym class because the other children were frightened by her bruised body. In another scene, her father shot his wife with a gun. In a third, her mother and father were fighting in the living room, knocking over a Christmas tree. "There was blood spurting everywhere." Yet, because they were so familiar with violence and bloodshed in the family, the children looked on in a detached and unemotional manner. The brother remarked that the blood was "gross." In yet another gruesome scene, the mother attempted suicide by slashing her wrists. (Some of these incidents are described in more detail below.) The family's neighbors, school officials, and so on were aware of the violence, but they seemed to look the other way. One reason for their refusal to intervene, Madeline surmises, was that her father was a very popular and socially powerful man in the community. He was a very gregarious and friendly man in public; he was a hard worker; he knew many people and knew how to help people when they needed help. For example, if somebody needed a new roof on a house, her father knew whom to call to get the job done for the best price. Many Native American families lived in this region. Many of these families were poor. But even compared to the other poor families, Madeline's family always stood out as different—as more dysfunctional and violent.

Madeline claims she was drinking heavily even as a young child. By third grade, she was taking whiskey to school in a thermos. From an early age, she was wild and incorrigible, seemingly always in trouble with school authorities (even though she liked school), and eventually running afoul of the law. By age 12, she was no longer living at home, though it is not clear exactly where she was. She apparently spent some time in foster homes. Early in her teenage years, she was arrested and incarcerated. She spent a great deal of time in jail during her teenage years. She does not detail her offenses, only saying that "I did everything." Drug abuse and alcoholism were obviously involved, and perhaps theft as well. She appears to have gotten into many physical fights, both in jail and on the streets. But she really does not disclose much about her criminal record. She is more explicit about what happened when she was in jail. Although she was a juvenile, she apparently was incarcerated with older women. Because she brutally beat a woman who was harassing her in jail, Madeline spent some time in solitary confinement. She was stripped naked and hosed down with water. For only 1 hour out of 24, she was led out of her cell so that she could walk around the yard. She spent a lot of time fantasizing about what life might have been like had she lived in a "perfect family," with "a dog and fish and loving friends and nice clothes." At some point in prison, she began to read books. This appears to have been something of a turning point. She became a voracious reader and began to educate herself. In and out of jail for many years, constantly in trouble and out of control, Madeline eventually resolved that she would go straight, that she would "never go back." She says that "after a really bad experience, I just decided I would never go back there again" (i.e., back to jail). To start a new life, she moved out of New Mexico to a prairie state.

Sometime around the age of 21, Madeline moved to "the middle of the prairie," got a job as a waitress, and began renting a little apartment. Like her dad, she proved to be a very hard worker. At some point in her 20s, she married a man, but they soon divorced. The relationship was never strong, she says, and it was based mainly on "good sex." Madeline began to take classes at a community college. She did some tutoring with an older illiterate man, experiencing tremendous joy in teaching him to read. She also met a college teacher who encouraged her to take more classes and to apply to a university. She was admitted to an Ivy League university, and eventually she received advanced degrees in social work and in law. At about the time of her undergraduate graduation (1993), Madeline met the man with whom she is currently romantically involved. She describes him as her "rock"—a solid foundation of support for everything she does. Although Madeline experienced some problems in obtaining a license to practice law (because of her criminal background), she has been spectacularly successful as a lawyer. Mainly she has worked with Native Americans, representing them in both civil and criminal cases. She is especially effective in communicating with jurors. As of January 2000, Madeline is scheduled to begin a new job as a defense lawyer with a prestigious law firm in Albuquerque. Apparently this firm is interested in expanding its base to include criminal defense of Native Americans, perhaps as a kind of pro bono effort.

Key Scenes

What follow are brief synopses of each of the key scenes Madeline identifies in her life story.

High Point

Madeline describes her high point as the day in May 1993 when she received her undergraduate degree. She had a party at her apartment. People from almost all walks of her life ("strippers, musicians, college professors," but not her family) were there. Everybody was having a good time. She felt triumphant. She had come so far, done so much after experiencing so much hardship. In the moment that stood out most clearly, she was standing on a balcony of her apartment looking down at the crowd of friends. "I did it right here, right now, and everybody helped me. I did it, and I'm gonna be okay."

Low Point

Visually, Madeline's low point was parallel to the high point. Again, she was standing up above, at the top of the stairs at home, looking down on the living room. She was perhaps 10 years old. She was walking down the stairs, with a pillow in her hands. She was going to suffocate her father: "I wanted to go into my father's room, to put it over his face, to kill him. I really needed to kill him." But she stopped halfway down, fell to her knees, and began sobbing. She realized she could not do it—not because she felt it was wrong, but because she felt she was not physically strong enough to kill him. She was devastated. She feared she would never get away from her father.

Turning Points

Madeline insists on describing three different events as turning points. The first was meeting a man with whom she fell in love, a few months before she graduated in 1993. But she was not ready to commit to him, and the relationship ended. It was a turning point because she learned how powerful romantic love can be. The second was when she was finally admitted to the bar, after struggling to win confirmation for many years. An older lawyer had sponsored her through this difficult period, and she presented him with an eagle feather as a sign of her gratitude at the confirmation ceremony. (It is this man's law firm in Albuquerque where Madeline will begin her new job in 2000.) The third event was falling in love with her current boyfriend; actually, this was a series of events in which he showed her how much he loves her, and she gradually became convinced that he is the right man for her. She attributes the success of this relationship to his goodness and to luck.

Early Memories

Madeline describes three early memories. In one, her father shot her mother. In another, they were fighting in the living room near the Christmas tree, as the children watched from a hole in the floor above. Her mother stabbed her father with scissors: "She took these scissors, and she stabbed him in the throat, and there's all this, like literally, blood spraying across the room, and I remember looking over at my brother and my brother looking at me going, 'Gross . . .' Then, like, just weird shit like that all the time."

In the third childhood memory, Madeline came home and learned that her mother was gone. Her father wouldn't tell her anything at first, but eventually she learned that her mother was in the hospital, having tried to kill herself by slitting her wrists. A day or two later, Madeline visited her in the hospital. A priest was there. It almost seemed as if the mother was going to die. Madeline had to go to school—"but I asked her if I could kiss her goodbye and she said, 'No.' So, another, that—that's kind of like, that's the capsule childhood memory. That's how close we were. Yeah. That's classic. So that's kind of how close my family was. So, love? Not a whole lot of love."

Adolescent Memory

Madeline's adolescent memory is of having a fight in prison with a fat woman. Madeline won the fight, but got thrown into solitary confinement. They stripped her and hosed her down. "They had just taken, like, a fire hose to me, you know, bang you against the walls and shit. And I'm just, like, sittin' there like a rat." In a remarkable epiphany, she realized she was becoming just like her father.

Adulthood Memory

Madeline recounts an adulthood memory of sitting on top of her car in Kansas just before a storm. She had been drinking a little, doing a little marijuana. She was feeling great. The sky was beautiful. She felt part of nature, exhilarated and inspired.

Greatest Challenge

Madeline describes her greatest life challenge as working hard to become a "better person." When she was a child, her father called her a "pinhead" and "the village idiot." At school, the other children knew she was from a "bad" family. Later, she was always in trouble with the law. Since she left prison, she has worked hard at becoming somebody who is good and who feels good about herself.

Greatest Positive and Negative Characters

The greatest positive character in her story is Madeline's boyfriend. The greatest negative character is her father, by far. He is described as a "fucking monster," among other things. A few years ago, she tried to explain to him why he needed to begin treating her like a human being, showing her some respect and consideration. Since then, he has not spoken to her. She has infrequent and very awkward interactions with her mother, who remains a mystery in this story. The mother appears to say and do little. The main thing she cares about is money, it appears.

Projection for Future Chapters

Madeline's projection for the future chapters of her story is very upbeat. She will be wildly successful at the new law firm. She will have a beautiful apartment in Albuquerque. She will continue her positive relationship with her lover. She will continue to represent members of the aboriginal community. She will develop more friendships. She has quit smoking recently, and she plans to stay nicotine-free. With her boyfriend's support, her new job, and her continued resolve to become a better person, "I can do anything." Only a few storm clouds appear on the horizon for her: What if she doesn't fit in with the blue-blooded lawyers in this establishment law firm? And what if she gets bored with life, or restless? She says that when she gets bored, she gets in trouble.

Basic Values and Beliefs

Madeline's religious/spiritual beliefs are a blend of traditional Indian spiritualism and rugged American individualism. She depends on her own powers, but she also feels connected to nature through her Navaho tribal heritage. She describes this heritage as believing that "there's a spirit in everything that's alive, and you are as important and as connected to that as it is to you, and you're respectful towards it and it's respectful back . . . and it's just understanding, coming to an understanding of where your place is . . . and knowing that all life must be in balance." It is not clear that these beliefs have as much influence on Madeline's private spiritual musings as they do on her professional work, in which her heritage serves her exceedingly well. Mainly, Madeline believes in herself. She sees herself as a positive force in the world, and she seems at times to suggest that she has almost superhuman powers. Politically, Madeline describes herself as a "bleeding-heart liberal," stating that "I will go to the wall" to help the poor, defend the underdog, and so on. These beliefs are translated into action every day in her work defending aboriginal clients. The most important value in living, she says, is trust.

Central Theme

Looking back over her entire life story at the end of the interview, Madeline says that the major theme in her story is "survival." She has survived, and she feels she is beginning to flourish.

INTERPRETATION

A full personological portrait of an individual must begin by addressing three different levels of personality description (McAdams, 1995, 2001). At the first level are dispositional traits, which are broad, decontextualized, and relatively stable dimensions of individual difference, such as Extraversion and Neuroticism in the five-factor model. At the second level are more contextualized and situated concepts, which spell out characteristic motivational, social-cognitive, and developmental adaptations to life challenges. At the third level are the integrative life stories that people construct as the unifying and purpose-giving identities organizing their entire lives. In brief, traits provide a dispositional sketch or outline of human individuality; characteristic adaptations fill in some of the details; and life stories speak to the narrative meanings that a person invokes to make sense of his or her life in time as a dynamic and integrated whole.

At the first level, Madeline's responses on the Big Five Inventory (BFI) suggest very high scores on the traits of Extraversion, Conscientiousness, and Openness to Experience. As is evident upon a first meeting, she is a very assertive, outgoing, and energetic woman (Extraversion). Even on the phone, she comes across as brash, dominant, and high-volume. Her high Openness to Experience becomes evident in the interview as she describes a wide range of experiences and relationships in very vivid and articulate ways. From early childhood, she has rebelled against the conventional norms represented by authorities, even as she now finds herself to be an integral part of the legal system. With respect to almost any reference group one can name, Madeline comes across as an adventurous experience seeker—distrustful of authority, open to new ideas, and eager to learn and know more. Evidence of high Conscientiousness outside the BFI scores is rather more indirect. In the interview, she certainly describes herself as hard-working, and since the time of her resolution to stay out of jail and turn her life around, she has set clear goals for her life and pursued them relentlessly. Yet as she describes it, she had no goals and no discipline as a child and teenager. Empirical evidence suggests that personality traits are relatively stable over the longitudinal life course. It is hard to imagine, however, that Madeline would have scored high on self-report measures of Conscientiousness when she was a child or teenager, but of course we will never know.

At the second level of characteristic adaptations, a more detailed picture begins to emerge. Explicit and implicit human motives are important factors here. Of the 10 personal strivings she has listed, 8 are explicit articulations of power goals. Madeline writes that she is typically striving to "impress other people," "win every argument," and "come in first in whatever I attempt." By contrast, she lists no goals that involve warm, close relationships. If the strivings give a sense of explicit motives, the TAT speaks more to implicit motivational trends in what people want in life. Here the picture gets more complicated. Her stories show high levels of both power motivation and intimacy motivation. Two of the stories suggest tender, romanticized moments of love and friendship. Still, agentic concerns seem to predominate, at the levels of both dispositional traits and characteristic motives. She is an energetic, hard-working, hard-driving, dominant, and outgoing woman who strives to have a large impact on others, to impress people, and to win. Indeed, in her Life Story Interview she boasts that she has won 53 legal cases in a row. At the same time, some communal aspects of personality certainly emerge. At the trait level, Agreeableness is moderate; however, a close look at the BFI items shows that she sees herself as caring and nurturant toward others, but as not especially cooperative and compliant in personal relationships. At the levels of motives and goals, her daily strivings do not seem to be related to warm and close relationships, but her TAT stories do suggest an implicit desire for warm, close, and caring interactions more generally. Put simply, Madeline is not "working on" intimacy goals in her daily life now, but she regards intimacy as an important general motive for her. She has strong needs to care for others, but she is not a nice and compliant do-gooder. She sees herself instead as a strong agent whose care and compassion come out in bold actions and in her valiant and usually victorious efforts to help others in need.

At the third level, we can account for Madeline's individuality from the perspective of the main themes and images in her self-defining life story. The Life Story Interview is merely a rough-and-ready tool for sampling aspects of Madeline's narrative identity. The interview gets at only pieces of a larger story, or set of stories, that Madeline is carrying around with her, implicit and evolving over time. Consistent with our analysis at the first two levels of traits and motives/goals, Madeline's life story contains a strong agentic theme. Many of the scenes she describes deal with the four main agentic themes identified in life stories—self-mastery, victory/status, achievement/responsibility, and empowerment (McAdams, Hoffman, Mansfield, & Day, 1996). Communal themes appear now and again as well, especially the theme of caring/help. The protagonist in this story eventually emerges in the third chapter, after childhood and prison, as a powerful agent who is capable of doing good things for others. As Madeline suggests, the fact that the protagonist even survived the harrowing experiences in the first two chapters speaks to her impressive agency.

Madeline's score on the Loyola Generativity Scale (LGS) is a 57 out of a possible 60. The mean score on this measure for adults in their mid-30s is about 41. Her score is at least two standard deviations above the mean; indeed, it is one of the highest scores we have ever obtained in our research. The LGS assesses individual differences in what Erik Erikson (1963) described as the central developmental task of middle adulthood—generativity. "Generativity" is the commitment to caring for and promoting the well-being of the next generation through such behaviors as parenting, mentoring, leadership, and a host of other activities and involvements aimed at leaving a positive legacy of the self for the future. In terms of the three-part model of personality I have described, generativity may be seen as a second-level construct—a characteristic adaptation linked to developmental concerns.

More importantly, though, research has shown that highly generative adults tend to construct certain kinds of life stories (McAdams, Diamond, de St. Aubin, & Mansfield, 1997). In particular, their stories tend to be structured as "commitment narratives." In a commitment narrative, the protagonist (1) experiences an early advantage or blessing, (2) witnesses the suffering of others at an early age, (3) establishes a set of clear values and beliefs in adolescence that continue to guide behavior over time, (4) redeems bad events into good outcomes, and (5) sets prosocial goals for the future. With one exception, Madeline's life story follows this format. At an early age, the protagonist witnessed a tremendous amount of suffering that was experienced by other people; indeed, she experienced it too. Once she left prison for good, she self-consciously articulated a set of values and beliefs according to which she would now live. She has remained steadfast in those beliefs, as they have also grown to encompass her Navaho Indian heritage and her liberal political outlook. The story is filled with "redemptive sequences," wherein bad events eventually yield good outcomes. Indeed, Madeline signals early in her account that hers is a redemptive story to tell: "All kinds of interesting things are happening now, born out of real shit."

In a redemptive sequence, bad events are eventually redeemed by good out-comes. For Madeline the "shit" happened early, but out of all that negativity she has emerged stronger, better, happy, and free. The story con-tains many redemptive moments. But there are also accounts of suffering and negative affect out of which nothing good seems to have come. And there is at least one example of the opposite sequence as well—a contami-nation sequence, wherein a good event turned suddenly and irrevocably bad. Highly generative people tend to emphasize redemption over contami-nation in their life stories. Madeline does this too, though the contamina-tion form does nonetheless appear. Looking to the future, the protagonist of Madeline's story sets forth goals and plans that aim to benefit both the self and the wider social world—again, a theme that is central to the com-mitment narratives often constructed by highly generative adults. The one exception to the model is the first theme, early advantage. Madeline's child-hood chapter is almost completely negative in emotional tone. She is not singled out as having had any kind of advantage at all. Only later, after prison, has she begun to see herself as special in a positive way.

Madeline's story is reminiscent of what Maruna (1997) has found in the life narratives of reformed criminals. In these narratives, early injury and suffering increase into late childhood, and the protagonist begins to spiral down into illegal activity and depravity. Eventually, the protagonist hits rock bottom. For Madeline, this happened when she was hosed down and thrown into solitary confinement, and she suddenly realized she was becoming her father—the man she still most hates. Like Maruna's exam-ples, Madeline experienced something of an epiphany and resolved to turn her life around. But such a comeback does not succeed unless the protago-nist finds viable outlets for meeting agentic and communal needs. In Madeline's case, some of this was accomplished through reading. She began to educate herself. Once out of prison, furthermore, she made new friend-ships in a new town, and began to experience small successes through her job, getting an apartment, and so on. Gradually, she has managed to inte-grate herself into the adult world of work and love. In the final chapters in Maruna's life stories, ex-cons find ways to be generative by sharing their re-form stories with others, so that others will not make the mistakes they have made. Although Madeline's story is not exactly like this, the work she has done with Native Americans—combining legal expertise and social work—appears to be a generative effort to make the world better for oth-ers, so that others will not have to experience the bad things that she, a Na-tive American herself, has suffered. Madeline's story also reflects themes a colleague and I have identified (McAdams & Bowman, 2001) in our stud-ies of highly generative African American adults. Most striking is Mad-eline's explicit identification of clear antagonists or enemies in her story (her father, certain legal authorities) and the way in which she sets her story up as a morality tale—the good protagonist (Madeline) battles the evil antagonists. As in the case of the African American stories we have studied, the protagonist will continue to fight the good fight. The battle is never over. No matter how many victories accrue, there always remains the possibility that the protagonist will ultimately be defeated. Consequently, the protagonist can never let up, but must always remain vigilant.

Madeline's identity integrates narrative forms common in contemporary American society. It is partly a rags-to-riches narrative, of the sort we all associate with upward social mobility among immigrants and others who come from humble backgrounds. This sort of progressive (constantly building, getting better, moving ahead) and ultimately redemptive life narrative is especially characteristic of life stories told by highly generative black adults in the United States, as I have suggested above. Madeline's is also partly a reform story, like the kind described by Maruna (1997) and characteristic of the life narratives promoted by Alcoholics Anonymous and other self-help groups. Reflecting a narrative move whose roots are in Christianity as much as anything else, she was "born again" in prison, as she resolved to turn her life around for good. The emphasis on the individual's relentless quest to expand the self and to discover the self anew is consistent with contemporary humanistic (and "New Age") thinking in our highly individualist society, and recaptures ancient narrative forms such as Joseph Campbell's (1949) myth of the hero. Like Campbell's hero, Madeline as the protagonist must battle a slew of dark forces and go on a journey of self-discovery. But she eventually returns home (to her Native American people), and brings to them a gift of some sort (what Campbell calls a "boon") to improve their lives.

Still, there are storm clouds on the horizon, as Madeline suggests toward the end of her interview. Redemption is not assured, given that the world will always be a dangerous place. Her partner provides a secure base for her; his love helps to give her the confidence she needs to fight the good fight. Another man who provides her with security and affirmation is the older lawyer whose firm she will soon be working for. Indeed, both the boyfriend (who is older than Madeline) and the lawyer seem to function as benevolent father figures in this story, though of course their roles are more complex as well. She has placed a great deal of trust in these two men. Should they fail her, she may become much more vulnerable. For example, Madeline worries that she may not fit in with the other lawyers at the new firm. Given her brash and earthy presentation, it makes sense to worry about this. Yet she feels that the older lawyer who has been her benefactor in the past will continue to teach her how to interact in this new context. But what if he fails? There is a sense in which Madeline's story for the future is too good to be true. She is "on a roll" now, but continued success is not assured. Furthermore, developmentally old and new issues are either not resolved or not addressed in the story. A coherent and psychologically satisfying life story aims to reconcile the past with the present and future.

But the protagonist in this story is now pretty much cut off from her family of origin. Her father will not speak to her. Her mother seems completely ineffectual. Madeline feels very distanced from her brother and sister. Of course, it is not necessary to make peace with the past in order to move forward. But the reader of her story may feel that too many damaging events and characters from the past have simply been sliced off from the main story line. The villains serve only as villains; there is little sense that their characters will evolve. Indeed, at one point in the interview, Madeline remarks on how she routinely slices off bad things and people from the past. She has no time to deal with that "shit." She feels that it is better not to look back, but to keep moving forward. As far as forward movement is concerned, the view of the future says little about whether or not she and her partner will start a family of their own. This is a highly generative woman; one might expect that she would want children very badly. On the other hand, her own experiences as a child were so toxic that she may worry about repeating aspects of the past. Furthermore, her generativity finds ample expression in her work.

What might go wrong? One could argue that Madeline's string of victories cannot go on forever. Should she encounter significant setbacks professionally, or should her relationship with her partner break up, perhaps she would lose focus. At the end of the interview, she remarks that she will probably be fine in life as long as she doesn't "get bored." As a highly extraverted and conscientious woman, open to new experiences, with very strong power motivation and values centered on prosocial action, Madeline has constructed a redemptive life story in which early suffering eventually gives way to victory in battle; she has made for herself a life that keeps her moving and focused, busy and engaged. The future surely looks bright. But even if things darken significantly, it is hard to imagine that life could ever return to the bleak depths Madeline experienced as a child and adolescent. The protagonist in this narrative is simply too strong now. The movement of the plot is strongly upward and progressive. The enemies have been irrevocably weakened. Even if the forces of evil manage to launch an aggressive attack as she moves into midlife, I would still put my money on Madeline.

8

Psychodynamic Assessment

REBECCA S. BEHRENDS
SIDNEY J. BLATT

In preparation for conducting a psychodynamic assessment of our research volunteer, we elected to obtain only the most minimal identifying information about her (i.e., her name, age, sex, and the fact that she has never been a patient in psychotherapy). Our purpose in this regard was to approach the test data with as few preconceived ideas about her as possible, in order to elicit the particular nature and quality of information that the psychodynamic orientation to psychological testing is uniquely suited to provide. Before we stated our intent to Jerry Wiggins, he did indicate that Madeline G is an attorney by profession. Beyond this, however, in formulating our interpretation of the test data, we knew nothing else of her background, except for the personal information that she herself chose to share spontaneously as a function of the testing situation itself.

ASSESSMENT METHODS AND RATIONALE

We hold the fundamental assumption that an understanding of the complexities of individual personality organization can best be achieved through an integration of (1) test scores; (2) content or themes of responses; (3) style of verbalization (i.e., the person's attitude and affective reactions toward his or her responses); and (4) the interpersonal relationship between the person and the tester, including the tester's empathic and introspective cues in the transaction (Allison, Blatt, & Zimet, 1988).

226

We also assume that these different sources of information need to be observed systematically under conditions that present different levels of organization or structure—from the well-structured, objective, reality-oriented context of an intelligence test, such as the Wechsler Adult Intelligence Scale—Third Edition (WAIS-III); to a somewhat less structured situation that emphasizes interpersonal relationships, such as the Thematic Apperception Test (TAT); to a relatively open-ended request to construct meaning in response to relatively ambiguous stimuli, such as the Rorschach. The goal of this type of assessment is to identify the organizational principles with which the individual functions across these three domains.

We supplement this more traditional ego-psychological approach to assessment (e.g., Allison et al., 1988; Rapaport, Gill, & Schafer, 1946) with an assessment of the content and structure of the representation of self and significant others by obtaining open-ended descriptions on the Object Relations Inventory (ORI; e.g., Blatt, Stayner, Auerbach, & Behrends, 1996). These sources of information, together, constitute the test data of our approach to psychological assessment. To this end, we have attempted to obtain, to the fullest extent possible, a verbatim recording of Madeline's verbalizations and emotional reactions, as well as observations of her behavior, from the outset of the testing encounter to its conclusion. We have also attempted to recreate the tester's ongoing thoughts, feelings, and impressions in relation to Madeline throughout the testing.

The assessment procedures were administered in the following order: WAIS-III, TAT, Rorschach, and ORI. The entire procedure took approximately 5½ hours. The TAT was somewhat abbreviated because Madeline overslept and was 1½ hours late for the testing session. Consequently, in the interest of time, the following TAT cards were presented: Card 1, Card 2, Card 3 GF, Card 14, Card 13 MF, Card 5, Card 10, Card 18 GF, and Card 17 BM. Because Madeline was so prolific in her responses, both to the TAT and throughout the entire test battery, we do not believe that the necessity of using fewer TAT cards than usual is likely to have seriously compromised the test results.

DIAGNOSTIC UNDERSTANDING

Madeline's personality and individuality are very much manifested in her striking physical presence. When she arrived for the testing session, her short, black, wavy hair was still wet from the shower. She wore a black turtleneck, black pants, and a plain black wristwatch. Her only jewelry was a diamond stud, worn high in the curve of one pierced ear. At one point, she referred to her physical appearance as having had an obvious impact when she first attempted to establish herself as an attorney in the courtroom. She went on to say with obvious pride that her "minority status" had been clear from the start, both as a woman and as a Navaho Indian. She has high cheekbones and strong features. Her skin appears medium to light in contrast to her black hair and clothing. She wore just the lightest touch of makeup. She has a medium frame, and her overall manner and stance can perhaps best be described as rather androgynous. Her gestures are highly expressive, and she inhabits her body fully, in a sensuous, cat-like way.

Madeline presents an extremely complex diagnostic picture. It is perhaps most fundamentally true of her that she is highly changeable from one moment to the next. She is action-oriented and highly emotional, with a flair for the dramatic. She is a free spirit and a bohemian, who prides herself on her own unconventionality and wears it for effect. She is intensely private, while at the same time being unashamedly exhibitionistic. Although she is headstrong and strives fiercely to be independent, she can, in the next moment, be achingly tender and vulnerable. And although she can be oppositional, there are also selflessness and generosity about her, as well as a remarkable capacity for empathy and mutuality.

Test findings reveal that underlying Madeline's compelling and highly variable presence is a serious vulnerability to intense depression. Madeline experiences a deep longing to be loved and admired by others. Coupled with this ever-present need is the largely unconscious fear that she will lose the others' love if she fails to meet their needs and expectations. Even more fundamental is Madeline's vulnerability to loneliness. At this level, what she most longs for unconsciously are the literal and direct nurturance and succorance that can only be provided by a primary caregiver or maternal figure. And because she feels that these basic, primary dependency needs have never been adequately met, she is vulnerable to a deep sense of loneliness and emptiness, together with a constant and overwhelming anxiety over the loss of others.

It is not only Madeline's vulnerability, however, that accounts for the range and variability of her personality functioning. Equally striking are her remarkable capacity for recovery and her ongoing struggle for mastery, in the face of a past history that she remembers as being violently traumatic and painfully depriving. Although her thinking is vulnerable to the intrusion of painfully disruptive associations, her openness to such experiences tends to enrich and enliven, rather than to disorganize, her overall functioning. Madeline attempts both to generate and to soak up whatever gratification she can in every conceivable circumstance. Her sensuousness, together with an active and continuous sensation seeking, work to fill her emptiness and loneliness and to protect her from succumbing to depression. Fundamentally, Madeline's mercurial nature is a sequence of strength, vulnerability, and progressive recovery. She has developed a remarkable capacity for creative mastery, and a resiliency that enables her to spring back, achieving even higher levels of development through ever-shifting processes of defense and sublimation.

FUNCTIONING WITHIN A HIGHLY STRUCTURED CONTEXT

Having established a basic framework for understanding the structure of Madeline's personality organization, we now describe the multiple and extremely complex forms of vulnerability and recovery that characterize her functioning across various circumstances. First, in the context of a highly structured situation, where the expectations are clear and the emotional climate is neutral, Madeline is stimulated on any number of developmental levels. She reactively manifests a complex array of defensive solutions, which tend to be highly action-oriented.

First, she anticipates the control that she imagines will be imposed upon her by the authority figure involved in such a structured setting, and she attempts to wrest control by taking over the situation herself. This identification with the anticipated aggressor was enacted quite dramatically in our very first contact with Madeline. When she was first called by the examiner (Rebecca Behrends) at her hotel to let her know that testing would begin at 8:30 the next morning, she protested. This was not what she had in mind at all! She had made plans for the evening, and this was just too early in the morning! A 10:30 starting time would suit her better. Thus, at the very outset of this highly structured and imposing situation, she became imposing and controlling herself. She was told that it would not be possible to complete the testing if we started later. Once a rationale was presented to her that related to our mutual needs and interests, her oppositionality and her sense of entitlement over the meeting time fell away, and she agreed to the earlier time, stating, "I'm a pretty flexible person." With regard to the latter comment, she was no doubt more comfortable with the idea of being able to define herself than she was at the anxiety-provoking prospect of being defined by the examiner and the testing procedure. She then quickly added, "It's Rebecca, right?" Thus she ended our conversation with the clearly enacted wish that this be a mutual collaboration between equals, expressed by calling the examiner by her first name in a familiar manner. She was momentarily able to relinquish her controlling and self-absorbed defenses, as well as her anxiety over being tested, and to express her affiliative needs by striving to establish an equal and more intimate working relationship.

It was both ironic and dynamically significant that the next morning, after she was already 45 minutes late, the examiner called her room but got no answer. Immediately thereafter, she phoned sounding frazzled and annoyed, but also rather sheepishly apologetic. Her alarm clock had failed to go off, and she had not received a wake-up call from the front desk. She promised to "jump in the shower" and hurry over as soon as possible. In the end, through this symptomatic enactment, she not only got her later morning appointment time, she also got the examiner to wake her up for the appointment (as would a mother whose child was late for school). And finally, she actually became more appealing in her tardiness—both because her demeanor was reminiscent of a "good kid," and also because she was genuinely empathic regarding the impact of her lateness on the examiner. Therefore, after quite a round of detours, she managed to recover on a higher developmental level, in the spirit of teamwork.

In a testing context, Madeline approaches highly structured tasks (such as those of the WAIS-III) with a sense of due diligence and earnestness. She shows persistence and manifests a disciplined ability to tolerate frustration as the tasks become increasingly difficult. Not only does she strive to do a good job, however, everything she says and does appears to be with the relationship in mind. For example, on the Picture Completion subtest of the WAIS-III, the question of "What is missing?" appears to elicit dependency longings, as she strokes and literally appears to feel the details of each picture with a sensuous pleasure that she exhibits freely. Such sensation seeking works to fill her emptiness over what is missing, as she simultaneously seeks to draw the examiner in to fill the void. This same sensation seeking is also motivated to impress, and ultimately to excite, both her and the examiner. Thus, even in this highly structured task, she is unable and unwilling to confine herself solely to verbal responses, even though her answers are largely correct. Also noteworthy is the finding that issues of personal concern are stimulated frequently and intrude into her verbal responses, even when the answers themselves are technically correct. For example, in relation to the item on the Picture Completion subtest of people jogging, she responds with "our footsteps"—a peculiar verbalization apparently merging her and the examiner, as well as merging the two of them with the joggers in the picture, while correctly identifying the footsteps as missing. Her only incorrect answer on this subtest is the final picture, where she fails to see the missing snow on the logs. She answers, instead, that it is "people" who are missing.

On other highly structured tasks that allow more free-ranging verbal expression (Vocabulary, Similarities, Comprehension), Madeline revels in her own unconventionality and wears it for effect. Indeed, she does not want to be conventional and follow the instructions. For example, on the Vocabulary subtest, instead of giving definitions of the words as instructed, she treats the task as though it were a word association test! Thus for the word "winter," her response is "cold," and with inquiry from the examiner, she elaborates it as "skiing." And to the word "assemble," she responds, "Ikea," and with inquiry, "Allen wrench." Only after repeated inquiry does she finally give the definition "put together." Even when she does relent and begins to define the words, she gives global, action-oriented, impulsive, and emotion-laden responses—responses that often characterize a hysterical character style. She is clearly functioning below her intellectual potential by striving to be clever, unique, and creative for the benefit of her relationship with the examiner.

Further examination of Madeline's thought, however, reveals that it is not just for dynamic reasons that the quality of her thinking is imprecise. Although Madeline is certainly intelligent in the sense of being extremely savvy and street-smart, she is still relatively unsophisticated and unschooled in her thought. She knows these vocabulary words on a visceral level, and at the level of action in terms of how they are used, but she does not think verbally on a highly abstract or conceptual level. This point is given additional support by Madeline's inability to render an abstract interpretation of the proverbs on the Comprehension subtest of the WAIS-III. For example, in response to the proverb "One swallow does not make a summer," she replies concretely, "A swallow as in a bird, or glass of water? I don't know. I never heard of it."

On other subtests of the WAIS-III, Madeline demonstrates additional intellectual weaknesses: in her fund of general information, and in her knowledge of the most basic arithmetic. In areas where she clearly has difficulty, she exhibits significant anxiety over her intellectual functioning, the latter of which is reflected in her relatively lowered score on the Digit Span subtest. Eventually, however, Madeline herself explains these puzzling findings in the context of the jury trial question on the Comprehension subtest. She volunteers that she herself is a highly successful trial lawyer who only represents clients with not-guilty pleas. She goes on to explain with pride that she has accomplished such success professionally, despite the fact that she went only as far as the sixth grade in school (before returning to college and going to law school as a young adult). She then confides poignantly, with the sweetness and vulnerability of a young child, "That's why I didn't know how to do the math. I never learned my times tables." She goes on to say that she left home at the age of 12, and subsequently lived in foster homes, which "did not work out." She acknowledges that she later worked, cryptically adding that she was "mainly in and out of jail after that." She states that she met with resistance when she applied for admission to the bar after her graduation from law school. Having taken the required exams, however, she fought for her rights and ultimately triumphed. It is no wonder, therefore, that she is anxious at the prospect of taking an intelligence test. She is all too aware of how her lack of formal schooling has presented obstacles in her life, in terms of truly fitting in. It is also not surprising that her thinking at times appears to be "unschooled," in light of the severe educational deprivation she has undergone in her life. What is surprising—even astonishing—is her ability to overcome such hardship, and to make of her life what she has. We explore this issue further as we relay additional findings later in this chapter.

To return to the WAIS-III, an additional point that bears mentioning is that on more verbally oriented tests such as the Vocabulary subtest,

Madeline repeatedly makes value judgments in relation to the words in the test questions. The words "remorse," "ponder," and "evolve" she pronounces as being "good" or "great" words. To the word "audacious," she states, "Piss and vinegar! It's underrated!" This need to pass judgment is one that we follow through the remainder of the chapter, as we attempt to understand her preoccupation with such valuations—which is later expressed in concerns about more cosmic issues of good and evil, as well as the question of guilt versus innocence.

Once Madeline has managed to establish both her independence and her tie to the other person, she strives to do a good job, and throws herself wholeheartedly into structured visual–motor and visual–spatial tasks where she can mediate verbally (e.g., Block Design, Matrix Reasoning, and Object Assembly). This is especially the case when the content of the work is something that piques her interest or offers a challenge that captures her imagination. Under these circumstances, she takes ebullient pleasure in the wonder of discovery, as she works to find the right solution to a given problem. Her childlike freshness and naiveté in doing this are completely without guile. She is not trying primarily to control or impress. Nor does she chafe against the structure. She is comfortable in the relationship, and lives fully in the moment. Remarkably, as she thinks her way through the various problems, she un-self-consciously does all her thinking *aloud*—like Vygotsky's young child, who uses "outer speech" as the natural precursor to an interior life characterized by "inner speech" or thought.

Under conditions of extremely high structure on a relatively routine task (e.g., the WAIS-III Digit Symbol subtest), where the only choice is total compliance or failure, Madeline complies, but with greatly diminished efficiency and disrupted functioning. When there is no room for self-expression, independent thought, or creativity, and the structure is so imposing that she is socially isolated, Madeline is vulnerable to a serious loss of efficiency, focus, and involvement as well as the threat of impaired functioning. This vulnerability is most clearly expressed on the Digit Symbol subtest. On this task she draws the symbols associated with an array of numbers in a strikingly disorganized manner, with several errors, and with pronounced psychomotor retardation suggestive of severe depression (see Figure 8.1). Thus, when Madeline is confronted with a banal, repetitive, unchallenging task, her functioning becomes badly impaired. Challenge, stimulation, and excitement all serve to enable Madeline to function at an impressive level. But without this stimulation, her functioning can seriously deteriorate.

OVERALL INTELLECTUAL FUNCTIONING

On the WAIS-III, Madeline's Verbal IQ is 110 and her Performance IQ is 113, resulting in an overall Full Scale IQ of 112. These scores place her in

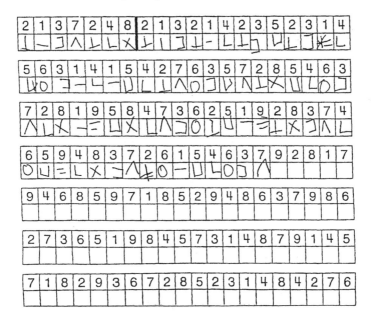

FIGURE 8.1. Madeline G's performance on the Digit Symbol subtest of the WAIS-III.

the high average range of overall intellectual functioning. As stated previously, however, these findings should be viewed as underestimates of Madeline's actual intellectual capacity—which is far better represented in less structured contexts, such as the TAT, the Rorschach, and the ORI.

Madeline's Verbal and Performance subtest scaled scores are presented in Table 8.1. In the Verbal realm, Madeline's vocabulary, fund of general information, and verbal concept formation ability are all in the high average range. She also demonstrates impaired verbal abstract reasoning ability in the form of concrete thinking when asked to interpret proverbs (Comprehension). All of these scores are certainly lower than would be expected for a law school graduate, and reflect a combination of these factors: (1) Madeline's prior impoverished educational history; (2) her determined unconventionality; and (3) the tendency for emotional and dynamic issues to intrude on her thinking, as previously discussed.

Somewhat higher is Madeline's performance on perceptual organizational tasks. Her ability to discriminate essential from nonessential detail is in the upper end of the high average range, as is her visual–motor integration ability when scores are adjusted for the time factor. Madeline shows psychomotor retardation on both visual–spatial and visual–motor integration tasks. For example, her performance on the Block Design subscale is only in the average range, due to motor slowing as a consequence of de-

TABLE 8.1. WAIS-III Scaled Scores of Madeline G

Verbal subtests		Performance subtests	
Vocabulary	12	Picture Arrangement	12
Similarities	12	Picture Completion	14
Information	12	Block Design	11
Comprehension	12	Matrix Reasoning	14
Arithmetic	12	Digit Symbol	9
Digit Span	9	Symbol Search	8
Letter–Number	10	Object Assembly	13

Verbal IQ = 110   Performance IQ = 113
Full Scale IQ = 112

pression as previously described. Even more impaired is her low average functioning on the Processing Speed Index (Digit Symbol and Symbol Search), which technically measures the speed and efficiency of visual–spatial processing. For example, on the Digit Symbol subscale (as noted earlier), Madeline produces crude, childlike renderings of the symbols associated with different numbers (see Figure 8.1). This lowered functioning does not appear to be due to organic factors; rather, it represents her depressed motor response in reaction to extremely high structure and to the interpersonal isolation that it entails, revealing her vulnerability to depression under such circumstances.

The Working Memory Index (Arithmetic, Digit Span, and Letter Number Sequence) of the WAIS-III shows intersubtest scatter. Madeline's capacity for sustained concentration appears to be quite good, as measured by her quick and efficient functioning on the first 16 items of the Arithmetic subscale. As indicated previously, her functioning on the final two items is hindered by the fact that she never learned her multiplication facts. In contrast to concentration, Madeline shows definite difficulty with attention, evidenced by a merely average Digit Span score, which reflects ongoing anxiety over intellectual insecurity arising from her educational background.

In the social arena, Madeline's ability to verbalize an intellectual understanding of social convention on the Comprehension subscale is measured only in the high average range. Here her score is lowered partially because of her concrete interpretation of proverbs on the same scale. In addition, however, she is genuinely puzzled over questions regarding social norms. Given her unusual childhood and adolescence, there is a sense in which Madeline comes to such questions as an outsider. Thus she does not know or own the rules, despite the fact that she specializes in the law! Finally, Madeline scores in the high average range in terms of the ability to anticipate, plan, and organize her experience in the social realm. Here again, she demonstrates a tendency at times to distort her perceptions of social interactions in terms of personal idiosyncratic concerns that are not inherent in the situation itself.

Finally, it is critical to note that there is relatively little variation among the various subtests (intersubtest scatter) on the WAIS-III, indicating relatively good cognitive efficiency and a basic intactness of Madeline's personality organization. This pattern of scores indicates that there is no serious disruption in her overall cognitive functioning, but rather some inefficiency due to dysphoric experiences.

FUNCTIONING WITHIN AN INTERPERSONAL CONTEXT

In less structured interpersonal situations, Madeline begins by being aggressive and attempting to exert control, just as at the outset of the testing encounter. Her predisposition in this regard is illustrated in striking fashion on the Picture Arrangement subtest of the WAIS-III. On the "shark" item, when the picture cards are placed in correct sequence, the story proceeds as follows: A man goes to the beach, only to find that it is extremely crowded with people. He leaves and goes to a store, where he buys a replica of a shark's head. Upon his return to the beach, he takes the shark's head into the water to scare away the other swimmers. He then has the water all to himself. In Madeline's own idiosyncratic arrangement of the pictures to this story, however, the man buys the shark's head from the outset, planning to scare away any other swimmers before he ever even sees the beach! Thus, in Madeline's world, it makes sense to be aggressive and controlling from the very beginning, given the presumed nature of people to thwart her needs. What is so remarkable about Madeline, however, is that she is every bit as ready to back down and literally to make friends as she is to do battle, once she encounters a person who is genuinely interested in relating to her with fairness and mutuality.

In the interpersonal domain, as best evidenced by the TAT, Madeline is endlessly curious, intrigued, and stimulated on every level imaginable (see Appendix A). Her evocative language, her subtle distinctions of affective nuance, and the complexity of her thought all suggest a keen intelligence—far more so than is demonstrated within a confining structure, such as that of the WAIS-III. Whereas a high degree of structure limits the free play of her imagination, the interpersonal arena gives full range to the richness of Madeline's fantasy life. She is deeply involved in the TAT stories that she tells, with themes rich in seduction and betrayal, guilt and innocence. It quickly becomes apparent that here above all else, Madeline is in her element. She exclaims that she loves the freedom the TAT gives her to "tell the story my way!"—remarkably, just as she has previously described telling

her clients' stories her way in court. As she becomes engrossed in the telling, it is as though she is finding the story that really exists in the picture,
allowing herself a momentary suspension of critical judgment and giving
herself permission to play. She runs the emotional gamut, from sheer ela-
tion to deep sadness and back again, as she draws the listener in. Here
again is an analogy to the courtroom; one finds it is easy to imagine
Madeline as a highly compelling and powerful presence, fully able to hold
the jurors in her thrall and to convince them of the innocence of her clients.

Not coincidentally, the theme of guilt and innocence is a major preoc-
cupying theme that infuses Madeline's experience of interpersonal relationships. The sensation seeking that she exhibits in structured situations becomes all the more intense and dramatic when she is with other people,
leading her directly into temptation that she sometimes finds impossible to
resist. For example, on Card 1 of the TAT, the boy with the violin has been
so overcome by his own curiosity and inquisitiveness that he impulsively
steals the violin. He knows he has done something that is morally wrong by
society's standards, and he is painfully aware of the consequences if he
should be caught. But, as Madeline is quick to reassure herself and the examiner, his motives are "not bad," and he is "not deceptive." After all, he
intends no harm to the owner. He is just so inquisitive and resourceful. He
knows that he can find a way to reverse the situation and return the violin
(which, by the way, is now broken), with no one ever being the wiser. So, in
the final analysis, he is not really guilty. This is merely a complicated situation that he may need some outside help to fix, but that he can essentially
undo.

Thus the trouble for Madeline, but also the pleasure, is that interpersonal relationships are just so tempting. And with many of the temptations
she encounters, she is highly conflicted over how to define her own moral
code. She is still haunted, more than she wishes to admit, by the moral and
legal transgressions of her past, as well as by the sexual and aggressive
urges she experiences in the present. Her TAT stories repeatedly suggest
that her curiosity and lust for literal experience may sometimes get the
better of her, making her vulnerable to impulsive action. For example, on
Card 13 MF, picturing a man standing with his arm over his eyes and a
woman on the bed before him, she tells the following story: "Oh, he's going
home to his wife! 'Thank you very much, mistress! That was great!' He's
happy and she's happy. She's smart, too. She loves the good sex—not the
trappings of a relationship. And he likes sex with her. If his wife ever found
out, his ass would be killed!" And on the next card presented (Card 5),
which pictures a woman simply looking into a room through a half-open
door, Madeline is compelled to continue with the sequel: "She's his wife!
She suspects something! She wasn't supposed to be home! She hears him!
He's [not pictured] got that look on his face—'I've been caught!' She wants
to know, but doesn't. If he did it, out he goes! The only one who has noth-

ing to lose is the beautiful mistress. He should have had a shower before he went home! She's gonna be able to smell that!" she exclaims, in an outburst of laughter.

Madeline takes an almost prurient interest in the sexual drama—both in its great pleasure, and in its capacity to ruin lives. The sexual male, with whom she partially identifies, is recklessly unfaithful. The stereotypic female, the wife, is a victim both of her husband's betrayal and self-indulgence, and of her own reluctance to face the truth because of her need for him. Madeline clearly identifies most strongly, however, with the smart, beautiful mistress who enjoys sex for its own sake and loses nothing in the bargain. It is noteworthy that in every TAT story, Madeline is able to empathize so fully with each of the characters in turn, whatever their motives. Although her cognitive style is global and impressionistic, she is not at all repressive like the classic individual with hysterical personality organization. Indeed, Madeline is a woman who has unusual tolerance for the entire spectrum of thoughts, feelings, and actions, both in herself and in others. Her ability to shift perspectives is so fluid, however, that there is almost an amoral quality about her at times. And Madeline herself sometimes doubts her own morality. However, the repeated theme of guilt versus innocence that runs through these stories leads to a different conclusion. Madeline has her own morality, which is defined differently from standard social convention. It can be summed up as follows: "First and foremost, do no harm; second, do not get caught or you will have to take the terrible consequences." Even on the WAIS-III, Madeline takes issue with questions of normative social convention. For example, she puzzles over why the state would require a license in order for people to get married. She simply cannot understand why someone would want marriage as a legally binding institution. She adds that she would never want to marry her long-time male partner, of whom she speaks with great respect and adoration on the ORI (see Appendix C). This is no wonder in light of her characterization of marriage on the TAT, not to mention her parents' violently abusive marriage as described in the ORI.

The issue of sexuality aside, Madeline's conflict over guilt versus innocence takes on desperate proportions when it comes to the issue of aggression. This conflict is powerfully represented in her response to Card 18 GF (a woman with her hands around the throat of another woman on a stairway) as follows: "They're having a scrap! This one's older [the woman being held], but this one's stronger in a way, emotionally. That [older] one's frail and weak. This [younger] one's physically stronger and really quite mean! As she [the older woman] deteriorates, the [younger] woman's frustration results in hitting her—beating her a lot. It's her [older woman's] house. She [younger woman] is a bad niece. . . . Nasty, nasty! This poor [older] woman's life is hellish." Madeline is very upset and completely lost in the story. To the inquiry "How does it end?," she responds: "It doesn't for a long time. She ends up dying in madness and mental hell. This one [older woman] is a bitter old witch. With any luck, she'll get hit by a bus. Okay. This [younger] one will die falling off a ladder—will break her neck! So *I* go in and *kick* it [exclaims with relish]! This poor woman dies all dirty . . . awful [barely audible]." Madeline then shakes her head as if to shake the experience away, and exclaims with a manic-like, defensive reaction (which is extremely characteristic), "Let's make a *happy* picture!"

This astonishing story of moral depravity, hellish suffering, and attempted deliverance through murderous revenge is hauntingly reminiscent of Madeline's descriptions of her parents and herself on the ORI. She describes how her mother, whom she describes as a greedy, phony, withholding "witch," was brutalized by her father, a charming but abusive alcoholic. She adds somewhat cryptically that he was "violent towards all of us." She relates a distinct memory of herself as walking down the steps with a pillow, thinking, "I gotta kill my father." She then remembers halting and beginning to sob, thinking, "He'll always be stronger." Here again, Madeline tolerates a great deal in herself. Rather than repress or deny her experience, she lives with the conscious recognition of the guilt that is inherent in fully intending to kill her father. And in the TAT story described above, she loses distance to such a degree that she enters the story herself, killing the sadistic perpetrator. Clearly, even in Madeline's own moral code, there are exceptions to this principle of doing no harm. Madeline lives not only with her guilt, however, but also with the pain of her own shattered innocence, and of her victimization by each of her parents. And in the end, she lives with the ongoing vulnerability to an excruciatingly painful depression that is the legacy of this traumatic past.

The "happy story" that Madeline tells in the last and final TAT card (17 BM—a man clinging to a rope) is truly Madeline's own. It represents her attempted antidote to her past and to the depression that she still carries in its wake. She exclaims exuberantly, "Well, well, ain't we a little naked trapeze artist! An inmate over the wall, getting away! He gets away successfully, too! Name's Herb. For days Herb is wearing women's pants, for 2 days! Gets a pretty bad rash on his scrotum [outburst of laughter]! He'll tell his *gynecologist* [emphasis added] about it later." (The issue of gender identity that this story raises is discussed later in the section on "Self and Others"). She continues: "He got pissed off one night. Got into some trouble. Landed in jail. Couldn't stand it! I like Herb! He does good for himself! Never goes back in again!" In this manic-like escape from all the imprisonments of her past, Madeline takes enormous pleasure. Fundamental to her life is the relish that she gets out of the idea of defying authority and "beating the system" (i.e., the legal system that resulted in her past incarceration, as well as the original parental authorities who hurt and deprived her as a child). The crowning achievement that is her professional life's work becomes explicable when viewed in this light. As an attorney who professes the innocence of her clients before the legal system, as well as her own innocence, she is symbolically able to redress her own past victimization, as well as to re-parent her victimized clients—like the nurturing mother and the strong and protective father she unconsciously still wishes for.

FUNCTIONING WITHIN AN AMBIGUOUS CONTEXT

In the context of a more ambiguous situation, such as the Rorschach, the predominant features of Madeline's functioning are extensive affective and ideational elaborations that often extend initially well-perceived, realistic responses in ways that are sometimes inappropriate and unrealistic (see Appendix B.1). These affective and ideational elaborations are often extremely positive, powerful, and strong, such as describing the frequently well-perceived figure of a woman in the center of Card I as "holding her hands up, got great big wings. Like she's professing. Very powerful. I like that. . . . Like her back is to you. She's facing a crowd. She'd have to be giving them information. . . . Someone important in front of all these people. Like she'd have something important to say." Another of these positive constructions is her response to Card V, which is also accurately perceived: "Looks like a butterfly in flight. Quite majestic, out for an afternoon flight." It is noteworthy, however, that these more positive, strong, and constructive elaborations tend to alternate with associative elaborations that are more negative, painful, and vulnerable. The majestic butterfly perceived on Card V, for example, is preceded by a response to Card IV of a "Scary monster! Great big scary monster, getting sick. Huge feet, small head, claws. Oh, it's like fire, burning this little person. Poor bugger. Very imposing figure! Tiny head. Not very smart, dangerous!" Madeline is very involved in this response and disturbed about the little person's being purposely burned. In reply to the examiner's inquiry about this response, Madeline elaborates, "The top is his head, looking down. Spraying from his mouth. First looks like he's getting sick. Then looks like fire, very dark." To the examiner's inquiry, "Burning?" Madeline replies, "Fire from guy's mouth. Burning him on purpose! Little bugger didn't stand a chance! . . . Like it wasn't accidental. Back is to us. He's inside of the fire. Little arms hanging down there." The examiner then inquires, "Poor little guy?" to which Madeline responds, "Don't you see that? God, I hope so! It's so obvious! I need to put some dancing pandas in that picture!" (referring back to one of her positive, more playful responses on Card II of the Rorschach).

These excessive affective and ideational elaborations are considered by Rapaport and colleagues (1946) as a form of disordered thinking—"confabulation," in which the distinction between the initial perception and one's personal reactions or associations to that perception is lost. Thus an initially accurate and well-perceived image is elaborated well beyond any justification existing within the stimulus. Of Madeline's total of 26 responses to the Rorschach, 6 are confabulations (2 with very positive, and 4 with very negative, content). These responses express the polarity of Madeline's experiences—from a sense of personal strength and power, to feelings that the world is a dangerous, destructive place in which a poor little person can be tortured and destroyed.

Given the frequency and intensity of this confabulatory thinking, and the ease with which it can be provoked, it is impressive that in a number of other aspects, Madeline's responses to the Rorschach indicate considerable psychological strength (see Appendices B.2 and B.3). Thus Madeline's Rorschach protocol is consistent with conclusions drawn from the WAIS-III and TAT, indicating that her functioning ranges across a very wide spectrum in terms of her capacity for adaptation. Overall, her protocol is quite intact, and usually her responses to aspects of the stimuli are congruent with conventional reality. Eight of her 26 responses are initially popular or very conventional images, though these popular responses are often marked by excessive associative elaborations. This expansive enrichment of her responses, indicating her inability or unwillingness to settle for clearly conventional responses, is a source of her creativity and uniqueness when it is well done, but it can also occasionally express her vulnerability to very painful thoughts and feelings. Generally she has a good capacity for cognitive control, as indicated by the fact that most of her responses are determined primarily by the form of the blot (F% = 54%) and these forms are usually reasonably well perceived (F+% = 64%). When she includes additional properties of the stimulus in her responses, such as chromatic color, achromatic color, or movement, these additional dimensions are most often secondary to the form in contributing to the construction of the response (Extended F% = 92%). Remarkably, as she includes these other dimensions in her responses, the accuracy of the perception of her responses increases even beyond the level when her responses are based on form alone (Extended F+% = 79%). Thus, though Madeline seems vulnerable to intensely powerful negative and positive associations to provocative stimuli, she is usually able to integrate these reactions in a constructive and sometimes very creative way—especially in the context of affect and interpersonal interaction (see Allison et al., 1988).

Madeline's capacity for adaptation, however, can become somewhat impaired, primarily around dysphoric issues. The sources of this dysphoria are feelings of abandonment and loneliness, issues of self-worth and sexual identity, and concerns about good versus evil. Madeline only occasionally experiences these intense dysphoric feelings, because they are strongly defended against by excessive activity, engagement with others, and stimulation seeking. These manic-like defenses are frequently channeled into constructive activities, but sometimes they are excessive and even off-putting and interpersonally jarring. These defenses are often successful in aiding Madeline to avoid the underlying depressive experiences. But when these defenses fail, Madeline can experience extreme feelings of depression, desolation, and hopelessness—even to the point of having thoughts of suicide, which are largely unconscious. Her two closing responses to the Rorschach on Card X communicate aspects of these struggles. She begins her responses as follows: "Looks like a party in a psychedelic aquarium. *Star Wars* meets Disney on acid. A party—they're having fun. Everybody's smiling. They live in an ecosystem, all in some way attached. Fine, no one's trying to get away. All enjoying themselves at the party. All so very, very, very different, but all work well together. Having a great time." Almost as an afterthought, Madeline then notes that there is a blue crab in the upper corner of the card and comments on this conventional response as follows: "That guy is forlorn, defeated. There is the eye. Big ole nose. Not so much sad as hopeless." And then, comparing this image on the one side of the card with a similar image on the other side, Madeline notes, "This is not a mirror image." (The examiner notes that she herself feels sad and tearful in reaction to Madeline's description of this closing response.) Madeline then concludes defensively with the hypomanic comment: "Otherwise, an underwater circus! A great thing going on!"

The underwater circus on Card X is in fact Madeline's second (or possibly even her third) transparency response. Several studies (e.g., Blatt & Ritzler, 1974; Fowler, Hilsenroth, & Piers, 2001; Hansell, Lerner, Milden, & Ludolph, 1988; Rierdan, Lang, & Eddy, 1978) provide empirical confirmation of the clinical observation (Roth & Blatt, 1974) of an association between transparent images and suicidal ideation and/or activity. Her prior transparency responses occur on Card IX of the Rorschach. She describes a "protective halo-aura" around a "special . . . person. Can't tell if it's a man or a woman. . . . Person part is really safe. Struggle here between good and evil. Evil part is really strong-muscled. Green part is extension of the person who's good. Evil is trying to influence the person, trying to get inside. But there's way too much good. It's not bad, because there's a little evil in all of us. Hands here are pushing the evil away. So looks like the person's very safe, well protected." In her reply to the examiner's inquiry, Madeline elaborates on the halo or aura: "The color is really rich, warm, comforting. Surrounds the person. Blanketing, but not suffocating, wrapping—just there." (Examiner: "Evil?") "Pushing itself onto the person, imposing and pushy, forcing itself in." Madeline then notes that a segment of this card "looks like a great big nose sneezing and all this splattering germs and bacteria against the glass. What a sneeze would look like, a lot of crap." In response to another inquiry, she elaborates further: "Nobody's nose. This is a visual of what a sneeze would be if you could see one. Colorful and messy. Could be fun to see a sneeze in color!" The sneeze response also has transparent features ("against the glass"), with the suggestion that the halo or aura is possibly also seen as transparent, like the psychedelic aquarium or underwater circus on Card X.

The fact that these transparency responses come late in the Rorschach adds further poignancy to Madeline's very painful struggles to find a place of safety and togetherness to ward off the intrusion of evil forces that she fears will contaminate or destroy her. These responses to Cards IX and X also illustrate dramatically the forced, manic-like activity in which these dysphoric experiences are embedded—activity that Madeline uses to defend against these very painful concerns. Again, most of the time these manic-like defenses are successful and result in constructive, imaginative, even creative activity; however, when these defenses are less successful, Madeline is left quite vulnerable to profound feelings of helplessness and hopelessness. When these dysphoric feelings are intense, they are often infused with overly symbolic moral concerns about good and evil and their power over her on a cosmic level. In an ambiguous context, these moral concerns are often accompanied by hypervigilance and paranoid-like ideation involving feelings of persecution.

SELF AND OTHERS

Drawing particularly from the data provided by the ORI (see Appendix C) makes it possible to glean a great deal of information about Madeline's representations of her self in relation to significant others in her life. We do not attempt to provide an exhaustive rendition of her ORI descriptions at this juncture. Rather, we encourage the reader to refer to the full transcript in Appendix C, to gain a more complete appreciation of Madeline's extremely rich and vivid experience of these primary relationships in her own words.

Madeline describes her mother as a greedy, phony, closed-off, and withholding "witch." Indeed, whenever the word "woman" is mentioned (whether it be on the WAIS-III, the TAT, or the ORI), Madeline's immediate response is "witch!" What comes through in Madeline's conscious description of her mother is how impossible that relationship is and has been for her, to such an extent that she tries not to think about her mother in her present life. She acknowledges with frustration that her mother has never been willing to share her own inner life or past history. Consequently, Madeline has tried to give up on ever getting to know her mother. What she does know comes from her observations (i.e., what she has seen and heard on the surface). As Madeline explains, "She won't let you know her, so your questions remain questions. If you ask her about her childhood, she just gets up and leaves! So I'm left with just blanks." And, indeed, this blank emptiness is what Madeline has been left with in the desolation and hopelessness of her depression.

At a deeper level even than the emptiness, however, is the aching yearning for her mother that Madeline has always carried with her, but needs to deny in its painfulness. This yearning for tender bodily contact comes through most poignantly in Madeline's later description of herself, where she states, "There was never a baby in our family. The first time I ever kissed my mother was when she was lying in the hospital, having just slit her wrists on the kitchen table. I saw my cousin brushing her hair, and I was green with envy." Thus Madeline will acknowledge this longing as a memory, but not as a fundamental aspect of who she is in the present.

The projective assessment sheds additional light on why Madeline needs to deny her ongoing longing for maternal nurturance. First, the Rorschach suggests that closeness to a stereotypic female (in this case, a mother figure) may stir erotic feelings, which for Madeline would be totally unacceptable. And on the TAT, conventional women—mothers and wives—are defensively viewed by Madeline with contempt as weak, banal, pathetic victims of the more powerful, sexual male. When two women are portrayed together, the situation inevitably becomes one of rancor, bitterness, brutality, and the ultimate destruction of them both. There are other data from the Rorschach suggesting that Madeline is able to conceive of a relationship with a female peer as collaborative and mutually satisfying. The woman would have to be approximately Madeline's own age, however, so that she would not be consciously reminded of the inherently destructive mother figure. In addition, a female friend would have to be the kind of woman Madeline sees herself as being (i.e., unconventional, powerful, and compelling, with both women possessing many of the positive characteristics of the traditional male).

Madeline describes her father as a "mean, violent monster," who is not smart, but whom she remembers as "an incredibly hard worker." Seen as the "life of the party" outside the family, her father was both popular and highly respected. For his family members, however, his violence and his alcoholism appear to have dominated their experience of him. Nowhere in Madeline's conscious description of her father is there the slightest suggestion of longing that so permeates her description of her mother. In recalling her father's own alcoholic parents' death in a fire, one is reminded of Madeline's horrific response to Card IV of the Rorschach, where the helpless "little bugger" is first vomited upon (referring to her father's alcoholism, perhaps), and then standing helplessly in flames as the monster purposely burns him. Madeline herself recalls the memory of intending to smother her father—and, presumably, the flames of his violence—with a pillow so as to kill him. Although there is no longing for this man, the foregoing description suggests that in her willingness to take up the violence and kill her father, she is in fact partially identified with him out of necessity, in order to try to save herself and the rest of her family. This identification with the strength and power of the male is contained in Madeline's ideal self-representation as the victor over her past, portrayed dramatically on Card I of the Rorschach, where a highly androgynous, extremely powerful woman is professing something of great importance before a crowd of listeners. It is this view of herself that she lives out in her professional life. On a deeper level, this idealized combination of both male and female characteristics may translate into some gender confusion or question (in a way that is less conscious) about how female or male she is, actually in a more literal sense. The most vivid example of these gender concerns is expressed in her response to the last TAT card, in which she describes a man wearing woman's pants and going to his "gynecologist" for the rash on his scrotum.

When it comes to describing herself, Madeline states that she is smart, but otherwise is completely unable to reflect on herself at a conceptual level, apart from seeing herself as a combination of both her parents. Throughout the testing, we know that she wrestles with powerful polarities in herself—good versus evil, strong versus weak, guilty versus innocent, and victor versus victim or even victimizer. Her descriptions from the ORI indicate that she feels neither of her parents had anything to give to her in the way of nurturance, so that she never had anyone to help her to think about herself. Though she portrays her parents in such highly negative terms, her resiliency and maturity suggest, however, that there must have been some constructive relationships early in her life. As she rightly says, she is closed—but most importantly to herself. She is so oriented toward others, and with such great ambivalence, that she has never had the stable mirroring required to form a mirror image of herself. Thus she is not able to engage in self-reflection at any depth. This long-unmet need to learn about and to understand herself is very likely one of the primary motivations compelling her to undergo this entire arduous, elaborate series of assessment procedures. Despite her desperate need to have primary relationships with others and a lack of an elaborate sense of self, interestingly, Madeline also has a capacity to tolerate and even enjoy solitude. Solitude is experienced by Madeline primarily in sensory–motor terms, especially in relation to nature.

It does appear that in Madeline's long-time relationship with her male partner, she has found in her adult life someone she can truly love and be loved by in return. She emphasizes that he is kind and not weak, saying, "I used to mistake kindness for weakness, but he has said to me that they are not the same thing!" She goes on to indicate that he is handsome, very loving, fair, funny, jealous, a good cook, and a good man. Clearly this very androgynous man has many of the characteristics of both the traditional male and female. For Madeline, their relationship appears to have been redemptive. As she herself acknowledges, "I can't ever leave my partner because he knows too much about me—warts and all!"

SUMMARY OF THE FINDINGS

Madeline is very intelligent, creative, savvy, and street-smart; she is highly sensitive and interpersonally perceptive. Yet she is relatively unschooled and unsophisticated in her thinking on a conceptual level. Also, she has had a very traumatic childhood and adolescence, and never had the opportunity to develop stable and consolidated feelings about herself and significant others that can sustain her during times of stress and loss. Because of the deprivation she has experienced, as well as brutality and abuse, aggression is a very powerful force with which she struggles in both adaptive and maladaptive ways. Both on the TAT and the Rorschach, we see marked variability in functioning—from extremely original and creative thought, to intense and overwhelmingly painful affects, and unrealistic and distorted ideation. She has experiences of strength and joy juxtaposed with feelings of desolation and hopelessness. She is aware of her vulnerability to depression and fears that something about her is badly damaged, giving her an unusual degree of access to very painful thoughts and feelings. She tries to avoid these painful experiences by her high level of activity, sensation seeking, and engagement with others, as well as in her professional accomplishments and career.

The juxtaposition of the intense dysphoria with her remarkable accomplishments suggests the possible meaning that her participation in this entire process of evaluation has had for Madeline, in terms of her willingness to reveal herself in repeated intrusive evaluations with five different sets of evaluators all over the country. She experiences the nagging question of whether there is something wrong with her and whether she has really been able to escape and overcome her painful and traumatic past. The answer to these questions, in light of our findings, must clearly be both yes and no. In this regard, one must have great admiration and respect for her ability to have established a career that is so personally meaningful and relevant for her, especially given the incredible interpersonal and educational deficits she has experienced. It is also remarkable, given the traumas she has suffered at the hands of the very people who were responsible for caring for her, that she has apparently been able to achieve a long-standing, committed relationship with a man—one that is deeply satisfying and stable. Though Madeline is impressive in her capacity to overcome adversity and to cope effectively with difficult situations, one should not underestimate her profound vulnerability to intense dysphoric feelings of helplessness and hopelessness around issues of professional disappointment and especially around issues of interpersonal loss and loneliness. Although Madeline is determined to stand free and independent, and she fiercely asserts and defends her autonomy, at the same time she very much seeks and needs interpersonal contact, care, and nurturance.

9

Interpersonal Assessment

AARON L. PINCUS
MICHAEL B. GURTMAN

OUR APPROACH TO ASSESSMENT

The approach we take to this assessment can best be described as application, at the level of the individual case, of a nomological net developed from the transactional evolution of interpersonal personality theory and a highly generative structural model, the interpersonal circumplex (Gurtman, 1992; Kiesler, 1996; Leary, 1957; Pincus, 1994; Wiggins, 1996b). This approach emphasizes understanding personality within an interpersonal or relational context. However, interpersonal assessment is not limited to explicit, overt behavior between two proximal people. Our interpersonal nomological net includes stable personality traits that can be understood in light of contemporary trait theory (e.g., Wiggins & Trapnell, 1996); covert social-cognitive processes within cycles of transactional influence (Kiesler, 1996) and self-fulfilling prophecy (Carson, 1982); and lawful patterns of interaction (e.g., complementarity) related both to self-definition (Leary, 1957) and to motivational needs, wishes, and fears (Benjamin, 1996). Pincus and Ansell (2003) have proposed that interpersonal theory is consistent with more explicit object relations theories of personality, and that the nomological net described above can be applied to the inner object world with some precision (Heck & Pincus, 2001; Pincus, Dickinson, Schut, Castonguay, & Bedics, 1999). Our interpretation of Madeline G's self-report responses to two interpersonal inventories and her partner's ratings of Madeline on these same two inventories are evaluated within this nomological net and within the specific context of her life story as formulated by McAdams (see Chapter 7).

One purpose of the assessment is to articulate Madeline's view of herself as an interpersonal being and to identify any interpersonal difficulties that she experiences. In addition, for an interpersonal assessment to be comprehensive, it is helpful to have a well-acquainted peer or partner also provide a view of Madeline's interpersonal functioning and difficulties. Such ratings can provide possible confirmation or disconfirmation of Madeline's view, leading to additional inferences regarding Madeline's personality. In utilizing the assessment data, we will attempt to understand the stable personality traits (McAdams's [1995] first level) that can be identified by the basic circular measurement procedures underlying the instruments used. In addition, Madeline's interpersonal diagnosis (Leary, 1957) or structural summary (Gurtman, 1994; Gurtman & Balakrishnan, 1998), and its convergence with or divergence from her partner's ratings of her, provide further information to describe Madeline's personality based on the interpersonal circumplex. This allows us to make McAdams's (1995) second-level inferences regarding potential interpersonal motives, needs, and adaptations, as well as Madeline's typical ways of thinking about self and other, and the impact she may have on others in a range of relationships and social roles. These inferences are based on an amalgam of interpersonal theory and empirical research utilizing the interpersonal circumplex as an organizing framework.

INTERPERSONAL ASSESSMENT METHODS

Madeline completed two interpersonal tests: the Interpersonal Adjective Scales (IAS; Wiggins, 1979, 1995) and the Inventory of Interpersonal Problems–Circumplex (IIP-C; Alden, Wiggins, & Pincus, 1990; Horowitz, Alden, Wiggins, & Pincus, 2000), each predicated on and intended to operationalize the interpersonal circumplex model of personality (see Figure 9.1; e.g., Kiesler, 1983; Wiggins & Trapnell, 1996). In addition, Madeline's common-law husband (hereafter called her "partner") completed informant versions of the two tests, thus providing a valuable "other" perspective to go along with Madeline's subjective self-ratings (Wiggins, 1973b).

Description of Tests

The IAS is a measure of interpersonal traits, providing scores on each of the eight "octants" of Wiggins's (1995) interpersonal circumplex. The test consists of 64 personality descriptors (e.g., "distant," "firm," "extraverted," "charitable") divided evenly into the eight scales. Test takers rate themselves on each descriptor, using a Likert scale from 1 ("extremely inaccu-

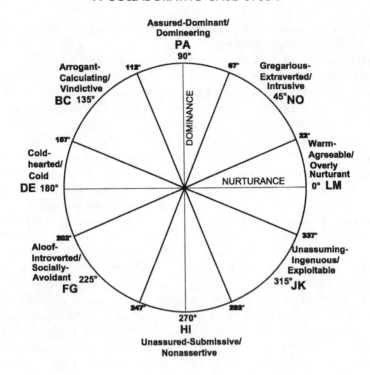

FIGURE 9.1. The interpersonal circumplex model of personality.

rate") to 8 ("extremely accurate"). Evidence for the reliability and validity of the test is summarized in the test manual (Wiggins, 1995).

The IIP-C is a 64-item circumplex measure of interpersonal problems, derived from the item pool of the original IIP (Horowitz, Rosenberg, Baer, Ureño, & Villaseñor, 1988). Items, in the form of problem statements, were developed on the basis of the presenting complaints of individuals seeking psychotherapy.

The IIP-C has two sections that assess forms of maladaptive interpersonal behavior consistent with the interpersonal perspective on maladjustment. The first section assesses enduring behavioral deficits and contains 39 items describing desirable behaviors that are hard to do (e.g., "It is hard for me to trust other people"). The second section assesses enduring behavioral excesses and contains 25 items describing undesirable behaviors that are done too much (e.g., "I fight with other people too much"). Test takers rate their degree of difficulty or distress on a Likert scale from 0 ("not at all") to 4 ("extremely"). Reliability and validity data appear in a number of sources, including Alden and colleagues (1990), Gurtman (1996), Gurtman and Balakrishnan (1998), and Horowitz and colleagues (2000).

Interpersonal traits and interpersonal problems converge in their basic circular structure. The relationship between interpersonal traits and interpersonal problems for the individual person requires further clarification. The interpersonal perspective on maladjustment emphasizes behavioral intensity and rigidity (Pincus, 1994), and interpersonal traits and problems correlate with each other in predictable ways (Alden et al., 1990). However, it is our view that while individuals exhibiting significant interpersonal problems are likely to be strongly "traited" along similar dimensions, the reverse is not inherently so (Pincus & Wiggins, 1990). Person–environment fit must also be considered. For example, a highly introverted individual who works the factory graveyard shift in a small rural town may not experience significant difficulties. But put the same person in a tension-filled advertising position for a Madison Avenue firm, and interpersonal problems are likely to ensue.

It should be noted that no IAS or IIP-C norms exist for Native Americans, and thus all scores were standardized using normative data from predominantly European American samples. Cultural sensitivity in personality assessment is a significant concern (Dana, 1993, 1994), and little assessment research has been done with regard to Madeline's Native American culture (Allen, 1998). Based on her life story, we assume that Madeline identifies strongly with both the majority culture and her Native American culture, thus achieving "bicultural immersion status" (Allen, 1998).

Analysis Approach

Madeline G's self-report IAS was scored for the eight octant scales of the Wiggins circumplex; each score's T-equivalent was obtained by applying the conversion table (norms for adult women) published in the test manual (Wiggins, 1995). Due to the lack of norms for IAS informant ratings, we used the same table to convert the partner's IAS ratings to T-scores.

The IIP-C octant scales were scored following Alden and colleagues (1990). At the time of this testing, a manual for the IIP-C (Horowitz et al., 2000) was in preparation, and hence adult norms were not available to us. Thus, to standardize raw scores to T-scores ($M = 50$, $SD = 10$), we used normative data from a study of married couples (Pincus, Boekman, & Laurenceau, 1994). These data were self-ratings and spouse ratings of IIP-C problems obtained from a sample of 110 husband–wife pairs.

Structural Summary

In the interpersonal tradition (e.g., Benjamin, 1996; Kiesler, 1996; Leary, 1957; Wiggins & Trapnell, 1996), interpersonal profiles are typically reduced to summary features that identify the individual's predominant interpersonal "trend" and the "intensity" or "extremity" of that trend. We follow a similar approach developed by Gurtman (1994; Gurtman & Bala-krishnan, 1998). This approach involves creating a "structural summary" of the profile by modeling the pattern of scores to a cosine-curve function. Accordingly, the profile is "decomposed" into two parts: a structured com-ponent (cosine function) reflecting the prototype for a circumplex, and a deviation component. As illustrated in Figure 9.2, the parameters of this curve are its (1) "angular displacement," or the peak shift of the curve, from 0°; (2) "amplitude," or peak value; and (3) "elevation," or mean level. (The coordinates in the analysis are the polar angles of the octant scales, as shown in Figure 9.1; e.g., LM at 0°, NO at 45°, etc.) The good-ness of fit of the modeled curve to the actual scores can also be calculated; the R^2 value essentially indicates the degree to which the profile can be re-duced to its summary features. Gurtman and Pincus (2003) provide a de-tailed description of the structural summary, as well as procedures for solv-ing for the various parameters.

Gurtman and Balakrishnan (1998) suggest interpretive guidelines that relate each of these summary features to clinical hypotheses. The angular displacement of the curve indicates the person's interpersonal "central ten-dency," signifying the individual's "typology" (Leary, 1957) or predomi-nant interpersonal "theme" (Kiesler, 1996). For example, based on the circumplex of Figure 9.1, a displacement of 135° suggests the central inter-personal qualities of distrust, exploitiveness, and vindictiveness (broadly, a hostile–dominant stance); 180° suggests lack of warmth and interpersonal distance; and so on. Amplitude is viewed as a measure of the profile's

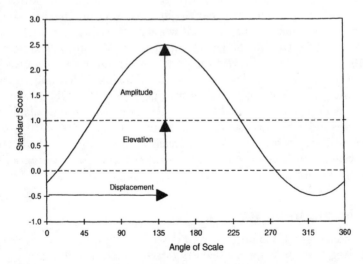

FIGURE 9.2. Illustration of the cosine-curve model. From Gurtman and Balakrishnan (1998). Copyright 1998 by Oxford University Press. Adapted by permission.

"structured patterning," or degree of differentiation, indicating the extent to which the predominant trend "stands out." An amplitude value of 0 indicates a flat (i.e., undifferentiated) profile; high amplitude indicates a profile with a clear interpersonal peak (and trough). Interpretation of elevation, or the mean level of the curve, depends in part on the circumplex model applied. Gurtman and Balakrishnan show that for an interpersonal-problems circumplex, elevation is an index of global interpersonal distress or maladjustment (high values indicating high overall distress); for an interpersonal-traits circumplex, elevation is probably best viewed as a response tendency (i.e., a nuisance factor that is not of substantive importance; see Gurtman, 1994).

RESULTS

Let us first look at Madeline's pattern of test responses—an indication of her general approach to the tests. On the IAS, she tends to respond with extreme answers—almost always (94%) endorsing either 1 or 8, depending on the octant category. Thus her cumulated octant scores tend to be quite high or quite low. On the IIP-C, she acknowledges difficulty (i.e., a nonzero response) on only 4 items out of the 64 (6%)—3 from the Overly-Nurturant (LM) octant and 1 from the Intrusive (NO) octant. On the other hand, her partner's ratings of her on the IAS and IIP-C are more typical in the range and usage of the response scales. In general, on both the IAS and IIP-C, he presents a more negative (i.e., hostile) picture of her interpersonal functioning than she does. Figures 9.3 and 9.4 show Madeline's IAS and

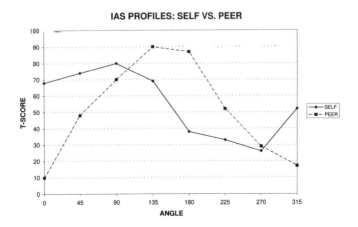

FIGURE 9.3. IAS profiles for Madeline's self-ratings and her partner's ratings of her (structural summary format).

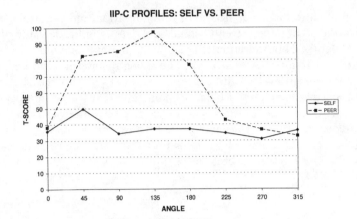

FIGURE 9.4. IIP-C profiles for Madeline's self-ratings and her partner's ratings of her (structural summary format).

IIP-C profiles, respectively; each figure also allows comparison of Madeline's self-ratings with her partner's perceptions. Table 9.1 presents the structural summary parameters that are based on these profiles.

As can be seen, with respect to the IAS, Madeline's self-reports indicate that she views herself as predominantly friendly–dominant. Her high amplitude and fit values suggest a well-defined interpersonal profile, with a clear peak (angular displacement) at 64° (on the border of the Assured–Dominant and Gregarious–Extraverted octants of the IAS). On the IIP-C, her resultant placement is again in the friendly–dominant region at 60°; however, her low elevation, low amplitude, and poor fit reflect her previously noted general denial of interpersonal problems.

Her partner's ratings of Madeline's interpersonal functioning provide a significantly contrasting view. With respect to interpersonal traits (the IAS), the partner perceives Madeline as predominantly hostile–dominant (at 146°); again, the profile pattern is well defined and has a single peak. Interestingly, he shares her view that she is dominant, but contrasts in his assess-

TABLE 9.1. Structural Summary for Self-Ratings and Partner Ratings on the IAS and IIP-C

Curve parameter	IAS		IIP-C	
	Self-rating	Partner rating	Self-rating	Partner rating
Displacement	64	146	60	115
Amplitude	26.5	39.8	4.3	33.7
Elevation	55.0	50.4	37.1	61.7
R^2 fit	.94	.97	.34	.93

ment of her along the hostile–friendly dimension. This pattern is replicated on the measure of interpersonal problems (the IIP-C): He reports that her interpersonal problems center in the hostile–dominant region (115°). With regard to global interpersonal adjustment, Madeline views herself as below average in interpersonal difficulty (elevation = 37.1), whereas her partner sees her as above average (elevation = 61.7).

Finally, it is worth noting the consistency observed in the assessments of interpersonal traits and interpersonal problems, suggesting further that the IAS and IIP-C are indeed tapping a common domain of personality. A useful measure of interpersonal correlation is the cosine difference, which is equal to the cosine of the difference between any two angles (see Gurtman, 1994, 1999). For Madeline's self-report IAS and IIP-C angles, the cosine difference is above .99; the partner's IAS and IIP-C angles agree .86. However, as expected from the previous descriptions, the agreement between self-ratings and partner ratings is much less, with an IAS correlation of .14 for the respective angles, and an IIP-C correlation of .57.

STANDARD IAS AND IIP-C PROFILES[1]

Figures 9.5 and 9.6 present the IAS profiles of Madeline's self-ratings and her partner's ratings of her, respectively, in the traditional format. Figures 9.7 and 9.8 present the traditional IIP-C profiles of Madeline's self-ratings and her partner's ratings of her, respectively.

INTERPRETATION

In the present case, there is some divergence in the ratings made by Madeline and her partner. Thus we must consider whether this arises because one person's or the other's responses are invalid, or because of personological reasons suggesting real differences in Madeline's experience of herself and her partner's experience of her. As will be detailed below, our view is that the "truth" may lie somewhere in between the two sets of responses. It is possible that neither respondent is without bias, and ultimately the interpersonal paradigm also recognizes that there are unique elements to specific relationships. This view does not imply that the most accurate result would be achieved by averaging the two sets of responses. It

---

[1] We have inserted these profiles into Pincus and Gurtman's original report for the benefit of those readers who are used to the "standard" format for presenting interpersonal profiles. It has been our experience that Gurtman's structural summary approach is most easily grasped in relation to standard profiles, at least for "old-timers."—K. K. T. and J. S. W.

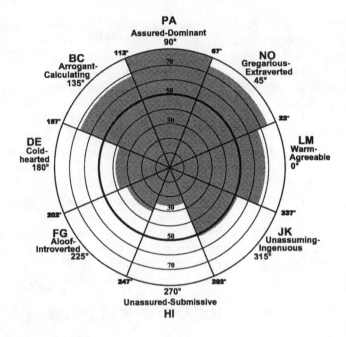

FIGURE 9.5. IAS profile for Madeline's self-ratings (standard format).

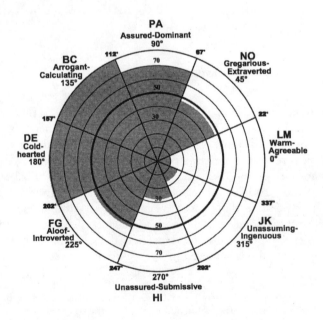

FIGURE 9.6. IAS profile for Madeline's partner's ratings of her (standard format).

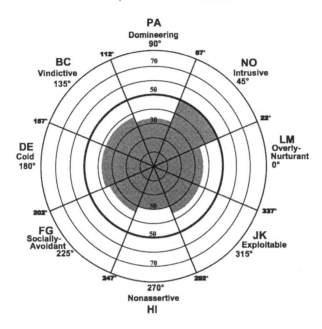

FIGURE 9.7. IIP-C profile for Madeline's self-ratings (standard format).

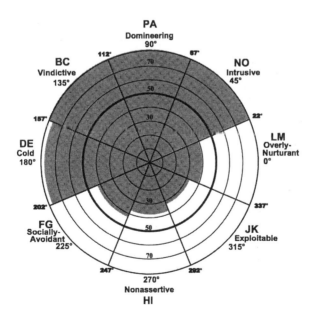

FIGURE 9.8. IIP-C profile for Madeline's partner's ratings of her (standard format).

merely suggests that interpretation proceed with the acknowledgment that neither set of ratings may be considered more accurate than the other. Madeline's responses are probably influenced by her own personality dynamics, and her partner's ratings of her may also be influenced by relationship issues at the time of the assessment.

We begin with item endorsement patterns (i.e., test-taking behavior). Madeline's partner endorses items in a fairly normative manner, utilizing the entire range of response scales. Madeline exhibits deviant item endorsement patterns on both tests. On the IAS, almost all items are endorsed as either 1, "extremely uncharacteristic" (typically descriptors reflecting submissiveness and hostility) or 8, "extremely characteristic" (typically descriptors reflecting dominance and nurturance). On the IIP-C, she denies any interpersonal difficulty or distress for the vast majority of problems assessed. Based on these response patterns, it appears likely that Madeline's profiles indicate a bias toward seeing herself in an overly positive light, reflecting a highly adjusted individual with strong agentic and caring qualities. This is consistent with her approach to the self-report testing reported in Chapter 7 by McAdams. In that testing, Madeline has also achieved high scores on the Big Five Inventory measures of Extraversion, Agreeableness, Conscientiousness, and Openness to Experience, and a remarkably high score on the Loyola Generativity Scale. It would be of interest to examine her item response patterns on those instruments.

We believe the congruence between Madeline's test-taking behaviors and her life story suggests that her responses reflect the ongoing process of how she sees herself, although this may be biased. That is, they may reflect the employment of security operations to maintain her experience of an idealized self-image (Sullivan, 1953b). Madeline's life story is permeated with themes of heroism, redemption, and reform. She appears so strongly committed (another identified theme) to progress in living out the third chapter of her life story that she cannot tolerate acknowledging personal qualities that are inconsistent with maintenance of her redeemed and reformed self. Madeline successfully began a new life after leaving jail for the final time. She was determined never to go back. Indeed, she hasn't gone back in a literal sense; nor does she "go back" in her self-ratings and incorporate much of her history in describing herself today. In Chapter 7, McAdams has noted Madeline's remark that she "routinely slices off bad things and people from the past" in her effort to keep moving forward. She also appears to "slice off," or selectively inattend to, that which is bad in herself (Sullivan, 1953b). The motives underlying Madeline's response biases make sense in the context of her life story. Therefore, instead of considering her responses invalid and restricting the remainder of our interpretation to her partner's ratings, we conclude that Madeline's self-ratings probably describe her ideal self, and her partner's ratings may better describe the typical interpersonal impacts Madeline has on others. However, as noted, her partner's ratings are also not free from potential biases. Therefore, we assume some generalizability from his ratings, while recognizing that they also reflect elements unique to this couple at this point in the relationship.

The fundamental dimensions of the interpersonal circumplex, dominance and nurturance, identify relatively enduring ways in which people perceive, think, feel, and behave in relational contexts. The structural summary parameters of angular displacement and amplitude are the most salient in this regard. In the present case, the most consistent information regarding Madeline is that she is a dominant person. Madeline's life story, her IAS and IIP-C self-ratings, and her partner's ratings of her converge in this regard. Her life is full of agentic themes, and the angular displacements of her interpersonal profiles also reflect this.

The discrepancies in angular displacements between Madeline's self-report ratings and her partner's ratings are due almost entirely to disagreement regarding Madeline's nurturance. Madeline's self-reports yield angular displacements that reflect the ideal of a strongly agentic and moderately nurturant woman with no interpersonal distress (i.e., low IIP-C elevation). Specifically, her amplitudes peak in the NO octant (bordering on PA), broadly reflecting a view of herself as "friendly–dominant." In contrast, her partner's angular displacements offer a view of Madeline as "hostile–dominant" and exhibiting some interpersonal adjustment difficulties (i.e., high IIP-C elevation), particularly with regard to being intrusive, domineering, vindictive, and cold.

The interpretive job here is a complex one. We must endeavor to account for the discrepancies while attempting to understand Madeline as an interpersonal being. Our approach is to interpret Madeline's responses as a description of her ideal self (the self she is striving to be) and her partner's responses as a description of Madeline's potential social impact. This places some limits on first-level interpretations and shifts emphasis toward second-level interpretations. Thus we limit first-level interpretations to the implications of Madeline's dominance—the trait that appears most consistently identified across observers and methods.

Madeline ideally sees herself as a woman who grants status and love to herself and to others (Wiggins & Trapnell, 1996), and reports being highly generative. She is a champion of Native Americans' legal rights and exerts her will to the fullest in furthering their causes. There appears no doubt that Madeline is an achiever with a strong will who is likely to take control of most situations. In most interactions, she typically expects to get what she wants and expects others to submit to her requests, follow her directions, and be convinced of her opinions. Professionally, this has led to a successful career as a defense attorney—where she is used to getting her way, winning, and enjoying victory. However, it is not clear that Madeline achieves these goals in ways that consistently grant love and status to others and that avoid interpersonal problems. Her partner's ratings are in agreement that she grants status and love to herself, but suggest that Madeline denies these social resources to others in her interpersonal interactions (Wiggins & Trapnell, 1996) and exhibits some interpersonal difficulties in relating to others. She clearly has the potential to deny others love and status, as her descriptions of her mother and father attest. Is this simply a case of Madeline being naively unaware of the impacts she has on others? We do not think it is that simple, and offer several hypotheses regarding this aspect of Madeline's assessment that suggest a more effortful use of security operations (Sullivan, 1953b). Notably, these hypotheses are not mutually exclusive, and we see them as potential complements rather than competitors.

One possibility is that Madeline's continuing view of the world as potentially dangerous, and her sense that she must always be on guard, vigilant, and ready to do battle, create a social context that normalizes a certain amount of hostility. In a doctoral dissertation some years ago, Foreman (1988) compared IAS self-ratings made by incarcerated prisoners and IAS ratings of the prisoners made by their guards. He found a consistent discrepancy similar to what we have observed in the present case. Guards and prisoners agreed that prisoners were dominant, but diverged with regard to nurturance. Guards saw prisoners as dominant and hostile, but prisoners simply saw themselves as dominant. In the prison context, where aggression and intimidation are normative, prisoners do not experience a basis for seeing themselves as particularly hostile. Madeline's history, which includes family violence, jail, and opposition to her strivings, may similarly have provided Madeline with a different normative context in which to evaluate herself. She appears to express care through competitive strivings rather than through interpersonal warmth. Thus championing her causes (self, Native Americans) is seen as an expression of nurturance, even if this is achieved through disaffiliative means.

There is additional evidence suggesting that the results of the assessment are best understood as reflecting Madeline's motives and adaptations, rather than naive lack of awareness of her social impact. Madeline herself hints at awareness of potential relational difficulties in disclosing anxiety about fitting in at her new law firm. She explicitly relates her anxiety to her interpersonal "presentation," suggesting that at some level she is conscious of the potential negative impacts she has on others. As noted previously, Madeline's test-taking behavior suggests that she is strongly motivated to progress in her fight to overcome her past and live out a successful life as a reformed and redeemed heroine. One adaptation she has made is to abandon her past by selectively inattending to all that reminds her of it. She enhances this by strongly identifying with her ideal self. Maintenance of her ideal self is an ongoing process. It is likely that in most situations, including her assessment, Madeline makes efforts to fight the good fight and strive toward her ideals. Thus, when presented with a series of trait descriptors and interpersonal problems, her responses reflect a somewhat unsophisticated effort to construct and reflect the ideal self. It does not appear that she is completely unaware of her potential interpersonal impacts and problems; rather, identification with her ideal self is simply a stronger motivation in the third chapter of her life. Given an opportunity to demonstrate this, for example, on objective personality tests, she follows through by using her adaptive strategy of slicing off attributes inconsistent with her ideal. It is notable that her partner sees Madeline as having significant interpersonal problems—specifically as being intrusive, domineering, vindictive, and cold. In her transformational epiphany in solitary confinement, Madeline realized she was becoming just like her father. In light of Madeline's description of her father in her life story, it is likely that these very same interpersonal problems would also apply to him. In order to live up to her ideal, Madeline is motivated to deny seeing any qualities in herself that might reveal similarity to that "fucking monster."

Ultimately, her partner's ratings and Madeline's own anxiety about fitting in at her new law firm suggest to us that as Madeline strives toward her ideal, she "comes on strong" and probably evokes a certain amount of frustration, hostility, competitiveness, distrust, and withdrawal in others. She is aware of this at a certain level, but is motivated to deny this impact most of the time. She may often experience such responses in others as indications of sought-after interpersonal "victories," given her preoccupation with agentic goals, while discounting her behavior's impact on intimacy goals (which are not currently salient for her).

A final hypothesis involves the possibility that Madeline exhibits a narcissistic character (Kernberg, 1996). We advance this hypothesis on the basis of the convergence of the present assessment results, research on narcissism and the interpersonal circumplex, and aspects of Madeline's developmental history. However, it is important to note that we are not pathologizing Madeline; nor are we proposing that she be seen as exhibiting narcissistic personality disorder. She is obviously a high-functioning woman with a successful career, a long-term relationship, and a satisfying social life. Nonetheless, perhaps the most integrative level of analysis of the present assessment can be made by considering the possibility that narcissistic personality dynamics underlie much of what we see.

Madeline's developmental history is consistent with Kernberg's (1984, 1992) description of the early environment of persons with narcissistic characters. Coldness, lack of love, and hostility are commonly responded to with the defensive development of a grandiose self-structure that protects such an individual from further psychological injury. However, the individual never develops a mature self that integrates idealized grandiose elements with negative elements and recognized limitations. This perpetuates an overly idealized view of the self; preoccupation with fantasies of unlimited success, perfect romance, and the like; and a tendency to ward off threat to this self-concept through cognitive splitting and alternately idealizing others who support the grandiose self, and devaluing others who challenge it. Finally, a common complaint of those with narcissistic personalities is boredom or emptiness. When life fails to provide sufficient support for the grandiose self, such individuals often complain of being bored, instead of articulating any personal affect such as depression, anxiety, or low self-esteem. When narcissism is viewed through the lens of the interpersonal circumplex, profiles very similar to those generated by Madeline's partner are typically recovered (Dickinson & Pincus, 2003; Gurtman, 1992, 1996; Pincus & Wiggins, 1990; Soldz, Budman, Demby, & Merry, 1993). Individuals with narcissistic personalities tend to be rated as hostile and dominant with respect to both interpersonal traits and problems.

Many of the preceding elements of narcissism are seen in Madeline's life history and interpersonal assessment. Her family environment was violent, unloving, and neglectful. Her early adjustment included acting out, drinking, and withdrawal. While in solitary confinement, Madeline fantasized about life in a perfect family. Her current predictions for her future also tend toward idealization—for example, predicting that she will be "wildly successful" at her new law firm. Her response biases on the IAS and IIP-C may reflect psychic splitting associated with an idealized grandiose self protected from acknowledgment of any weakness or problems. This is similar to her tendency to describe others as either completely devalued (e.g., her parents) or highly idealized (her partner). It is notable that she describes her partner as her "rock," providing solid support for everything she does. This may be quite true, but it lacks acknowledgment of the significant discrepancy of opinion between Madeline and her partner regarding her interpersonal functioning. Is this something she truly is unaware of, or does she selectively inattend to problematic aspects of her relationship, just as she selectively inattends to such things within herself? The apparent lack of integration in her experience of self and others seems rather pervasive. Finally, one concern Madeline expresses for her future is that she may become bored, which she describes as a warning signal of potential but unarticulated problems.

In offering the three foregoing hypotheses, we attempt to make sense of our interpersonal assessment results at the level of Madeline's motives and adaptations. In considering the future, we emphasize those issues most relevant to Madeline's interpersonal functioning: her new job, her relationship with her partner, and her future adjustment. We predict occupational success for Madeline. In fact, her interpersonal style is a good fit with the role requirements of a successful defense attorney, even if she fails to acknowledge some of the very qualities about herself that may ultimately contribute to her legal victories. However, there may also be pitfalls ahead. Indeed, she may not make the hoped-for positive interpersonal impacts on others at the law firm. A period of mutual adjustment may be necessary as both she and her colleagues negotiate their relationships through cycles of transactional influence. Hostile–dominant impacts may evoke competitive, hostile, or unsupportive responses in others. It is not clear how Madeline will handle critical feedback from others if it occurs. Will she accommodate and change, or will she devalue and ignore the opinions of others? Madeline has rarely if ever lost in court. How will she respond if a case does not go her way? Will she be able to accept such interpersonal feedback and profit from it, or will her passion for Native American rights and her need to maintain a positive self-image lead to externalizing blame (judges, juries, other attorneys) and pursuing endless appeals with little chance of legal success?

Madeline reports that her relationship with her partner is a very important source of support. However, Madeline's partner clearly holds a view of her that is divergent from the view she holds of herself. This divergence may become problematic in the future if it is not addressed. How will Madeline respond to such feedback from her partner? We simply do not know. However, if he communicates his views, will she accept them as part of the ongoing negotiation of their relationship? Or will such feedback be so dystonic that it will be ignored or devalued in order to maintain commitment to her ideal self-view and fulfill the need to see her partner in an idealized way? Madeline and her partner are likely to butt heads about this at some point, and its resolution will be critical to the stability of their relationship.

Finally, we predict that Madeline will continue to achieve, strive toward her agentic personal and professional goals, and successfully live out this third chapter in her life. However, the same basic concerns discussed with reference to occupational and relationship adjustment may remain a continuing challenge. In one sense, Madeline shows remarkable adjustment for someone with her background. Yet, in our opinion, this "adjustment" is a bit too constructed to be a certainty as yet. Madeline's redemption and reform thus constitute a work in progress. She will continue to rely on her dominance to achieve her agentic goals. If, in the future, she turns more of her attention toward intimacy goals, a more balanced view of her interpersonal self may be required. Thus the interpersonal domain of communion may be where Madeline's most difficult future challenges will be encountered.

10

Multivariate Assessment
NEO PI-R Profiles of Madeline G

PAUL T. COSTA, JR.
RALPH L. PIEDMONT

Our case study subject, Madeline G, provided a self-report on the Revised NEO Personality Inventory (NEO PI-R); her significant other completed Form R, the parallel observer form of the NEO PI-R. Unfortunately, there are no Navaho or even general Native American norms at present for the NEO PI-R. So Madeline's scale and domain scores are evaluated with respect to the adult female and/or combined norms in the NEO PI-R manual (Costa & McCrae, 1992). Although we have no evidence to indicate that using these norms leads to any particular errors of interpretation, it is possible that her standing on the various dimensions might change.

Madeline G answered all 240 inventory items, but did not answer Items A, B, and C on the bottom of the answer sheet. Items A, B, and C provide simple validity checks and alert the interpreter as to whether the test taker has completely and accurately completed the 240 items. Normally, when the respondent endorses "disagree" or "strongly disagree" to Item A (which asks whether the respondent has answered the items in an honest and accurate manner), the clinician would discuss with the respondent the reasons for a negative response to this item. Clinicians can in certain cases determine that the data are valid and interpretable, despite this response. (Items B and C are meant to remind and prompt the respondent to complete missing items and to double-check missing items on his or her answer sheet.) It is suggested that the professional clinician may wish to discuss with the respondent the reasons for the response or lack of response to determine whether or not the data are valid.

Madeline G's answers on Form S were entered into the NEO Software System (Costa, McCrae, & PAR Staff, 1994), which automatically screens the protocol for acquiescence (i.e., it counts the number of "agree" and "strongly agree" responses across all 240 items). Respondents with 150 or more acquiescent responses are indicated, and the report indicates to the interpreter that caution should be exercised because a strong acquiescence bias may have influenced the results. Madeline's protocol passed the acquiescence screen. Similarly, the computer program checks the answers for "nay-saying" responses and random responding; it also determines whether the same response option has been used over a long series of items. Although Madeline's protocol did not indicate excessive nay-saying or random responding, the NEO Software System provided a summary of the following responses: "strongly disagree" at 33.75%, "disagree" at 6.25%, "neutral" at 0.83%, "agree" at 10.42%, and "strongly agree" at 48.75%. Fewer than 18% of her responses are not extreme (i.e., either "disagree," "neutral," or "agree"). One of the things to note is that she has responded to the NEO PI-R with a great preponderance of extreme responses, which may overstate her standing on the various personality traits. Visual examination of her answer sheet did not reveal any changed answers, or any noticeable pattern of careless, random, or fixed responding.

TWO PERSPECTIVES ON MADELINE G

One of the unique strengths of the NEO PI-R is a parallel observer form, which we are fortunate to have on Madeline; it was completed by her significant other. The observer, her common-law husband, indicated that he answered all of the 240 items in an honest and accurate manner, and he placed his answers correctly on the answer sheet. The NEO Software System did not detect any acquiescence, nay-saying, or random responding. Visual examination of his answer sheet did not reveal anything remarkable.

Table 10.1 presents the self-report (Form S) and significant other's (Form R) ratings of Madeline. It is clear from an examination of her self-report domain scores that her profile is a very extreme one, and that impression is sustained from the observer's perspective. Both agree that Madeline exhibits high Extraversion, Openness to Experience, and Antagonism (low Agreeableness). Certainly we can be confident that Madeline has a strong, assertive personality that can easily imagine possibilities and move toward them in ways that may seem calculating and brusque, especially to her common-law husband.

As can be seen from Table 10.1, there are two domains in which Madeline's self-report diverges sharply from her significant other's view of

TABLE 10.1. Self-Report (Form S) and Significant Other's (Form R) Ratings of Madeline G

Scale	Madeline's self-report ratings (Form S)			Common-law husband's ratings (Form R)			Combined T-score	r_{pa}
	Raw score	T-score	Range	Raw score	T-score	Range		
Factors								
(N) Neuroticism	—	34	Very low	—	57	High	45	−1.26*
(E) Extraversion	—	89	Very high	—	61	High	79	1.75
(O) Openness to Experience	—	80	Very high	—	60	High	73	1.73
(A) Agreeableness	—	16	Very low	—	4	Very low	4	9.82
(C) Conscientiousness	—	57	High	—	41	Low	49	−0.55*
Neuroticism facets								
(N1) Anxiety	3	27	Very low	17	55	Average	40	−1.69*
(N2) Angry Hostility	21	67	Very high	30	78	Very high	76	3.25
(N3) Depression	0	27	Very low	13	53	Average	38	−1.30*
(N4) Self-Consciousness	4	26	Very low	17	60	High	42	−2.99*
(N5) Impulsiveness	25	69	Very high	24	72	Very high	74	2.97
(N6) Vulnerability	1	25	Very low	13	58	High	40	−2.65*
Extraversion facets								
(E1) Warmth	29	64	High	15	26	Very low	44	−4.20*
(E2) Gregariousness	32	82	Very high	24	59	High	74	1.37
(E3) Assertiveness	32	85	Very high	30	74	Very high	84	5.33
(E4) Activity	28	73	Very high	29	74	Very high	77	3.85
(E5) Excitement-Seeking	32	82	Very high	28	81	Very high	86	6.65
(E6) Positive Emotions	32	75	Very high	22	56	High	68	0.71
Openness facets								
(O1) Fantasy	28	74	Very high	24	71	Very high	74	3.24
(O2) Aesthetics	30	73	Very high	22	58	High	68	1.21
(O3) Feelings	32	77	Very high	22	54	Average	68	0.24
(O4) Actions	27	78	Very high	18	55	Average	69	0.32
(O5) Ideas	31	76	Very high	19	52	Average	66	−0.19*
(O6) Values	31	78	Very high	26	65	High	75	2.71
Agreeableness facets								
(A1) Trust	27	63	High	12	26	Very low	44	−3.89*
(A2) Straightforwardness	3	5	Very low	9	22	Very low	8	7.79
(A3) Altruism	27	58	High	10	10	Very low	32	−5.47*
(A4) Compliance	3	10	Very low	0	15	Very low	7	9.36
(A5) Modesty	5	11	Very low	1	13	Very low	6	9.48
(A6) Tender-Mindedness	26	66	Very high	11	24	Very low	44	−5.07*
Conscientiousness facets								
(C1) Competence	24	56	High	23	44	Low	50	−0.14*
(C2) Order	27	69	Very high	21	53	Average	63	0.22
(C3) Dutifulness	26	57	High	14	15	Very low	34	−4.10*
(C4) Achievement Striving	29	74	Very high	25	61	High	70	1.67
(C5) Self-Discipline	32	73	Very high	13	28	Very low	51	−6.24*
(C6) Deliberation	7	26	Very low	8	23	Very low	21	4.36

Note. *, significant discrepancy between self-report and significant other's ratings. Overall profile agreement: r_{pa} = .948 (very good agreement).

her (Neuroticism and Conscientiousness). Although observer ratings provide a unique source of information about a target individual, they should not be considered as the "gold standard" for interpreting those instances when discrepancies arise. Observer ratings generally agree with self-reports, but differences or disagreements can occur. Research on normal volunteers (McCrae, Stone, Fagan, & Costa, 1998) indicates that the reasons for such discordant perceptions are often idiosyncratic, frequently involving different interpretation of words or items, idiosyncratic or different behaviors that are considered, and unavailability of covert experience to the observer. On other occasions, such disagreements may speak more to the divergent perceptions of the two raters than to any inaccuracies in the self-report. An observer may only have access to a small spectrum of a target individual's life, observing the person only at home or at work. Nonetheless, an observer is able to comment on an individual's public self or reputation, to indicate how he or she may be perceived, and to suggest the interpretations that the social world may be making of the target's behavior. These types of insights are unobtainable from a self-report. Comprehensive assessment requires a judicious integration of both sources of information.

On the Neuroticism domain, the observer sees Madeline as being significantly higher on the Anxiety, Depression, Self-Consciousness, and Vulnerability facets. Clearly this person observes much more negative affect than Madeline has noted. There may be two interpretations here. First, the observer, given his intimate position, may see more of the distressed side of Madeline either than she is aware of or than she displays in her larger social world. She may not realize the extent of her own emotional distress, given her very strong dominance or social presence. If his ratings are based only on their own relationship and do not consider this broader picture, he may be overemphasizing these feelings. A second interpretation of his ratings of Self-Consciousness and Vulnerability may be that he interprets this negative affect as an inability to cope rather than as a manipulation tactic on her part, which may be her way of getting others to do things she wishes done.

The significant other perceives Madeline as being significantly lower on the Conscientiousness domain overall, and specifically on the facets of Competence (C1), Dutifulness (C3), and Self-Discipline (C5). Taken together, this pattern indicates that the observer believes that Madeline is not very resourceful or capable, that she really does not follow through on things as completely as she might, and is easily distracted and lacking in motivation. Madeline may not always be counted on to follow through on her commitments, even though she initially brings a creative vision, high energy, focus, and persuasiveness to the task. His very low rating of her on Self-Discipline (C5) suggests that he sees Madeline as very lacking in persistence and unable to complete her personal tasks in a timely manner. This conveys a sense of the important divergences between Madeline's views of herself and her significant other's views of her. Obviously, if we recognize her accomplishments—including graduating from law school and assuming a position in a prestigious law firm—we might regard the informant's low ratings on Self-Discipline and Competence as problematic. Madeline's significant other may have as his focus the intimate and personal contexts of their relationship, and he may not be attuned to the legal arena, which is so central to her self-concept. She may in fact be highly conscientious in the legal context, but may have only depleted resources of Self-Discipline and Competence in her intimate interpersonal context (see Muraven & Baumeister, 2000). Under this latter interpretation, the best estimate of her true Conscientiousness might be midway between her self-report rating and the observer's rating.

AN INTEGRATED PORTRAIT

Ideally, as McCrae (1993) has pointed out, when there is such a level of significant disagreement, the next step would be to go back to both sources and get further information to help resolve the discrepancies, as well as to help understand the distinct picture each source paints. But in this case, as so often is the case, that is not possible. In the absence of additional information, neither the self-report ratings nor the observer ratings can be given priority. Instead, we recommend the psychometrically based approach of aggregation or combining discrete sources of data: namely, averaging the two sets of ratings. This procedure is justified because, despite occasional divergences, the coefficient of profile agreement (r_{pa}; McCrae, 1993) indicates that the personality profiles of the self and the observer show very good overall agreement; both are obviously describing the same person. The best estimate of the true personality profile is thus the average of the two sets of ratings (adjusted to compensate for the reduced variance of averaged variables; see Appendix A in McCrae et al., 1998).

Figure 10.1 plots these adjusted average T-scores. If we start at the extreme left of Figure 10.1, considering Madeline G's standing on the Big-Five domains, Extraversion (E) and Agreeableness (A) are clearly her most extreme or distinctive features. An especially salient feature of Madeline's personality is her antagonistic interpersonal orientation to others. Her score on A (T-score = 4) is 4.6 standard deviations below the normative mean; the extreme lowness of this score can be appreciated from the fact that fewer than 3 out of 100,000 NEO PI-R test-takers would get A scores lower than hers. Briefly, Madeline is exceedingly antagonistic. She is characteristically suspicious of other people and skeptical of others' ideas and opinions. She can be callous in her feelings, and her attitudes are tough-minded in most situations. She prefers competition to cooperation, and she expresses hostile feelings directly with little hesitation (e.g., physical fights

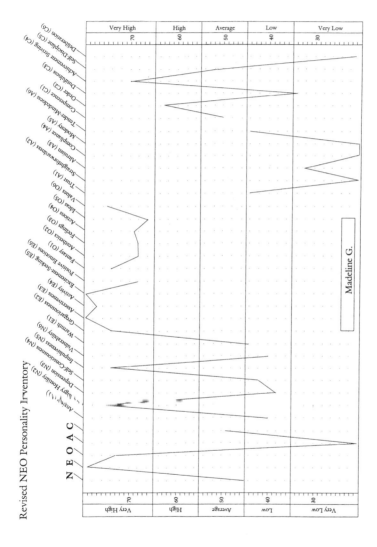

FIGURE 10.1. Combined Revised NEO Personality Inventory (NEO PI-R) profile of Madeline G. N, Neuroticism; E, Extraversion; O, Openness to Experience; A, Agreeableness; C, Conscientiousness. Profile form is reproduced by special permission of the publisher, Psychological Assessment Resources (PAR), Inc., 16204 North Florida Avenue, Lutz, FL 33549, from the Revised NEO Personality Inventory, by Paul T. Costa and Robert R. McCrae. Copyright © 1978, 1985, 1989, 1992 by PAR, Inc. Further reproduction is prohibited without permission of PAR, Inc.

in jail). People might describe her as relatively stubborn, critical, manipulative, or selfish. Although antagonistic people are generally not well liked by others, they are often respected for their critical independence, and their emotional toughness and competitiveness can be assets in many social and business roles.

Madeline is also extremely high in E. She is active and energetic. Extraverts greatly enjoy the company of others and the stimulation of social interaction, and Madeline is no exception. She prefers large parties and events to more intimate gatherings, and is often a group leader, taking the responsibility for initiating group activities. She is typically forceful, energetic, and fast-paced in style, and cheerful and enthusiastic in mood. Madeline likes excitement, and those who know her would describe her as very sociable, energetic, fun-loving, talkative, and joyful, but not warm or affectionate.

Next, let us consider Madeline's level of Openness to Experience (O). She is interested in experience for its own sake, seeking out novelty and variety. She has a very heightened awareness of her own feelings and can be perceptive in recognizing the emotions of others. Madeline is very responsive to beauty in art and nature, and is strongly attracted to new ideas and alternative value systems. She has difficulty passively accepting authority and honoring tradition; she prefers to see herself as a social maverick, finding unconventional attitudes and values congenial to her ways of thinking. Her common-law husband (the fact that they are not legally married may itself be a reflection of her resistance to convention and social custom) shares this view of Madeline, rating her as imaginative, daring, independent, and creative.

Madeline is average in Neuroticism (N). She is generally calm and able to deal with stress, but sometimes experiences feelings of guilt, anger, or sadness. She experiences a normal amount of psychological distress and has a typical balance of satisfactions and dissatisfactions with life. Madeline is neither high nor low in self-esteem, and her ability to deal with stress is as good as the average person's.

Finally, although Madeline is rated in the average range in overall Conscientiousness (C), her Achievement Striving scores are very high, and her need for Order is high. That is, she has very high aspiration levels and a clear sense of purpose and direction in life. She is also neat and well organized. Interestingly, Madeline is very low in matters dealing with ethical principles and moral obligations, as shown by her low ratings on Dutifulness. Also very low is her standing on Deliberation: She often speaks and acts in a hasty fashion without considering the consequences. At times, this appears as spontaneity and an ability to make snap decisions when necessary; at other times, this high level of impulsivity may be very problematic and maladaptive.

PERSONALITY STYLES: FACTOR PAIRS

But personality traits interact with each other and with other features of the person and the environment to account for the individual's actions and experiences. As the manual supplement for the NEO-4 (Costa & McCrae, 1998) indicates,

> Broad personality factors are particularly pervasive influences, and combinations of factors provide insight into major aspects of people's lives, defining what can be called *personality styles*. For many years, psychologists have noted that interpersonal interactions can be conceptualized in terms of a circular ordering or circumplex, defined by the two axes of Dominance versus Submission and Love versus Hate (Wiggins, 1979). Regarded as personality traits, these two axes are intermediate between the two personality factors of Extraversion and Agreeableness (McCrae & Costa, 1989). E and A thus define a personal style that is directly relevant to interpersonal relations; here it is called *Style of Interactions*. (p. 3; emphasis in original).

Figures 10.2 to 10.6 contain the 10 personality styles that result from combinations of the five domains. Let's consider the combination of the factors in terms of those that are most distinctive or salient for Madeline. As indicated at the top of Figure 10.2, Madeline's Style of Interests (E and O) is that of a Creative Interactor; she is interested in the new and the different, and enjoys meeting people from different backgrounds (recall that strippers joined musicians and college professors at her graduation party). Her Style of Interactions (E and A), as the bottom of Figure 10.2 indicates, is that of a Leader; she enjoys social situations, prefers to give orders, and believes that she is particularly well suited to make decisions. Such people "may be boastful and vain, but they also know how to get people to work together."

From the top of Figure 10.3, it can be seen that Madeline's Style of Well-Being (N and E) is that of an Upbeat Optimist; she is usually cheerful and has a keen appreciation of life's pleasures, but when faced with frustration she may become angry, although she puts these feelings behind her, preferring to concentrate on the future. She presents her Style of Defense (N and O) as that of an Adaptive individual who is keenly aware of conflict, threat, and stress, but uses these situations to stimulate creative adaptations (see bottom of Figure 10.3).

As can be seen from the top of Figure 10.4, Madeline's Style of Anger Control (N and A) is Cold-Blooded. Cold-blooded people "don't get mad, they get even." They often take offense, but instead of immediately reacting, they keep accounts; they then express their animosity and seek revenge at times and in ways that suit them. And from the bottom of Figure 10.5, it

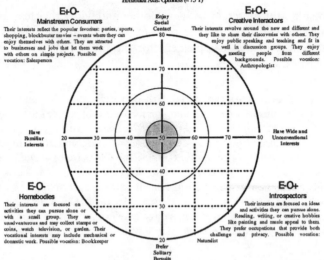

Style of Interests

Vertical Axis: Extraversion (= 79 T)
Horizontal Axis: Openness (= 73 T)

E+O-
Mainstream Consumers

Their interests reflect the popular favorites: parties, sports, shopping, blockbuster movies – events where they can enjoy themselves with others. They are attracted to businesses and jobs that let them work with others on simple projects. Possible vocation: Salesperson

Enjoy Social Contact

E+O+
Creative Interactors

Their interests revolve around the new and different and they like to share their discoveries with others. They enjoy public speaking and teaching and fit in well in discussion groups. They enjoy meeting people from different backgrounds. Possible vocation: Anthropologist

Have Familiar Interests

Have Wide and Unconventional Interests

E-O-
Homebodies

Their interests are focused on activities they can pursue alone or with a small group. They are unadventurous and may collect stamps or coins, watch television, or garden. Their vocational interests may include mechanical or domestic work. Possible vocation: Bookkeeper

Prefer Solitary Pursuits

E-O+
Introspectors

Their interests are focused on ideas and activities they can pursue alone. Reading, writing, or creative hobbies like painting and music appeal to them. They prefer occupations that provide both challenge and privacy. Possible vocation: Naturalist

Style of Interactions

Vertical Axis: Extraversion (= 79 T)
Horizontal Axis: Agreeableness (= 4 T)

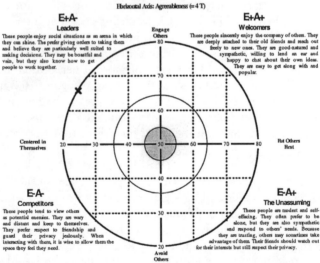

E+A-
Leaders

These people enjoy social situations as an arena in which they can shine. They prefer giving orders to taking them and believe they are particularly well suited to making decisions. They may be boastful and vain, but they also know how to get people to work together.

Engage Others

E+A+
Welcomers

These people sincerely enjoy the company of others. They are deeply attached to their old friends and reach out freely to new ones. They are good-natured and sympathetic, willing to lend an ear and happy to chat about their own ideas. They are easy to get along with and popular.

Centered in Themselves

Put Others First

E-A-
Competitors

These people tend to view others as potential enemies. They are wary and distant and keep to themselves. They prefer respect to friendship and guard their privacy jealously. When interacting with them, it is wise to allow them the space they feel they need.

Avoid Others

E-A+
The Unassuming

These people are modest and self-effacing. They often prefer to be alone, but they are also sympathetic and respond to others' needs. Because they are trusting, others may sometimes take advantage of them. Their friends should watch out for their interests but still respect their privacy.

FIGURE 10.2. NEO PI-R style graphs of Madeline G: Style of Interests (above) and Style of Interactions (below). The style graphs here and in Figures 10.3–10.6 are reproduced by special permission of the publisher, Psychological Assessment Resources (PAR), Inc., 16204 North Florida Avenue, Lutz, FL 33549, from the NEO PI-R Interpretive Report, by Paul T. Costa, Robert R. McCrae, and PAR Staff. Copyright © 1985, 1988, 1992, 1994, 2000 by PAR, Inc. Further reproduction is prohibited without permission of PAR, Inc.

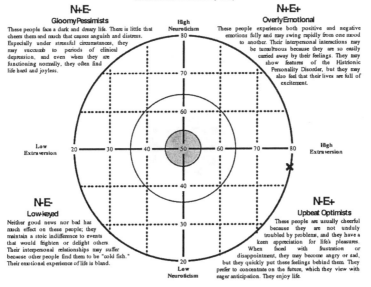

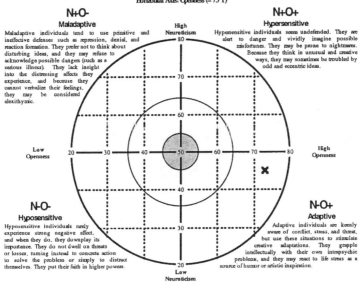

FIGURE 10.3. NEO PI-R style graphs of Madeline G: Style of Well-Being (above) and Style of Defense (below).

can be seen that her Style of Attitudes (O and A) is that of a Free-Thinker. She is swayed neither by tradition nor by sentimentality, and is willing to disregard others' feelings in pursuing her own idea of truth. No single Style of Impulse Control (N and C) is indicated, because her N and C scores are average, and thus she is likely to show some features of each style (see bottom of Figure 10.4).

For the remaining styles Madeline is less prototypical, occupying two descriptors. Thus, from the top of Figure 10.5, it can be seen that Madeline's Style of Activity (E and C) is that of a Funlover and to a lesser degree that of a Go-Getter. As a Funlover, she is full of energy and vitality, but sometimes finds it difficult to channel her energy in constructive directions. As a Go-Getter, she is productive and can be eager to pitch in and follow her goals with zeal.

Figure 10.6 shows that Madeline's Style of Learning (O and C) is that of both a Dreamer (she is attracted to new ideas and can develop them with imaginative elaborations, but may get lost in flights of fantasy, is less successful in completing projects, and needs help in staying focused) and a Good Student (combining a real love of learning with diligence and organization to excel; she has a high aspiration level and often uses creative approaches to solving problems). Madeline's Style of Character (A and C) can be both Undistinguished (more concerned with her own comfort and pleasure than with the well-being of others) and that of a Self-Promoter (concerned first and foremost with her own needs and interests, effective in pursuing her own ends, and highly successful in business and politics because of her single-minded pursuit of her own interests).

FACET-LEVEL INTERPRETATION

It is precisely because broad domains are heterogeneous with respect to content that we need to focus on particular components or facet scales of the NEO PI-R (see Table 10.1). The most interesting thing about Madeline's N is the great deal of scatter among the facet scales, most notably the twin peaks on the Angry Hostility and Impulsiveness facets. In terms of negative affect, she scores low in Anxiety and Depression. Similarly, her Self-Consciousness and Vulnerability scores are in the low range, suggesting that her self-esteem and emotional hardiness are good. Her high elevation on N2 (Angry Hostility) highlights the fact that she readily experiences anger and related states, such as frustration and bitterness. Her high score on N2 indicates that she is temperamental and quick to anger, and her Style of Anger Control would clearly be Temperamental if one were to substitute N2 for the overall N score. If we focus on Anxiety and Depression, combined with her low A scores, we see how she fits the Cold-Blooded style. The high hostility in the context of her extremely antagonistic interpersonal

Style of Anger Control

Vertical Axis: Neuroticism (= 45 T)

Horizontal Axis: Agreeableness (= 4 T)

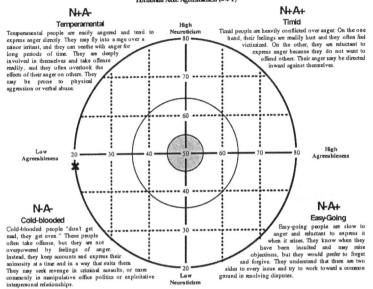

N+A-
Temperamental

Temperamental people are easily angered and tend to express anger directly. They may fly into a rage over a minor irritant, and they can seethe with anger for long periods of time. They are deeply involved in themselves and take offense readily, and they often overlook the effects of their anger on others. They may be prone to physical aggression or verbal abuse.

N+A+
Timid

Timid people are heavily conflicted over anger. On the one hand, their feelings are readily hurt and they often feel victimized. On the other, they are reluctant to express anger because they do not want to offend others. Their anger may be directed inward against themselves.

Low Agreeableness

High Agreeableness

N-A-
Cold-blooded

Cold-blooded people "don't get mad, they get even." These people often take offense, but they are not overpowered by feelings of anger. Instead, they keep accounts and express their animosity at a time and in a way that suits them. They may seek revenge in criminal assaults, or more commonly in manipulative office politics or exploitative interpersonal relationships.

N-A+
Easy-Going

Easy-going people are slow to anger and reluctant to express it when it arises. They know when they have been insulted and may raise objections, but they would prefer to forget and forgive. They understand that there are two sides to every issue and try to work toward a common ground in resolving disputes.

Style of Impulse Control

Vertical Axis: Neuroticism (= 45 T)

Horizontal Axis: Conscientiousness (= 49 T)

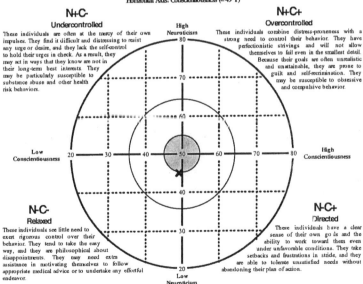

N+C-
Undercontrolled

These individuals are often at the mercy of their own impulses. They find it difficult and distressing to resist any urge or desire, and they lack the self-control to hold their urges in check. As a result, they may act in ways that they know are not in their long-term best interests. They may be particularly susceptible to substance abuse and other health risk behaviors.

N+C+
Overcontrolled

These individuals combine distress-proneness with a strong need to control their behavior. They have perfectionistic strivings and will not allow themselves to fail even in the smallest detail. Because their goals are often unrealistic and unattainable, they are prone to guilt and self-recrimination. They may be susceptible to obsessive and compulsive behavior.

Low Conscientiousness

High Conscientiousness

N-C-
Relaxed

These individuals see little need to exert rigorous control over their behavior. They tend to take the easy way, and they are philosophical about disappointments. They may need extra assistance in motivating themselves to follow appropriate medical advice or to undertake any effortful endeavor.

N-C+
Directed

These individuals have a clear sense of their own goals and the ability to work toward them even under unfavorable conditions. They take setbacks and frustrations in stride, and are able to tolerate unsatisfied needs without abandoning their plan of action.

FIGURE 10.4. NEO PI-R style graphs of Madeline G: Style of Anger Control (above) and Style of Impulse Control (below).

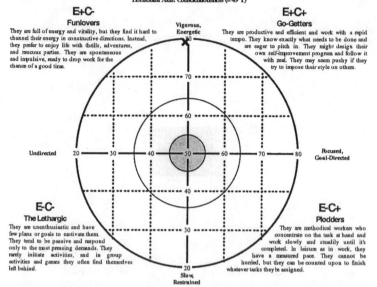

Style of Activity

Vertical Axis: Extraversion (= 79 T)

Horizontal Axis: Conscientiousness (= 49 T)

E+C-
Funlovers

They are full of energy and vitality, but they find it hard to channel their energy in constructive directions. Instead, they prefer to enjoy life with thrills, adventures, and raucous parties. They are spontaneous and impulsive, ready to drop work for the chance of a good time.

Vigorous, Energetic

E+C+
Go-Getters

They are productive and efficient and work with a rapid tempo. They know exactly what needs to be done and are eager to pitch in. They might design their own self-improvement program and follow it with zeal. They may seem pushy if they try to impose their style on others.

Undirected

Focused, Goal-Directed

E-C-
The Lethargic

They are unenthusiastic and have few plans or goals to motivate them. They tend to be passive and respond only to the most pressing demands. They rarely initiate activities, and in group activities and games they often find themselves left behind.

Slow, Restrained

E-C+
Plodders

They are methodical workers who concentrate on the task at hand and work slowly and steadily until it's completed. In leisure as in work, they have a measured pace. They cannot be hurried, but they can be counted upon to finish whatever tasks they're assigned.

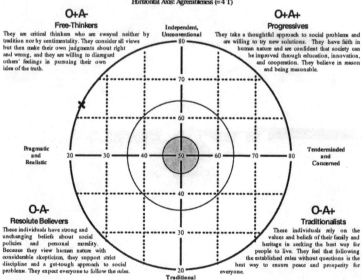

Style of Attitudes

Vertical Axis: Openness (= 73 T)

Horizontal Axis: Agreeableness (= 4 T)

O+A-
Free-Thinkers

They are critical thinkers who are swayed neither by tradition nor by sentimentality. They consider all views but then make their own judgments about right and wrong, and they are willing to disregard others' feelings in pursuing their own idea of the truth.

Independent, Unconventional

O+A+
Progressives

They take a thoughtful approach to social problems and are willing to try new solutions. They have faith in human nature and are confident that society can be improved through education, innovation, and cooperation. They believe in reason and being reasonable.

Pragmatic and Realistic

Tenderminded and Concerned

O-A-
Resolute Believers

These individuals have strong and unchanging beliefs about social policies and personal morality. Because they view human nature with considerable skepticism, they support strict discipline and a get-tough approach to social problems. They expect everyone to follow the rules.

Traditional

O-A+
Traditionalists

These individuals rely on the values and beliefs of their family and heritage in seeking the best way for people to live. They feel that following the established rules without questions is the best way to ensure peace and prosperity for everyone.

FIGURE 10.5. NEO PI-R style graphs of Madeline G: Style of Activity (above) and Style of Attitudes (below).

Style of Learning

Vertical Axis: Openness (= 73 T)
Horizontal Axis: Conscientiousness (= 49 T)

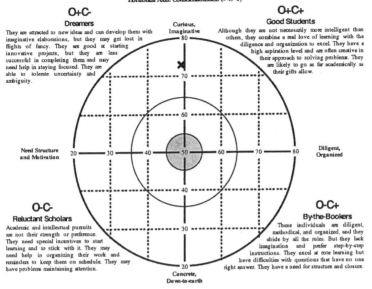

O+C-
Dreamers

They are attracted to new ideas and can develop them with imaginative elaborations, but they may get lost in flights of fancy. They are good at starting innovative projects, but they are less successful in completing them and may need help in staying focused. They are able to tolerate uncertainty and ambiguity.

Curious,
Imaginative
— 80 —

O+C+
Good Students

Although they are not necessarily more intelligent than others, they combine a real love of learning with the diligence and organization to excel. They have a high aspiration level and are often creative in their approach to solving problems. They are likely to go as far academically as their gifts allow.

Need Structure
and Motivation

Diligent,
Organized

O-C-
Reluctant Scholars

Academic and intellectual pursuits are not their strength or preference. They need special incentives to start learning and to stick with it. They may need help in organizing their work and reminders to keep them on schedule. They may have problems maintaining attention.

O-C+
By-the-Bookers

These individuals are diligent, methodical, and organized, and they abide by all the rules. But they lack imagination and prefer step-by-step instructions. They excel at rote learning but have difficulties with questions that have no one right answer. They have a need for structure and closure.

Concrete,
Down-to-earth

Style of Character

Vertical Axis: Agreeableness (= 4 T)
Horizontal Axis: Conscientiousness (= 49 T)

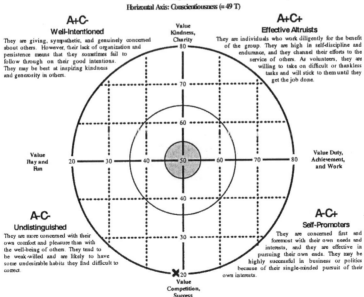

A+C-
Well-Intentioned

They are giving, sympathetic, and genuinely concerned about others. However, their lack of organization and persistence means that they sometimes fail to follow through on their good intentions. They may be best at inspiring kindness and generosity in others.

Value
Kindness,
Charity
— 80 —

A+C+
Effective Altruists

They are individuals who work diligently for the benefit of the group. They are high in self-discipline and endurance, and they channel their efforts to the service of others. As volunteers, they are willing to take on difficult or thankless tasks and will stick to them until they get the job done.

Value
Play and
Fun

Value Duty,
Achievement,
and Work

A-C-
Undistinguished

They are more concerned with their own comfort and pleasure than with the well-being of others. They tend to be weak-willed and are likely to have some undesirable habits they find difficult to correct.

A-C+
Self-Promoters

They are concerned first and foremost with their own needs and interests, and they are effective in pursuing their own ends. They may be highly successful in business or politics because of their single-minded pursuit of their own interests.

Value
Competition,
Success

FIGURE 10.6. NEO PI-R style graphs of Madeline G: Style of Learning (above) and Style of Character (below).

style (low A) indicates the potential problem that conflicts can occur easily and escalate rapidly. It would not be surprising to learn that her history of relationships is replete with incidents of bitterness, acrimony, and physical fighting.

A potential concern is that of inappropriate anger episodes and displays and her personal resources to control them. Consider Madeline's score on N5 (Impulsiveness); such a high level signifies that she has frequent and intense urges and impulses. Again we want to be alert to other aspects of her personality profile that might help restrain or modulate their activation or expression (especially C5, Self-Discipline, and C6, Deliberation). Persons who are high in Impulsiveness experience a great deal of difficulty in controlling their desires and urges, and situations that require them to resist temptations may further exacerbate tendencies to feel hostility and bitterness. We have some indication that she has had experience with drugs and alcohol, but whether this history points to a characteristic pattern of problems is unknown.

The most striking things about Madeline's E facets are the consistent and extremely high scores on Assertiveness, Excitement-Seeking, Activity, Gregariousness, and Positive Emotions. She greatly prefers the company of others (the more the merrier), is forceful and dominant with others, is rarely a wallflower, is energetic and busy, does things with gusto and a rapid tempo, and craves thrills and stimulation. Her high E6 (Positive Emotions), score indicates that she often bubbles over with cheer, joy, and happiness. Her average N, and particularly her low N3 (Depression), along with her high E6 (Positive Emotions), indicates that she is a happy person and would be unlikely to seek treatment. By contrast, her score on E1 (Warmth), seems low, but it is on the cusp between average and low. The picture one gets is that she is forceful, active, voluble, and venturesome—in an "in-your-face" manner—but at the same time she is somewhat detached and formal, keeping others at somewhat of an emotional distance, including her common-law husband.

Madeline scores very high on all six O facets, indicating that she has a vivid imagination and an active fantasy life; she is responsive to beauty as found in art or nature; and she experiences feelings and emotional reactions that are both varied and important to her. Madeline enjoys new and different activities. She is interested in intellectual challenges and in unusual ideas and perspectives, and is generally liberal in her social, political, and moral beliefs.

As her profile reveals, the A facets demonstrate a similar, if reverse, pattern of peaks and valleys. We see four very low scores (T-scores less than 35) on the facets of A2 (Straightforwardness), A3 (Altruism), A4 (Compliance), and A5 (Modesty), and two low scores (T-scores between 35 and 44) on the A1 (Trust) and A6 (Tender-Mindedness) facets. Her extremely low A2 (Straightforwardness) scores, in conjunction with her cynical and suspicious views of others (A1, Trust), suggest that she is more than willing to manipulate, con, or flatter people into doing what she wants. Direct or straightforward communication is not her preferred interactional style; deception and manipulation are not infrequent parts of her daily interactions. She is characteristically shrewd and cunning in dealing with others.

Madeline is not thoughtful and considerate of others (very low A3, Altruism). She is self-centered and can be exploitative, nasty, and/or aggressive when it suits her purposes. As undesirable as these interpersonal traits may be, her tendency to be self-centered and selfish has its adaptive or beneficial aspects. Persons with these traits can protect themselves and others from exploitation and victimization, and are less likely to lose in conflicts or struggles because they are so self-focused. When we consider her high levels of assertiveness and activity, we add fuel to her "egocentric fire." They support her supporting her own adaptation and needs. On the other hand, her extremely low A4 (Compliance) scores reflect a predisposition for aggression. Persons with very low A4 scores tend to be argumentative, contentious, stubborn, and belligerent, and can be physically aggressive. High scorers on A5 are humble and self-effacing. Her standing on A5 (Modesty), however, is very extreme and exceedingly low. She often appears to others as conceited, arrogant, boastful, and even pompous, as her significant other concurs. She is so immodest that others may see her as narcissistic. Compared to other people, then, Madeline is hard-headed and tough-minded, and her social and political attitudes reflect her pragmatic realism.

Madeline is perceived as being reasonably efficient and generally sensible and rational in making decisions (C1, Competence). She is described as very neat, punctual, and well organized (C2, Order); but her low to very low score on C3 (Dutifulness) indicates that she is not very dependable and reliable, and is more likely to bend the rules than the average person. She has a high aspiration level and strives for excellence in whatever she does (C4, Achievement Striving). Madeline is average in C5 (Self-Discipline) and generally finishes the tasks she starts. She tends to be quite hasty, careless, and impetuous and sometimes acts without considering all the consequences.

POTENTIAL PROBLEMS IN LIVING

Personality disorders can be conceptually characterized by a prototypic profile of NEO PI-R facets that are consistent with the definition of the disorder and its associated features. McCrae's (1993) coefficient of profile agreement can be used to assess the overall similarity of a patient's personality to each of the 10 *Diagnostic and Statistical Manual of Mental Disorders*, fourth edition (DSM-IV) personality disorder prototypes. In clinical settings, it is possible to develop hypotheses about personality disorders. If Madeline were a treatment-seeking patient, then her profile might suggest several DSM-IV Axis II disorders, particularly antisocial (APD), histrionic (HST), and narcissistic (NAR) personality disorders. It is even possible to see some of the features of these disorders in her life history. For example, we can see evidence in her life narrative for APD in her jail experience (including fights), explosive and irritable temperament (low A and low C), and immaturity leading to physically aggressive ways of dealing with conflict. Evidence for HST includes her strong self-focus, overdramatizing behaviors, and need to be the center of attention. Finally, we see evidence for NAR in Madeline's low Modesty, Straightforwardness, and Compliance traits—all of which contribute to a very self-focused, ego-expansive orientation.

PERSONALITY AND THE LIFE COURSE

Whereas personality has been shown to be relatively stable and displays great continuity in the decades from adulthood to old age (the 30s to 90s), there are significant developmental changes and shifts in the five dimensions from the early teens to the late 20s and 30s, which are being documented by findings of cross-cultural maturational patterns (McCrae et al., 1999; McCrae, Costa, Ostendorf, et al., 2000). It is also of interest to note that basic tendencies, whether they are stable or changing, influence and find expression in characteristic adaptations or maladaptations (McCrae & Costa, 1996). It is particularly instructive in this regard to consider Madeline's extreme scatter on the Agreeableness–Antagonism facet scales. In an earlier period of her life, these motivations may have contributed more to characteristic maladaptations (fights, drinking, etc.); in later periods, as an adult, these same enduring aspects of her personality appear to have fostered more successful characteristic adaptations (her law career). What better career for a person with this antagonistic profile to channel her aggressive tendencies into socially directed ways, than as a lawyer securing the civil rights of underdogs? It is interesting to consider that the enduring personality traits that were earlier maladaptive now seek adaptive expression and foster socially desirable projects and aims. What factors might have led to this turnabout? In addition to the themes of redemption and of significant interactions with mentors (e.g., her common-law husband) that McAdams identifies in Chapter 7, one possibility resides in age-related changes in personality traits—namely, declines in thrill seeking and negative affectivity, and corresponding increases in aspects of Conscientiousness, especially her Achievement Striving and Self-Discipline (McCrae, Costa, Ostendorf, et al., 2000).

As a mature adult, Madeline is unquestionably a socially dominant and forceful individual, very much her own woman with a clear set of goals and purposes. We know that she sees herself more positively than her significant other sees her; this might be an operational definition for narcissism (i.e., overstating one's own positive attributes), but it is also part of her enduring experiential style. Her experience is extremely intense and vivid; she is open and unconventional; and she may be perceived as quite unpredictable and perhaps unstable, and lacking in self-direction. But there is no question that when external events that occupy her attention coincide with her own aims, she has the wherewithal, energy, and focus to be a very powerful person. At the same time, these attributes, which are strengths in certain contexts, may contribute to problems in living in other contexts—especially those involving intimacy, nurturance, acceptance, tolerance, and forgiveness.

In Chapter 7, McAdams describes the central dynamic of Madeline as both power and intimacy motivation. Her NEO PI-R profile is consistent with the notion that power motivation is a cardinal characteristic. On the other hand, her profile does not suggest that she has strong intimacy motives. Clearly underexpressed or latent aspects of her personality have to do with what Wiggins, in Part I of this book (see especially Chapter 6), calls "communion goals." Intimacy or communion for Madeline is expressed only in abstract forms as embodied in victorious legal rulings and case law, and not in the more direct, concrete, and personal forms. Warmth and caring take a back seat to her high levels of Gregariousness and Assertiveness. Close relationships are not characteristic parts of her personality; rather, they are expressed more attitudinally and cognitively as high levels of Altruism, Tender-Mindedness, and Trust. Interestingly, her very high Loyola Generativity Score (57 out of 60) is consistent with these cognitive or attitudinal expressions. Her "generativity" is strained through more abstract filters, and with respect to her personality profile (Figure 10.1), her low Warmth, high Angry Hostility, and low Compliance (or aggressiveness) make sustained personal expressions of warmth unlikely.

As Madeline prepares to move into a new phase of her professional and perhaps personal life, she may wish to consider some issues as she goes forward, given her NEO PI-R profile. First, we would expect that she is unlikely to desire to become a mother and have children. Given her passion for her work, it seems that she would have trouble balancing the needs of her career with those of a family. Relatedly, intimacy and submitting to a traditional husband would be problems for her; if she were to be in a traditional relationship, it could be fiery and tempestuous.

Other continuing concerns relate to her health behaviors and health habits. Her NEO PI-R profile indicates an impulsive orientation: high N5 (Impulsiveness), high E5 (Excitement Seeking), and low C6 (Deliberation). These characteristics can put people at risk to engage in potentially harmful, addictive behaviors (see Piedmont, 1998). As such, she should be careful to avoid drugs, limit consumption of alcohol, and watch what she eats. Temper and anger control will be important, especially as she moves into her new law office. It is noted in her life narrative that she has just given up smoking; this is a positive step, but one that may require much effort and energy if she is to continue to be successful.

Madeline needs to have safeguards from her own impulsiveness. Her legal career and her significant other are important to her and provide those kinds of safeguards. Depending upon how different situational factors may impinge upon her, the elements of her personality that reflect impulsive sensation seeking (e.g., high Impulsiveness, Angry Hostility, and Excitement-Seeking; low Compliance, low Deliberation) will need to be constrained. If not, then it is possible that provocative events may interact to create a situation, like the action of a full moon or a hurricane producing abnormally high tides, where a concatenation of her worst traits could occur and lead to real problems. As noted in her life narrative, she too intuits this potential and evidences realistic concerns about it. However, she does have temperamental resources to draw on to manage this stressor. Her levels of Openness to Experience provide flexibility and a capacity to respond to challenges that come her way in creative ways. Madeline's high Activity and Positive Emotions, and low Vulnerability (to stress), are other assets that should propel her on a positive life trajectory.

ACKNOWLEDGMENTS

We wish to express appreciation to Paul Jurica and R. Bob Smith for their assistance in scoring the NEO PI-R and granting permission to present the results in this chapter. Special thanks are also happily given to Jeffrey Herbst, Robert McCrae, and Thomas Widiger for critical comments on earlier versions of this chapter, and especially to Krista K. Trobst and Jerry S. Wiggins for their invitation.

11

Empirical Assessment
The MMPI-2 Profile of Madeline G

YOSSEF S. BEN-PORATH

Madeline G's basic Minnesota Multiphasic Personality Inventory—2 (MMPI-2) profile is reproduced in Figure 11.1, following the revised format of the recent MMPI-2 manual update (Butcher et al., 2001). MMPI-2 interpretations typically provide a description of the test taker without reference to the specific sources for interpretive comments. For the benefit of readers unfamiliar with the intricacies of MMPI-2 interpretation, an annotated analysis (identifying the specific MMPI-2 sources of interpretive statements) is provided. This is followed by a summary description containing typical interpretive comments in narrative format. In the final part of this chapter, the MMPI-2 data are considered in the context of McAdams's life story analysis of Madeline (see Chapter 7).

Prior to proceeding to interpret Madeline's MMPI-2 profile, it is important to consider what impact her status as a Native American might have on this process. Use of the MMPI (and to a lesser extent the MMPI-2) with minority group members has in the past been criticized. Detailed consideration of this topic runs beyond the scope of this chapter; however, research with African Americans has provided consistent findings that the MMPI-2 is equally valid for African Americans and European Americans (Graham, 2000).

Research on the MMPI-2's validity with Native Americans is much

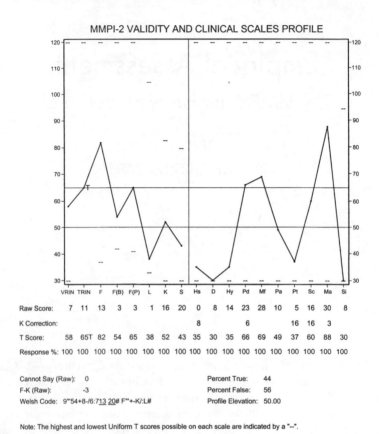

FIGURE 11.1. Madeline G's MMPI-2 profile. From Butcher et al. (2001). Copyright 2001 by the University of Minnesota Press. Reprinted by permission.

more scarce. However, the MMPI-2 has been translated and adapted successfully into a large number of languages and in a broad array of cultures. Butcher (1996) provides chapters describing effective MMPI-2 translation and adaptation projects written by authors from 22 different countries. The test's robustness across countries and cultures as different as Japan, China, Chile, Argentina, Mexico, Iceland, and Turkey (to name just a few) is consistent with the assumption that the MMPI-2 should provide valid information when used in the United States with Native Americans. It is under this assumption that Madeline's MMPI-2 profile is interpreted.

AN ANNOTATED MMPI-2 INTERPRETATION

This section provides a detailed interpretation of Madeline's scores on the MMPI-2 validity, clinical, content, and supplementary scales. For illustrative purposes, each set of scales is interpreted separately, and specific MMPI-2 scales are identified as the sources for various interpretive statements. Readers interested in learning more about the MMPI-2 and its scales are referred to the comprehensive textbooks of Butcher and Williams (2000) and Graham (2000).

The MMPI-2 Validity Scales

The MMPI-2 validity scales provide the test interpreter with a comprehensive picture of the respondent's test-taking attitude. In addition to identifying the number of items left unanswered (or answered both "true" and "false"), the validity scales provide information about response inconsistency, infrequency, and defensiveness. The inconsistency indicators, Variable Response Inconsistency (*VRIN*) and True Response Inconsistency (*TRIN*), can identify random or fixed (i.e., acquiescent and counter-acquiescent) response sets. The response infrequency indicators, Infrequency (*F*), Back-Infrequency (*Fb*), and Infrequency–Psychopathology (*Fp*), are used to screen for exaggeration or fabrication of problems. The defensiveness scales, Lie (*L*), Correction (*K*), and Superlative Self-Presentation (*S*), convey information about attempts to deny or minimize psychological difficulties or undesirable characteristics.

Madeline responded to all of the test items (CNS = 0), suggesting a cooperative approach to the evaluation. Her scores on the MMPI-2 consistency scales, VRIN and TRIN, are well below a level that would suggest possible carelessness or a pervasive fixed response style. Her score on TRIN ($T = 65T$) indicates a moderate pattern of acquiescence; however, this level of yea-saying is not sufficient to generate concern about overall profile validity.

Madeline has produced an unusual pattern of scores on the infrequency scales. Her score on *F* ($T = 82$) is unexpectedly high for an individual with no history of involvement with the mental health system. Her score on *Fb*, a measure of infrequent responding to the second part of the MMPI-2 booklet, is substantially lower ($T = 54$). A difference of this magnitude between the two scales, with *F* being substantially higher than *Fb*, is quite unusual. Her score on *Fp* is moderately elevated ($T = 65$), indicating that Madeline has provided a number of responses that are given rarely by individuals with significant psychopathology.

There are several reasons (not mutually exclusive) why an individual might produce an elevated score on *F*. These include random or fixed responding, exaggeration or fabrication of problems, and accurate reporting of significant psychopathology and/or psychological distress. The relatively low scores on *VRIN* and *TRIN* rule out random or fixed responding as possible sources for Madeline's elevated score on *F*. Individuals who fabricate mental health problems tend to do so pervasively, throughout the test, and are therefore unlikely to score well within normal limits on *Fb*, as Madeline has done in this case. Individuals experiencing substantial psychological distress score at least as high on *Fb* as they do on *F* (in fact, they often score considerably higher on *Fb* than on *F*).

Having ruled out random or fixed responding, outright fabrication of problems, and accurate reporting of significant psychological distress, we must next consider the possibilities of accurate reporting of significant psychopathology and exaggeration of existing problems. Moderate elevation on *Fp* is found typically only among individuals who have a significant history of mental illness. Given that Madeline lacks such a history, it is likely that she has exaggerated or embellished (but has not fabricated) her self-described problems or characteristics. The most likely interpretation of this pattern of scores on the response frequency indicators, then, is that Madeline has openly reported a number of psychological problems or undesirable psychological characteristics, and that in doing so she has probably embellished their extent and significance. This response pattern does not compromise the validity of the resulting test scores. It indicates that the respondent is quite willing to acknowledge problems and shortcomings, but may be overly dramatic in describing some of these features.

Madeline's scores on the MMPI-2 defensiveness scales are consistent with the interpretation of her infrequency scale pattern. Her low score on *L* (*T* = 38) indicates that Madeline has made no effort to deny minor faults or shortcomings, and in fact has acknowledged more of these characteristics than do most people. She apparently has little interest in being perceived as a person who subscribes to traditional societal morals. The within-normal-limits scores on *K* (*T* = 52) and *S* (*T* = 43) reflect an open and forthcoming approach to the MMPI-2.

The MMPI-2 Clinical Scales

The MMPI-2 clinical scales are unparalleled in the quantity and quality of the empirically generated information available to guide their interpretation. Clinical scale interpretation typically begins with an examination of the overall pattern of scores and proceeds to consideration of scores on the individual scales that make up the profile. Interpretation of elevated scores on the clinical scales can sometimes be facilitated by examination of scores on their subscales, when these are available.

Examination of Madeline's MMPI-2 clinical scale profile reveals a considerable amount of scatter, with *T*-scores ranging from a high of 88 on Scale 9 to a low of 30 (the floor for all MMPI-2 *T*-scores) on Scales 2 and 0. The very low scores on Scales 1, 2, 3, and 7 indicate that Madeline presents with little or no psychological distress at this time. In fact, there is a noteworthy absence of any report of anxiety. Because there are no indications on the validity scales of a defensive approach to the test, these uncommonly low scores on the MMPI-2 psychological distress indicators suggest that, overall, Madeline perceives herself as being free of psychological distress at this time.

Among the elevated scales on Madeline's MMPI-2 clinical scale profile, Scale 9 stands out as being dramatically elevated—nearly five standard deviations above the normative mean, and well beyond the remaining scales on the profile. Therefore, let us begin our identification of characteristics indicated by Madeline's profile by examining the empirical correlates of elevated scores on Scale 9. Graham (2000) begins his description of individuals who produce elevated scores on Scale 9 as follows:

> Extreme elevations ($T > 80$) on scale 9 may be suggestive of a manic episode. Patients with such scores are likely to show excessive purposeless activity and accelerated speech; they may have hallucinations and/or delusions of grandeur; and they are emotionally labile. Some confusion might be present and flight of ideas is common. (p. 82)

Madeline's life story does not contain information suggestive of a history of manic or hypomanic symptoms, however. It is possible that her highly elevated score on Scale 9 is in part a product of the embellishment suggested by Madeline's elevated score on F, and that in the absence of this tendency to be overly dramatic, she might have scored somewhat lower than 80 on Scale 9. Graham (2000) provides the following description for individuals who score above 65, but below 80, on this scale:

> Persons with more moderate elevations are not likely to exhibit frankly psychotic symptoms, but there is a definite tendency toward over-activity and unrealistic self-appraisal. High scorers are energetic and talkative, and they prefer action to thought. They have a wide range of interests and are likely to have many projects going at once. However, they do not utilize energy wisely and often do not see projects through to completion. They may be creative, enterprising, and ingenious, but they have little interest in routine or details. High scorers tend to become bored and restless very easily, and their frustration tolerance is quite low. They have great difficulty in inhibiting expression of impulses, and periodic episodes of irritability, hostility, and aggressive outbursts are common. An unrealistic or unqualified optimism is also characteristic of high scorers. They seem to think that nothing is impossible, and they have grandiose aspirations. Also, they have an exaggerated appraisal of their own self-worth and self-importance and are not able to see their own limitations. High scorers have a greater than average likelihood of abusing alcohol and drugs and getting into trouble with the law. (pp. 82–83)

In describing their interpersonal relationships, Graham (2000) has the following to say about individuals with elevated scores on Scale 9:

> High scorers are very outgoing, sociable, and gregarious. They like to be around other people and generally create good first impressions. They impress others as being friendly, pleasant, enthusiastic, poised, and self-confident. They tend to try to dominate other people. Their relationships are usually quite superficial, and as others get to know them better they become aware of their manipulations, deceptions, and unreliability. (p. 83)

Finally, Graham (2000) adds the following caveats regarding the appearance of confidence and poise in persons scoring high on Scale 9:

> In spite of their outward picture of confidence and poise, high scorers are likely to harbor feelings of dissatisfaction concerning what they are getting out of life. They may feel upset, tense, nervous, anxious, and agitated, and they describe themselves as prone to worry. Periodic episodes of depression may occur. (p. 83)

Madeline has produced moderate elevations on two additional clinical scales, 4 and 5. Interpretation of moderate elevations on the clinical scales is sometimes aided by examination of the relevant subscales (see Table 11.1). Madeline has produced significant elevations on two of the subscales for Scale 4, *Pd1* (Familial Discord) and *Pd2* (Authority Problems). Interpretation of Madeline's moderate elevation on Scale 4 ($T = 66$) will focus on these features. Characteristics associated with this level of elevation on Scale 4 include rebelliousness toward authority figures, stormy interpersonal and familial relationships, a tendency to blame family members for one's difficulties, histories of underachievement, a tendency to experience marital problems, striving for immediate gratification of impulses, and failure to plan and consider possible consequences of one's actions. Other features associated with this score include poor judgment, risk taking, interpersonally manipulative behavior, and an absence of deep emotional experiences. Several characteristics of individuals who score high on Scale 4 are consistent with features associated with elevations on Scale 9. These include being viewed by others as likeable and creating a good first impression; having shallow, superficial relationships; being extraverted and outgoing; and a proclivity to become bored and, as a consequence, depressed.

Madeline's elevated score on Scale 5 indicates that she probably lacks stereotypically feminine interests, and that she may have interests and engage in activities that are typically associated with a masculine gender role. This score does not necessarily reflect confusion or uneasiness in the area of gender identity.

Low scores on the MMPI-2 clinical scales are typically not interpret-

TABLE 11.1. Madeline G's Scores on the MMPI-2 Harris–Lingoes Subscales

Scale/subscale	Raw score	T-score	Resp %
Depression subscales			
Subjective Depression (*D1*)	1	34	100
Psychomotor Retardation (*D2*)	0	30	100
Physical Malfunctioning (*D3*)	3	48	100
Mental Dullness (*D4*)	1	43	100
Brooding (*D5*)	0	37	100
Hysteria subscales			
Denial of Social Anxiety (*Hy1*)	6	61	100
Need for Affection (*Hy2*)	4	38	100
Lassitude–Malaise (*Hy3*)	0	39	100
Somatic Complaints (*Hy4*)	0	37	100
Inhibition of Aggression (*Hy5*)	2	39	100
Psychopathic deviate subscales			
Familial Discord (*Pd1*)	5	68	100
Authority Problems (*Pd2*)	7	84	100
Social Imperturbability (*Pd3*)	6	64	100
Social Alienation (*Pd4*)	4	49	100
Self-Alienation (*Pd5*)	3	48	100
Paranoia subscales			
Persecutory Ideas (*Pa1*)	3	57	100
Poignancy (*Pa2*)	2	46	100
Naivete (*Pa3*)	3	41	100
Schizophrenia subscales			
Social Alienation (*Sc1*)	5	57	100
Emotional Alienation (*Sc2*)	1	49	100
Lack of Ego Mastery, Cognitive (*Sc3*)	2	55	100
Lack of Ego Mastery, Conative (*Sc4*)	1	44	100
Lack of Ego Mastery, Defective Inhibition (*Sc5*)	3	59	100
Bizarre Sensory Experiences (*Sc6*)	2	50	100
Hypomania subscales			
Amorality (*Ma1*)	5	79	100
Psychomotor Acceleration (*Ma2*)	8	65	100
Imperturbability (*Ma3*)	7	75	100
Ego Inflation (*Ma4*)	5	62	100
Social Introversion subscales			
Shyness/Self-Consciousness (*Si1*)	0	36	100
Social Avoidance (*Si2*)	0	37	100
Alienation—Self and Others (*Si3*)	5	49	100

Note. Uniform *T*-scores are used for *Hs, D, Hy, Pd, Pa, Pt, Sc, Ma* and the content scales; all other MMPI-2 scales use linear *T*-scores.

able at the individual scale level. The exception to this rule is Scale 0, where Madeline's score is at the floor ($T = 30$). Graham (2000) states:

> Low scorers on Scale 0 tend to be socially extroverted. They are outgoing, gregarious, friendly, and talkative. They have a strong need to be around other people, and mix well with other people. They are seen by others as verbally fluent and expressive. They are active, energetic and vigorous. They are interested in power, status, and recognition, and they tend to seek out competitive situations. (p. 85)

The MMPI-2 Content Scales

The MMPI-2 content scales were inspired by and fashioned after the content scales developed by Jerry Wiggins (1966) for the original MMPI. Content-based MMPI-2 interpretation is predicated on the notion that though we need not accept a test taker's self-presentation at face value, we may still learn a great deal about the individual by acquiring a comprehensive view of the picture the person has sought to paint in responding to the test items. The MMPI-2 content scales serve this purpose. Their interpretation is not based solely on item content. A number of studies that have established these scales' empirical correlates can guide the content scales' interpretation, along with item content.

Madeline has produced a highly elevated score on the content scale Antisocial Practices (*ASP*) (see Figure 11.2). Many of the items on this scale are worded in the past tense. As a result, an individual with a history of antisocial behavior may produce an elevated score on *ASP*, regardless of his or her current behavioral tendencies. However, at her level of elevation on this scale, Madeline must have endorsed items reflecting both past and current antisocial behavioral tendencies. As I have noted earlier in considering her highly elevated score on Scale 9, it is possible that the overall level of elevation on *ASP* partly reflects Madeline's tendency to embellish or dramatize her self-presentation. Because of their intentionally transparent nature, the content scales are particularly susceptible to embellishment. However, even if we discount the overall level of elevation, Madeline's score on *ASP* indicates the presence of significant antisocial proclivities.

Individuals who score this high on *ASP* are likely to have been in trouble with the law. They report a history of acting-out behavior beginning during their childhood or adolescence. They believe that most people share their antisocial attitudes, and they tend to have a rather cynical view of others. These individuals are also resentful of authority, blame others for their difficulties, and tend to be self-centered. Others may view them as dishonest, not trustworthy, and not believable. They are at increased risk for having substance abuse problems, tend to act out impulsively, and tend to be angry and aggressive in interpersonal contexts.

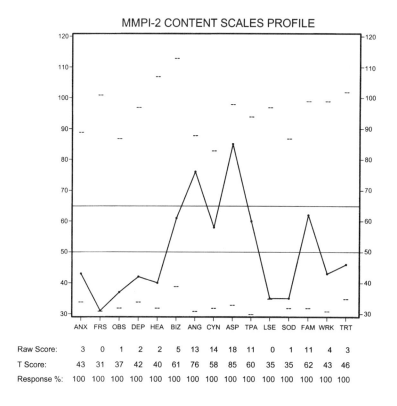

FIGURE 11.2. Madeline G's pattern of scores on the MMPI-2 content scales. From Butcher et al. (2001). Copyright 2001 by the University of Minnesota Press. Reprinted by permission.

Madeline has also produced an elevated score on the content scale Anger (*ANG*). When individuals produce moderately elevated scores on the content scales, the content component scales—subscales we have developed (Ben-Porath & Sherwood, 1993) for the MMPI-2 content scales—may help identify particular areas of focus for the interpretation. In this case, Madeline produced very disparate scores on *ANG*'s two content component scales. As seen in Table 11.2, Madeline produced a highly elevated score on the content component scale Explosive Behavior (*ANG1*; *T* = 84) and a much more moderate score on Irritability (*ANG2*;

TABLE 11.2. Madeline G's Scores on the MMPI-2 Content Component Scales

Scale/subscale	Raw score	T-score	Resp %
Fears subscales			
Generalized Fearfulness (FRS1)	0	42	100
Multiple Fears (FRS2)	0	30	100
Depression subscales			
Lack of Drive (DEP1)	1	45	100
Dysphoria (DEP2)	0	40	100
Self-Depreciation (DEP3)	0	40	100
Suicidal Ideation (DEP4)	0	45	100
Health Concerns subscales			
Gastrointestinal Symptoms (HEA1)	0	43	100
Neurological Symptoms (HEA2)	1	45	100
General Health Concerns (HEA3)	0	40	100
Bizarre Mentation subscales			
Psychotic Symptomatology (BIZ1)	1	54	100
Schizotypal Characteristics (BIZ2)	3	60	100
Anger subscales			
Explosive Behavior (ANG1)	6	84	100
Irritability (ANG2)	5	59	100
Cynicism subscales			
Misanthropic Beliefs (CYN1)	9	59	100
Interpersonal Suspiciousness (CYN2)	5	59	100
Antisocial Practices subscales			
Antisocial Attitudes (ASP1)	12	70	100
Antisocial Behavior (ASP2)	5	90	100
Type A subscales			
Impatience (TPA1)	4	58	100
Competitive Drive (TPA2)	5	64	100
Low Self-Esteem subscales			
Self-Doubt (LSE1)	0	39	100
Submissiveness (LSE2)	0	39	100
Social Discomfort subscales			
Introversion (SOD1)	0	37	100
Shyness (SOD2)	0	35	100
Family Problems subscales			
Family Discord (FAM1)	3	47	100
Familial Alienation (FAM2)	5	86	100
Negative Treatment Indicators subscales			
Low Motivation (TRT1)	0	41	100
Inability to Disclose (TRT2)	2	53	100

$T = 59$). This pattern indicates that interpretation of Madeline's elevated score on ANG should focus on external expressions of anger. Specifically, Madeline's score on ANG indicates that she has a short temper, that she is inclined to be easily provoked to experience anger, and that she is likely to act out and expresses her feelings of anger when they occur. She probably has poor impulse control and poor tolerance for frustration. She may become physically aggressive when she believes that she has been wronged.

Madeline has produced moderate elevations on three additional content scales: Bizarre Mentation (BIZ), Cynicism (CYN), and Family Problems (FAM). Examination of her scores on the BIZ content component scales does not point to the presence of any significant psychotic symptoms or schizotypal characteristics. This pattern of scores on BIZ is sometimes seen in individuals who use (or have used) drugs and describe some unusual experiences associated with this behavior. The moderate elevation on CYN is consistent with other indications that Madeline tends to view others as untrustworthy and probably has difficulties establishing trusting relationships. Examination of the content component scales associated with FAM indicates that Madeline does not report a great deal of discord in her current family relationships; however, she feels quite alienated from her family and is not likely to view family members as possible sources of warmth or support.

The MMPI-2 Supplementary Scales

The MMPI-2 supplementary scales are a collection of measures developed in largely independent research projects over the course of the test's history. Most were developed with the original MMPI and maintained on the MMPI-2 because of the wealth of empirical evidence available to guide their interpretation. Others were introduced with, or shortly after, publication of the MMPI-2.

Madeline has produced noteworthy scores on several MMPI-2 supplementary scales (see Figure 11.3). Most of the interpretations suggested by her supplementary scale scores have already been identified on the scales previously analyzed. These findings can be viewed as corroborating the previous interpretations. Her moderately elevated score on Ego Strength (Es) indicates that Madeline does not report any current significant emotional problems, and that she tends to be energetic and have many interests. Individuals who produce this score present as confident and outspoken. They have a good sense of reality and tend to be competitive and work-oriented. These individuals create favorable first impressions and are able to win the cooperation of others. They may be rebellious toward authority figures and can be sarcastic and cynical. Madeline's elevated score on the Gender Masculine (GM) scale, coupled with her very low score on the Gender Feminine

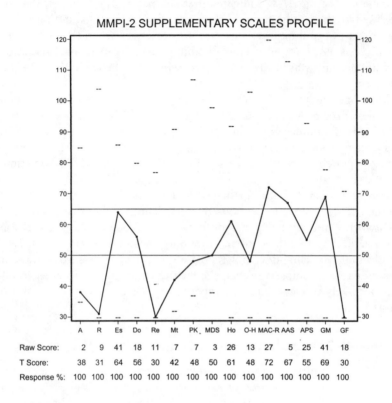

MMPI-2 SUPPLEMENTARY SCALES PROFILE

	A	R	Es	Do	Re	Mt	PK	MDS	Ho	O-H	MAC-R	AAS	APS	GM	GF
Raw Score:	2	9	41	18	11	7	7	3	26	13	27	5	25	41	18
T Score:	38	31	64	56	30	42	48	50	61	48	72	67	55	69	30
Response %:	100	100	100	100	100	100	100	100	100	100	100	100	100	100	100

Note: The highest and lowest Uniform T scores possible on each scale are indicated by a "--".

FIGURE 11.3. Madeline G's profile on the MMPI-2 supplementary scales. From Butcher et al. (2001). Copyright 2001 by the University of Minnesota Press. Reprinted by permission.

(*GF*) scale, indicates that she presents as favoring traditional masculine interests and rejecting traditional feminine interests.

   Madeline's scores on the MMPI-2 substance abuse scales indicate that she possesses personality characteristics placing her at significant risk for developing substance abuse problems, and that she acknowledges a history of such difficulties. Her score on the MacAndrew Alcoholism—Revised (MAC-R) scale indicates that Madeline's sensation-seeking and risk-taking characteristics increase the likelihood that she may abuse alcohol and/or drugs. Her score on the Addiction Acknowledgment scale (AAS) scale indicates that she indeed confirms a history of substance abuse. These scales cannot indicate whether Madeline presently engages in substance abuse; however, they do suggest an increased probability that Madeline may currently or in the future abuse substances.

AN MMPI-2 NARRATIVE INTERPRETATION

Madeline has produced a valid MMPI-2 profile. She was able to understand and respond relevantly to the test items, and did so in a forthcoming manner. Her scores indicate that she has openly acknowledged some psychological problems or undesirable personality characteristics, and that she may have exaggerated or embellished the significance of these features of her personality. She has little or no interest in being perceived as a person who conforms to societal norms or morals. Her scores on the substantive scales of the MMPI-2 are likely to yield an accurate portrayal of Madeline's psychological functioning, though they may also reflect an attempt to amplify the significance of her self-identified negative characteristics.

Madeline feels rather positive about her current situation and denies presently experiencing any negative emotions. She is likely to present as a socially outgoing, energetic, confident, and poised individual. She gives the impression of having a very positive self-view. She is probably creative and enterprising; she may be particularly effective at developing new projects and ideas, but less effective at seeing them through to completion. Madeline does not adhere to, and may in fact reject, traditional social and moral values. She also rejects the stereotypically feminine gender role. She has very little tolerance for frustration or delay, and may act out impulsively against perceived injustice. She may have difficulties with time management and planning. She may be preoccupied with activities designed to prevent herself from becoming bored—a situation she finds particularly aversive. Madeline is at risk for developing substance abuse problems, and she acknowledges past and possible current problems in this area.

Madeline reports a significant tendency toward past and present antisocial behavior. She has probably experienced difficulties with the law and does not report much remorse about these experiences. She views people as selfish, deceitful, and dishonest, and may be viewed similarly by others. She harbors anger and resentment, and she tends to act out impulsively when angry at others. She may occasionally resort to physical aggression in such instances. Madeline feels very alienated from members of her family and probably blames them for many of her difficulties.

In spite of her problems with anger, Madeline is likely to create a favorable first impression; people may find her to be charming and engaging, although a bit domineering. She may have difficulty maintaining deeply rooted social relationships, however, and some may view her as being interpersonally manipulative. Madeline's outward presentation of social poise and confidence may mask long-standing doubts and fears about inadequacy. Finally, Madeline's MMPI-2 profile indicates the possibility that she is at risk for experiencing manic or hypomanic symptoms.

MADELINE'S MMPI-2 PROFILE IN THE CONTEXT OF HER LIFE STORY

Madeline's MMPI-2 profile can assist in illuminating some of the issues identified in McAdams's analysis of her life story (see Chapter 7), and vice versa. In light of her extraordinarily difficult childhood, Madeline's current alienation from family members is quite understandable. It may also help explain her difficulties in forming and maintaining warm interpersonal relationships. Madeline's turbulent years as a teenager and young adult probably account for the MMPI-2 findings of a significant history of antisocial behavior. Her substance abuse, beginning in childhood, is consistent with indications throughout her profile that Madeline is at significant risk for difficulties in this area. The story about brutally beating a female inmate who had harassed her is consistent with MMPI-2 indications that Madeline harbors a great deal of anger and aggression, which, when triggered, may result in physically violent reactions.

McAdams's description of Madeline's current life view is consistent with MMPI-2 findings that she presents as poised, confident, self-assured, and currently free of significant emotional discomfort. However, it is possible that Madeline's self-view that she is a "spectacularly successful lawyer" who has "won 53 legal cases in a row," and her expectation that she will be "wildly successful," may reflect some of the excessive optimism and the tendency toward presenting in an unrealistically positive manner typical of individuals who produce highly elevated scores on Scale 9.

In describing Madeline's dispositional traits, McAdams notes that on the Big Five Inventory she scores very high on Extraversion, Conscientiousness, and Openness to Experience, and moderately on Agreeableness. The MMPI-2 findings on Scales 0 and 9 are consistent with Madeline's high scores on Extraversion and Openness to Experience, respectively. However, the very high score on Conscientiousness is quite inconsistent with MMPI-2 findings. Not surprisingly, McAdams struggles somewhat when attempting to incorporate the high Conscientiousness score into Madeline's life story. Madeline's moderate score on the Big Five Inventory's Agreeableness scale is also contradicted by MMPI-2 findings suggesting that Madeline harbors significant anger and is likely to act out on these feelings in interpersonal contexts. Here too, there appears to be greater consistency between the MMPI-2 findings and Madeline's life story.

Finally, McAdams notes that Madeline herself suggests there may be a few "storm clouds" on her horizon. Will Madeline be able to fit in at her new law firm? Will the two father figures in her life live up to her expectations? Will she be able to avoid feelings of boredom and the trouble that in the past has followed such feelings? These concerns are consistent with MMPI-2 indications that Madeline's outward presentation of confidence and poise may mask some underlying insecurity. In light of her history, Madeline's concerns about these issues appear more realistic than the picture of bluster and assurance she projects. The fact that she is aware of these issues, and is able to articulate them toward the end of her interview, increases the likelihood that she will be able to navigate successfully through the setbacks she may experience.

12

Constructive Alternativism in Personality Assessment

Madeline G from Multiple Perspectives

KRISTA K. TROBST
JERRY S. WIGGINS

Historically, personality assessment has been employed for a variety of purposes under a number of different rationales. Within the personological paradigm, assessment may be directed toward achieving what might be considered an "understanding" of a person (McAdams, 1993). In applied situations, personality assessment may be directed toward "evaluating" a person's suitability for a placement or treatment (Wiggins, 1973b). Another such purpose has been described by Kenneth Craik (1986) as learning to "appreciate" persons. This third purpose was the principal rationale behind having graduate students serve as assessors in the intensive live-in assessments that were held at the Institute of Personality Assessment and Research (IPAR).

Whether focused on understanding, evaluation, or appreciation, personality assessment that involves multiple measures and multiple assessors will almost inevitably involve the resolution of apparently contradictory findings about those who are assessed. George Kelly (1955) suggested that persons will be seen differently when they are viewed from within different construct systems, advocated a relativistic approach to understanding persons. Within the area of personality psychology, this position has been formalized by the following proposition: "Personality is best considered from

296

many, often conflicting points of view" (Wiggins, Renner, Clore, & Rose, 1971, p. 7).

As discussed in the Introduction, the five different paradigms have different ranges and foci of convenience (see Table Int.2 of the Introduction), and the most comprehensive assessment of an individual is often achieved by an integration of apparently conflicting findings from multiple paradigms. Although there are some points of divergence across the assessments of Madeline G, on the whole we are mostly struck by their remarkable convergence in capturing her character, despite the vastly different measures, methods, and assumptions of the various paradigms. In proceeding to "integrate" and discuss the findings, we have chosen to focus on some highlights within each of the paradigms; the most notable points of convergence and divergence among the paradigms; and what we loosely term "validity assessment." With respect to this third category, we provide a description of Madeline that has been obtained by summarizing the views of a few of her friends, in order that the formal assessment results may be compared with informal assessments provided by those who know her well. Finally, we provide an update regarding the significant events that have occurred in Madeline's life in the 3 years since the assessments occurred, and we review how those events correspond with the predictions and concerns offered by her assessors.

SOME HIGHLIGHTS WITHIN EACH OF THE PARADIGMS

Madeline G underwent a series of assessment procedures in an effort to enhance our understanding, evaluation, and appreciation of her as the subject of this collaborative case study. Only two of the assessors within the various assessment paradigms actually met Madeline (i.e., personological and psychodynamic), the assessors representing the other paradigms relied on self-report data (i.e., empirical) and a combination of self-report and peer report data (i.e., interpersonal and multivariate). Two things are worth noting in this regard: (1) Those assessors who met Madeline appeared to find her fascinating and likeable; and (2) those assessors who didn't meet Madeline were reliant upon McAdams's personological assessment (Chapter 7) for further information about Madeline and her history in formulating their reports.

Madeline G and the Psychodynamic Paradigm

As stated near the beginning of Chapter 8, the psychodynamic paradigm as implemented by Behrends and Blatt gathers information from test scores, content or themes of responses, verbalization style, and the interpersonal relationship between the person and the tester, *"including the tester's empathic and introspective cues in the transaction"* (emphasis added). In this last context, Rebecca Behrends's description of her empathic and introspective reactions to Madeline must rank among the most perceptive accounts of interpersonal dynamics in the testing situation since Schafer (1954) first described these phenomena.

One means of discussing the distinction between "objective" and "projective" tests is to refer simply to the reliability of scoring responses. On this basis, Exner's approach to Rorschach testing is one that tends, among other things, to make the scoring of Rorschach responses more "objective." However, the distinction between the psychodynamic paradigm and the other paradigms discussed in this book is perhaps best illustrated by the manner in which Behrends and Blatt rely upon observation and introspection within an object relations framework in their case formulations.

These authors note that "Madeline's personality and individuality are very much manifested in her striking physical presence." Behrend's vivid descriptions of Madeline's physical appearance, dressing style, overall manner, and stance are unforgettably *visual*: " . . . she inhabits her body fully, in a sensuous cat-like way." In the context of a highly structured situation, where the expectations are clear, "First, she anticipates the control that she imagines will be imposed upon her by the authority figure involved in such a structured setting, and she attempts to wrest control by taking over the situation herself." Behrends's interpretations of the telephone conversations with Madeline G prior to the actual testing session (e.g., "It's Rebecca, right?") are every bit as revealing as the test protocols themselves; once again, they illustrate the importance of the tester's use of empathic and introspective cues within the psychodynamic paradigm. Within the object relations perspective, the *relationship* between subject and tester is of considerable importance, as is the openness of the examiner to cues that suggest the nature of this relationship.

Madeline is seen as "every bit as ready to back down and literally to make friends as she is to do battle, once she encounters a person who is genuinely interested in relating to her with fairness and mutuality." And there is every reason to believe that Rebecca Behrends has been such a person for Madeline in the testing situation. For example, on the "jogger picture" of the Wechsler Adult Intelligence Scale—Third Edition (WAIS-III) Picture Completion subtest, Madeline refers to "our footsteps" (hers and the examiner's), indicating the substantial degree of rapport achieved in this testing session. From the standpoint of evaluation, this rapport may not always be to Madeline's advantage: "She is clearly functioning below her intellectual potential by striving to be clever, unique, and creative for the benefit of her relationship with the examiner."

Madeline G and the Interpersonal Paradigm

In Chapter 9, Aaron Pincus and Michael Gurtman illustrate the application, at the level of an individual case, of a richly substantiated nomological net focused on the circular representation of interpersonal behavior. The stable personality traits assessed by the interpersonal circumplex correspond to those McAdams has classified as "first-level." The structural summary of Madeline's circumplex (Gurtman & Balakrishnan, 1998) yields an interpersonal diagnosis that is compared to the one obtained from her partner's ratings, and that allows for inferences concerning Madeline's motives and adaptations ("second-level").

The parallel circumplex structures of the Interpersonal Adjective Scales (IAS) and the Inventory of Interpersonal Problems—Circumplex (IIP-C) allow Pincus and Gurtman to make relatively precise comparisons of Madeline's characteristic patterns of adapting to her social environment and of her perceived interpersonal problems as reported by *both* Madeline and her partner. On a very general level, Madeline and her partner are in agreement that Madeline is a highly agentic individual, but they strongly disagree about her communal inclinations. Pincus and Gurtman interpret Madeline's extreme response style as "a bias toward seeing herself in an overly positive light, reflecting a highly adjusted individual with strong agentic and caring qualities."

Although not intending to "pathologize" Madeline, Pincus and Gurtman assemble an impressive array of evidence suggesting similarities between Madeline's interpersonal test results and life story on the one hand, and those of individuals diagnosed as having narcissistic personality disorder on the other. They also make the subtle point that Madeline expresses care through competitive strivings (defending Native Americans) rather than through warmth. Overall, their chapter is an excellent illustration of the diagnostic use of test results within the interpersonal paradigm.

Madeline G and the Personological Paradigm

The early description by Dan McAdams of Madeline G as "amazing" (see the brief introduction to Part II), suggests that the Life Story Interview went quite well. There is little doubt that McAdams appreciates the value of a good life story: "I believe that coming to a conscious understanding of the details of your self-defining personal myth can markedly enrich your life and promote your development as a person" (McAdams, 1993, p. 264). Nor is there doubt that Madeline G enjoyed the opportunity to relate her life story to an interested and sympathetic listener.

Upon completing the assessment session in Evanston, Illinois, Madeline G called us in a euphoric state. She "absolutely loved" Professor

McAdams and felt that the session had been of great personal value to her. It is not surprising that Madeline enjoyed 3 hours of uninterrupted focus on her favorite subject (her!), given her narcissistic tendencies, but there was more to it than that. She found that the Life Story Interview procedure (the division of her life into chapters; the identification of high points, low points, and turning points; imagining future chapters; etc.) gave a new "focus" to her life and allowed her to put things "in order." But most of all, she felt that the interview experience had clarified how much her partner is an indispensable source of love and support in her life, and she vowed to treat him more kindly.

The life story approach to assessment augments the traditional life history by placing that history in a thematic context that has additional predictive value. Recognition of the "contours of a person's identity" allows for comparisons with other narrative forms in contemporary American society. Thus, in Chapter 7, McAdams identifies Madeline's story as a "redemptive life narrative" reflecting a contemporary "born-again" quality and an ancient "myth of the hero"; these qualities permit predictions regarding the possible outcomes of such a story. Although clearly recognizing "storm clouds on the horizon," McAdams considers the future to be a bright one. As he puts it in life story terminology,

> The protagonist in this narrative is simply too strong now. The movement of the plot is strongly upward and progressive. The enemies have been irrevocably weakened. Even if the forces of evil manage to launch an aggressive attack as she moves into midlife, I still would put my money on Madeline.

Madeline G and the Multivariate Paradigm

In Chapter 10, Costa and Piedmont describe their multivariate assessment employing the Revised NEO Personality Inventory (NEO PI-R). This instrument is notable for the high-bandwidth/high-fidelity approach (see Chapter 4), providing information regarding a broad array of characteristics. Madeline's extreme response style tendency (which is apparent in her responses to the interpersonal inventories) is also evident in her NEO PI-R protocol (fewer than 18% of her responses are not extreme). Also, as found within the interpersonal paradigm, there is significant disagreement between Madeline and her partner in rating Madeline's personality. Madeline and her partner agree that Madeline exhibits high Extraversion, Openness to Experience, and Antagonism (low Agreeableness). However, Madeline and her partner disagree regarding her Neuroticism and Conscientiousness; her partner rates Madeline as being higher on the Anxiety, Depression, Self-Consciousness, and Vulnerability facets of Neuroticism, and as being lower on the Conscientiousness domain in general and lower on the specific facets of Competence, Dutifulness, and Self-Discipline. In her partner's view, Madeline is at least somewhat apprehensive; prone to worry, sadness, and hopelessness; and quite vulnerable to stress—all of which Madeline denies. He also sees her as not sensible, prudent, or effective; not governed by conscience; and subject to boredom and other distractions—which she also denies. It is not that Madeline's partner views her as lacking in motivation to succeed; rather, he ascribes to her more "sociopathic" characteristics associated with low Conscientiousness. Costa and Piedmont also emphasize Madeline's antagonistic view of the world, her suspiciousness of others, and her callousness and tough-minded attitudes toward others: "People might describe her as relatively stubborn, critical, manipulative, or selfish."

Additional information is provided in the form of NEO PI-R style graphs (see Figures 10.2–10.6 in Chapter 10), from which we learn, for example, that Madeline is a Leader, a Creative Interactor, a Free-Thinker, and an Upbeat Optimist, and that she is Cold-Blooded and Adaptive. On the whole, Madeline is seen as having the potentialities to be a very powerful person, although it is noted that the same attributes that act as strengths in certain contexts may undermine her abilities in achieving intimacy, nurturance, tolerance, acceptance, and forgiveness in other contexts.

Madeline G and the Empirical Paradigm

Any doubt about the diagnostic utility of the Minnesota Multiphasic Personality Inventory—2 (MMPI-2) is dispelled by Ben-Porath's didactic illustration in Chapter 11 of the power of this newer version of a venerable instrument. An impressive use of both original and new validity scales in concert serves to identify Madeline's tendency to exaggerate or embellish (but not to fabricate) her self-described problems or characteristics, as well as her indifference to traditional societal mores. That interpretation of the MMPI-2 clinical scales is empirically based is clearly illustrated by the lengthy quotes from Graham's (2000) classic textbook surveying the research literature on the MMPI-2. Perhaps equally impressive are the clear diagnostic "hits" generated by this research-based approach.

Also impressive is the *range* of assessment tools available from a single instrument. The MMPI-2 content scales provide an alternative view of self-report (e.g., Wiggins, 1966), as well as providing incremental validity to the clinical scales in psychodiagnosis (e.g., Barthlow, Graham, Ben-Porath, & McNulty, 1999; Wiggins, 1966). And the supplementary scales preserved in the MMPI-2, as well as those developed for this revision, extend even more the range of assessment questions that can be explored with the MMPI-2 (Graham, 2000, pp. 146–187).

Within the empirical paradigm, we come to know of Madeline as an individual who reports little or no psychological distress; rather, she has marked hypomanic characteristics and is likely to be unrealistically optimistic, with grandiose aspirations and an exaggerated sense of self-worth. Madeline's significant antisocial history and tendencies are highlighted, as is her propensity for anger, her alienation from her family, and her heightened risk for substance abuse.

CONVERGENCES AND DIVERGENCES
ACROSS THE ASSESSMENTS

Agency and Communion

As noted in Chapter 6, Bakan's (1966) metaconcepts of "agency" (strivings for mastery and power that differentiate the individual) and "communion" (strivings for intimacy, union, and solidarity within a social entity) are central to all paradigms of personality assessment under various guises. As such, all of the present assessors might be expected to comment about characteristics related to Madeline's propensities for agentic and communal actions, although not all of them would necessarily reach the same conclusions, given the use of different methods and sources of information in different paradigms.

Agency

That Madeline is a highly agentic individual is apparent from the remarkable convergence across the paradigms (and, where relevant, across Madeline's and her partner's reports) with respect to such characteristics as dominance, control, and power motivations and goals. It is, in fact, Madeline's agency that is the most common and repeated theme across the various assessments.

Madeline's Agency within the Personological Paradigm. Our first introduction to Madeline occurs within McAdams's personological assessment in Chapter 7, and it is here that Madeline begins to emerge as a highly agentic individual. From her life story, it becomes apparent that "She sees herself as a positive force in the world, and she seems at times to suggest that she has almost superhuman powers." McAdams also describes Madeline as highly assertive and notes, "Even on the phone, she comes across as brash, dominant, and high-volume." The most compelling evidence within the personological paradigm of Madeline's agency comes, however, in the form of her personal strivings. McAdams notes that "Of the 10 personal strivings she has listed, 8 are explicit articulations of power goals. Madeline writes that she is typically striving to 'impress other people,' 'win every argument,' and 'come in first in whatever I attempt.' " Madeline's Thematic Apperception Test (TAT) stories also contain a preponderance of agentic themes, although some communal themes are also apparent. Finally, agentic themes predominate in McAdams's summary comments regarding Madeline, including references to Madeline's "impressive agency" and her need to "fight the good fight," "remain vigilant," and "battle a slew of dark forces."

Madeline's Agency within the Psychodynamic Paradigm. Although Madeline's agency is not the predominant theme within Behrends and Blatt's psychodynamic assessment report in Chapter 8, the view of Madeline as a highly agentic individual occurs from her very first interaction with Behrends while arranging a time for meeting. As we have quoted earlier, "she anticipates the control that she imagines will be imposed upon her by the authority figure involved in such a structured setting, and she attempts to wrest control by taking over the situation herself." Also, with respect to the Picture Arrangement subtest of the WAIS-III, Madeline's arrangement of the pictures for one of the items leads the assessor to conclude: "Thus, in Madeline's world, it makes sense to be aggressive and controlling from the very beginning, given the presumed nature of people to thwart her needs." Madeline's Rorschach responses also demonstrate "a sense of personal strength and power," and there is a suggestion, given Madeline's responses to the Object Relations Inventory (ORI), that she partially identifies with her father—"identification with the strength and power of the male."

Madeline's Agency within the Interpersonal Paradigm. The interpersonal paradigm provides our first introduction to the views of Madeline's partner, and in Chapter 9 we see that although Madeline and her partner disagree a great deal regarding Madeline's communal tendencies, they agree that Madeline is a highly agentic individual: "In the present case, the most consistent information regarding Madeline is that she is a dominant person." In her partner's view, Madeline's agentic tendencies not only suggest that she is highly dominant, but also suggest that she has interpersonal *problems* of being domineering. Although strong trait tendencies will not necessarily be associated with allied interpersonal problems, individuals whose trait tendencies (in any given direction) are as extreme as Madeline's are more likely than not to have some related negative interpersonal impacts. It is perhaps primarily in this regard that Madeline's partner's report begins to appear more trustworthy than Madeline's self-report. Madeline reports being very dominant, but denies being domineering, despite the likelihood that as such a highly agentic individual she is likely perceived as domineering by those with whom she interacts (and as her partner reports). As Pincus and Gurtman note, "In most interactions, she typically expects to get what she wants and expects others to submit to her requests, follow her directions, and be convinced of her opinions."

Madeline's Agency within the Multivariate Paradigm. As Costa and Piedmont (Chapter 10) note in their multivariate assessment of Madeline, significant discrepancies occur between Madeline's and her partner's ratings regarding some aspects of her personality; however, those discrepancies occur primarily within the NEO PI-R domains of Neuroticism and Conscientiousness. These authors indicate that Madeline and her partner agree that Madeline is highly antagonistic and assertive: "She prefers competition to cooperation, and she expresses hostile feelings directly with little hesitation." Also, she "is often a group leader taking the responsibility for initiating group activities." Through the use of the style graphs, we also come to know that Madeline's Style of Interaction is that of a Leader, and as such she prefers giving orders to taking them and feels particularly well suited for making decisions.

Madeline's Agency within the Empirical Paradigm. Ben-Porath begins the discussion of Madeline's MMPI-2 clinical scale profile in Chapter 11 by noting her extremely elevated Scale 9, which is associated with (among other things) an exaggerated sense of self-importance, grandiose aspirations, and a tendency to try to dominate other people. Furthermore, Madeline's extremely low ($T = 30$) Scale 0 score is associated with being competitive and interested in status and power. Within the content scales, Madeline's high Antisocial Practices score is associated with being self-centered and aggressive, and her high Anger score suggests that she is prone to anger outbursts and aggression. Within the supplementary scales, Madeline's Ego Strength score is suggestive of someone who is confident, outspoken, competitive, and work-oriented. The combination of Madeline's Gender Masculine and Gender Feminine scores also suggest that she favors masculine characteristics and interests.

Communion

As previously noted, communion is another metaconcept common to all paradigms of personality assessment—but, unlike the reports regarding Madeline's agency (on which there is remarkable convergence), there is much less consensus regarding Madeline's communal tendencies. Discrepancies clearly exist between paradigms in this respect. On the whole, in forms of assessment where Madeline's self-view is the basis for interpretation (i.e., face-valid assessment), Madeline generally emerges as a highly communal individual (e.g., Madeline's self-report on the IAS within the interpersonal paradigm and her Loyola Generativity Scale [LGS] score within the personological paradigm). In forms of assessment where Madeline's partner's views are considered, though, Madeline emerges as decidedly noncommunal in orientation (e.g., Madeline's partner's IAS within the interpersonal paradigm). The discrepancies continue, however, beyond the relatively straightforward level of disagreement between Madeline and her partner. The interpretation of Madeline's behavior and responses within the psychodynamic paradigm (where face-valid self-report is decidedly not the basis for interpretation) is also suggestive of some communal tendencies, needs, and motives, possibly lending credence to her self-view. However, Madeline's self-report within the multivariate paradigm suggests an overall *very low* score on Agreeableness, possibly lending credence to her partner's view. Here, we discuss the various perspectives and some possible means of reconciliation.

Madeline's Communion within the Personological Paradigm. As previously mentioned in discussing Madeline's agency, Madeline's responses regarding personal goals are primarily agentic in nature, and McAdams notes in Chapter 7 that "she lists no goals that involve warm, close relationships." However, McAdams goes on to say that with respect to the TAT stories, where more implicit (rather than explicit) motivations should arise, "Here the picture gets more complicated. Her stories show high levels of both power motivation and intimacy motivation." With respect to her Big Five Inventory scores, McAdams indicates that Madeline "sees herself as caring and nurturant toward others, but as not especially cooperative and compliant in personal relationships." Madeline's LGS score is also extraordinarily high, suggesting strong interests in caring for others. However, it seems that Madeline's form of caring may be decidedly agentic (rather than nurturant) in quality: "She sees herself instead as a strong agent whose care and compassion come out in bold actions and in her valiant and usually victorious efforts to help others in need."

Madeline's Communion within the Psychodynamic Paradigm. Madeline's potential capacity for, and need for, communion are perhaps nowhere more apparent than within the psychodynamic assessment. From the beginning of Chapter 8, Behrends and Blatt emphasize Madeline's more caring and vulnerable qualities: "Although she is headstrong and strives fiercely to be independent, she can, in the next moment, be achingly tender and vulnerable. And although she can be oppositional, there are also selflessness and generosity about her, as well as a remarkable capacity for empathy and mutuality." Furthermore, when arrangements were being made for Behrends and Madeline to meet, "She was momentarily able to relinquish her controlling and self-absorbed defenses, as well as her anxiety over being tested, and to express her affiliative needs by striving to establish an equal and more intimate working relationship." Also suggestive of a strong desire for communion, "in relation to the item on the Picture Completion subtest of people jogging, she responds with 'our footsteps,' a peculiar verbalization apparently merging her and the examiner." Unfortunately, as noted earlier, it appears that some of Madeline's desire for connectedness with the examiner works to her detriment with respect to her performance on the WAIS-III: "She is clearly functioning below her intellectual potential by striving to be clever, unique, and creative for the benefit of her relationship with the examiner."

It becomes increasingly apparent in the description of Madeline within the psychodynamic paradigm that however striking her agentic tendencies may be, Madeline regularly "overcomes" those needs in order to establish a communal connection: "What is so remarkable about Madeline, however, is that she is every bit as ready to back down and literally to make friends as she is to do battle, once she encounters a person who is genuinely interested in relating to her with fairness and mutuality." However, in the summary of the psychodynamic assessment's results, we also catch a glimmer into her "inner workings" suggesting that communion may be more a *need* for her than it is a *capacity*: "Although Madeline is determined to stand free and independent, and she fiercely asserts and defends her autonomy, at the same time she very much seeks and needs interpersonal contact, care, and nurturance." It seems clear that Madeline strives for *having* communion, but it is less clear to what extent she is willing and able to *provide* communion.

Madeline's Communion within the Interpersonal Paradigm. Madeline's communion is clearly in dispute within the interpersonal paradigm; Chapter 9 makes it clear that Madeline's and her partner's views diverge dramatically regarding her propensity for warmth and nurturance. Whereas Madeline's self-ratings suggest that she is well above average in nurturance and below average in coldness, her partner's ratings suggest that Madeline is strikingly non-nurturant and extraordinarily cold. As noted earlier, neither Madeline's nor her partner's ratings are necessarily free of bias. Madeline's self-ratings may reflect her "ideal self," and her partner's ratings may be affected by current issues within the relationship. It may well be that the truth lies somewhere between their two sets of ratings, but in the absence of additional information, Madeline's level of communion remains unclear.

Madeline's Communion within the Multivariate Paradigm. Discrepancies between Madeline's self-views and her partner's views with respect to Madeline's communal tendencies are not highlighted within the multivariate assessment. However, the examination in Chapter 10 of Madeline's Agreeableness facet scores and the Extraversion facet of Warmth suggests a pattern of disagreement between Madeline and her partner similar to that observed within the interpersonal paradigm. With respect to the Agreeableness facets, Madeline agrees with her partner that she is decidedly *not* high in Straightforwardness, Compliance, or Modesty. However, whereas her partner also describes her as decidedly *not* high in Trust, Altruism, or

Tender-Mindedness, Madeline disagrees, rating herself as high or very high in these characteristics. The same pattern of disagreement occurs on the Extraversion facet of Warmth. The Warmth and Altruism facets bear the closest resemblance to items assessing nurturance within the IAS; as such, it appears that Madeline and her partner demonstrate the same diverging views regarding Madeline's communal tendencies within the multivariate paradigm as they do within the interpersonal paradigm (i.e., he rates her very low, and she rates herself high).

Madeline and her partner clearly disagree regarding Madeline's communal tendencies, both within the interpersonal paradigm and, to a lesser extent, within the multivariate paradigm. The resolution of this disagreement is unclear. One possibility is, as Pincus and Gurtman note in Chapter 9, that Madeline is tending to describe her "ideal self"—but one wonders then why she would rate herself as very low in Compliance, Straightforwardness, and Modesty. Another possibility is that because of Madeline's admittedly immodest, noncompliant, and manipulative tendencies, it may be understandably difficult for her partner to conceive of her as having warm, altruistic, and tender-minded orientations, although both sets of characteristics may be true. More specifically, it may well be that Madeline likes most people and builds strong emotional attachments with friends (Warmth), is sympathetic to the plights of others (Tender-Mindedness), and tries to help others (Altruism)—while also being self-aggrandizing (low Modesty), competitive and stubborn (low Compliance), and deceptive (low Straightforwardness). However, it also seems likely that, given her strong agentic tendencies, Madeline shows her caring and assists others in highly agentic ways. Although Madeline sees this as caring, intimates may expect and desire more tender forms of care.

Madeline's Communion within the Empirical Paradigm. Little of the information provided in the empirical assessment relates directly to Madeline's communal tendencies or lack thereof, although we are left with the impression that she is probably not a particularly warm individual. Ben-Porath notes in Chapter 11, for example, that "Madeline is likely to create a favorable first impression; people may find her to be charming and engaging. She may have difficulty maintaining deeply rooted social relationships, however, and some may view her as being interpersonally manipulative."

On the whole, it is likely that Madeline is at most average in her communal tendencies, and that her less agreeable characteristics interfere with her being seen as particularly warm and nurturing by others, whatever her sympathetic thoughts and altruistic motives may be. It is likely that when Madeline expresses caring she does so through highly agentic actions; however welcome these actions may be, they probably leave intimates feeling more *assisted* than *nurtured*.

Other Common Themes

Several other common themes emerge across the various assessments. Although many, if not all, of these themes may be argued to have communal and agentic underpinnings (or, at least communal and agentic implications; see Wiggins & Trapnell, 1996), we have categorized them separately here because they provide a finer-grained level of analysis and understanding of Madeline. It is also beyond the scope of this chapter to discuss all of the themes that have arisen across the five assessments, so we have selected only a few that we deem to be most common and/or central (whether agreed upon or not among the paradigms).

Narcissism

The most thorough discussion of Madeline's possible narcissistic tendencies occurs within the interpersonal paradigm. In Chapter 9, Pincus and Gurtman discerningly synthesize aspects of Madeline's developmental history, self-presentation style, and partner-reported characteristics to venture the hypothesis that the most integrative description of her might suggest underlying narcissistic personality dynamics (rather than narcissistic personality disorder per se). Other evidence for narcissistic tendencies is readily available within the multivariate assessment; Costa and Piedmont indicate in Chapter 10 that Madeline is "more concerned with her own comfort and pleasure than with the well-being of others," and that "she is so immodest that others may see her as narcissistic." Costa and Piedmont also note that if Madeline were a treatment-seeking client, evidence for narcissistic personality disorder would be found in "Madeline's low Modesty, Straightforwardness, and Compliance traits—all of which contribute to a very self-focused, ego-expansive orientation." Ben-Porath, in the empirical assessment (Chapter 11), refers to Madeline's very high MMPI-2 Scale 9 score as indicating a likely tendency to have grandiose aspirations and an exaggerated sense of self-worth; with respect to her high Antisocial Practices score, she is described as likely to be self-centered. The personological paradigm says little with respect to the presence or absence of Madeline's narcissistic tendencies, although McAdams does note in Chapter 7 that "Indeed, in her Life Story Interview she boasts that she has won 53 legal cases in a row," and "There is a sense in which Madeline's story for the future is too good to be true." Madeline's narcissistic tendencies are also not a primary subject of discussion within the psychodynamic paradigm, although Behrends and Blatt do refer in Chapter 8 to Madeline's "self-absorbed defenses" and note that "She volunteers that she herself is a highly successful trial lawyer." It is likely that Madeline does demonstrate significant narcissistic tendencies, particularly with respect to being boastful.

Antisocial Behavior

We first come to know of Madeline's history of antisocial behavior within the personological paradigm (Chapter 7), where Madeline tells of having spent much of her youth in jail. Having spent time in jail is also mentioned by Madeline when she is interacting with Rebecca Behrends during the psychodynamic assessment (Chapter 8). Within the interpersonal paradigm (Chapter 9), we also come to know that both Madeline and her partner describe her as well above average in BC (Arrogant–Calculating) characteristics—characteristics that are generally associated with (although not necessarily indicative of) a propensity for antisocial practices and psychopathy. Costa and Piedmont also indicate in Chapter 10 that antisocial personality disorder would be one potential diagnosis worthy of further exploration, were Madeline a treatment-seeking client. The most information regarding Madeline's antisocial behavior (past) and antisocial tendencies (current) is presented in Chapter 11 within Ben-Porath's empirical assessment of Madeline. In particular, we learn that Madeline's highly elevated score on the Antisocial Practices content scale is suggestive of not only a history of antisocial behaviors, but also current antisocial inclinations.

Mania

The strongest evidence suggesting manic or hypomanic tendencies in Madeline's character has also emerged within the empirical paradigm (Chapter 11). Madeline's extremely elevated Scale 9 score on the MMPI-2 is considered by Ben-Porath to be somewhat of an exaggeration in light of Madeline's history (which does not suggest manic or hypomanic behavior that would be as problematic as her score suggests) and her validity scale profile (which suggests a tendency toward exaggerating and being overly dramatic). The likely manifestations of Madeline's hypomanic tendencies are summarized by Ben-Porath in quotations from Graham (2000, pp. 82-83), and are not reiterated here. Suffice it to say, for the current purposes, that an unrealistic vision of the future and a grandiose self-concept are associated features (see the discussion of narcissism above), as are a high energy level and a propensity for preferring action to thought. Madeline's NEO PI-R profile within the multivariate assessment (see Chapter 10) also shows some signs of a potential for hypomania, in that she is seen as "energetic and busy, does things with gusto and a rapid tempo, and craves thrills and stimulation." And, although references to Madeline's hypomanic potential are very indirect within the psychodynamic assessment, Behrends and Blatt do note in Chapter 8 that "She reactively manifests a complex array of defensive solutions, which tend to be highly action-oriented."

Boredom

Madeline's fear of boredom (and the negative effects boredom has on her) becomes apparent from her first assessment. In speaking with Dan McAdams (see Chapter 7), Madeline "remarks that she will probably be fine in life as long as she doesn't 'get bored.' " Within the psychodynamic paradigm (Chapter 8), we see how her cognitive functioning declines when she is understimulated: "Thus, when Madeline is confronted with a banal, repetitive, unchallenging task, her functioning becomes badly impaired. Challenge, stimulation, and excitement all serve to enable Madeline to function at an impressive level. But without this stimulation, her functioning can seriously deteriorate." The NEO PI-R profile within the multivariate paradigm (Chapter 10) elaborates that Madeline likes excitement, craves thrills and stimulation, and "is interested in experience for its own sake, seeking out novelty and variety." Madeline's MMPI-2 clinical scale profile (i.e., an extremely elevated score on Scale 9 and an elevated score on Scale 4) within the empirical paradigm (Chapter 11) suggests that she has "a proclivity to become bored and, as a consequence, depressed," and that "she may be preoccupied with activities designed to prevent herself from becoming bored—a situation she finds particularly aversive." Lastly, further insight into Madeline's propensity for, and fear of, boredom is found in Pincus and Gurtman's discussion within the interpersonal paradigm (Chapter 9) of Madeline's possible narcissistic personality structure: " . . . a common complaint of those with narcissistic personalities is boredom or emptiness. When life fails to provide sufficient support for the grandiose self, such individuals often complain of being bored, instead of articulating any personal affect such as depression, anxiety, or low self-esteem."

Distrust

A good deal of information is also provided across the various assessments suggesting that Madeline is distrustful in general, and probably distrustful of authority figures in particular. Given her background, and the tremendous harm she suffered at the hands of those who had control over her as a child, this is hardly surprising. In the personological assessment (Chapter 7), McAdams indicates from the start that Madeline is distrustful of authority; however, much more explicit evidence of his having formed a view of Madeline as highly self-protective and distrustful comes toward the end of his assessment, when he notes that "The battle is never over. No matter how many victories accrue, there always remains the possibility that the protagonist will ultimately be defeated. Consequently, the protagonist can never let up, but must always remain vigilant." Within the psychodynamic paradigm (Chapter 8), we see Madeline "preparing for battle" from her very first contact with the assessor: "First, she anticipates the control that she imagines will be imposed upon her by the authority figure involved in such a structured setting, and she attempts to wrest control by taking over the situation herself." With regard to the interpersonal paradigm, both Madeline and her partner rate her as well above average in hostile–dominant qualities, and Pincus and Gurtman suggest in Chapter 9 that "Madeline's continuing view of the world as potentially dangerous, and her sense that she must always be on guard, vigilant, and ready to do battle, create a social context that normalizes a certain amount of hostility." The multivariate assessment (Chapter 10) also indicates that Madeline is likely to be "characteristically suspicious of other people and skeptical of others' ideas and opinions." And within the empirical assessment (Chapter 11), we come to know of Madeline as rebellious against authority, with a cynical view of others as being selfish, dishonest, and untrustworthy. It should be borne in mind, however, that whatever Madeline's propensities for feeling distrustful, every indication suggests that she does not feel this way toward her partner (see her discussions of her partner in Chapters 7 and 8). This implies that Madeline is able to overcome her suspiciousness and distrustful inclinations in some circumstances, in order to forge deeper communal connections.

Neuroticism and Vulnerability

Madeline's current experience of, and potentiality for, negative emotions constitute another common topic of discussion. Where the emphasis is placed upon *current* experience of psychological distress, the answer seems clear: Madeline is decidedly *not* distressed. That Madeline feels that she is currently experiencing few, if any, feelings of distress is readily apparent within her self-reports (i.e., very low scores on the Anxiety, Depression, Self-Consciousness and Vulnerability facet scales of Neuroticism on the NEO PI-R [Chapter 10] and on Scales 1, 2, 3, and 7 of the MMPI-2 [Chapter 11]). Her partner's views of her Neuroticism on the NEO PI-R are, however, somewhat discrepant from her self-views; they suggest that her partner sees her as average with respect to Anxiety and Depression, and as in the high range with respect to Self-Consciousness and Vulnerability.

Whatever her current level of distress may be, however, her potentiality for experiencing significant vulnerability in the future is related not only to what her trait tendencies might be (e.g., her NEO PI-R scores on the related facets of Neuroticism), but also to the possibility of fragility in her overall character structure. It is in the latter regard that Behrends and Blatt (Chapter 8) suggest that Madeline is at risk for depression and possibly suicidality. Madeline's vulnerabilities are, in fact, the predominant theme of the psychodynamic assessment, in which much more implicit forms of information (i.e., not self-report information) provide the bases for conclusions. It is clear that Madeline has overcome a great deal and is apparently very "well defended," but Behrends and Blatt note that many painful issues also remain unresolved for Madeline:

> Madeline only occasionally experiences these intense dysphoric feelings, because they are strongly defended against by excessive activity, engagement with others, and stimulation seeking. These manic-like defenses are frequently channeled into constructive activities, but sometimes they are excessive and even off-putting and interpersonally jarring. These defenses are often successful in aiding Madeline to avoid the underlying depressive experiences. But when these defenses fail, Madeline can experience extreme feelings of depression, desolation, and hopelessness—even to the point of having thoughts of suicide, which are largely unconscious.

A PEER REVIEW OF MADELINE G

In this section, we provide a summary of the views of some of Madeline's friends. These individuals did not formally participate in the assessment process, but their more informal views provide another source of information against which all of the assessment results can be compared. A great deal of information about Madeline has been obtained and presented, and both Madeline's self-views and the views of her partner have been conveyed, albeit in response to the particular questions that form the bases of the inventories employed. The accuracy or *validity* of the information obtained is a difficult thing to determine; it is dependent upon the validity of the instruments and the honesty, insight, and correctness of the respondents (in this case, Madeline and her partner). One means of "checking" on this information, however, is to obtain much more information about Madeline, from other persons who know her, and then to examine how their information and impressions compare with what has been gleaned from the tests completed by Madeline and/or her partner. We therefore have compiled additional information about Madeline, obtained through discussions with some of the people who know her and consider her a friend. It should also be noted that the vast majority of this section, surveying the views of her friends, was written *prior* to obtaining the knowledge gleaned from the assessment reports. This section was not written to address or refute the assessment results, but in retrospect, its contents therefore probably lend further validity to what became apparent to her assessors.

Madeline G is a highly unusual woman in many respects, and it is in part those qualities that led to her being chosen as the subject for the present multifaceted case study; she is generally thought of as a "colorful character" and as having "a lot of personality." In addition, however, we wanted the case study to involve the description of a "normal" person (i.e., one who is not seeking treatment, or easily diagnosed and dismissed), and Madeline has not now or in the past sought psychological intervention.

Providing a nutshell description of Madeline is difficult, given the complexity of her personality, but it may be facilitated by a consideration of some of the predominant themes that have arisen in discussions with individuals who know her well. Madeline is an extremely extraverted and exhibitionistic woman. She is audacious, brash, and brazen, and being out in public with her can be highly embarrassing for the weak of heart. In addition to regularly engaging complete strangers in conversations, she is apt to making sexually suggestive remarks and to flaunt her own considerable sexuality. She also appears to have a fondness for doing so with individuals who are made uncomfortable by such actions, playfully mocking their prudishness. Episodes of "flashing" (flaunting her nudity) are not uncommon party behaviors for her, and on at least one occasion she reportedly bit the buttons off the shirt of a man she had just met. To some, these antics are amusing; to others, they are highly offensive. Despite these idiosyncracies, an invitation to one of her infamous parties is considered a social coup, and she has a truly remarkable ability to bring together large groups of highly disparate individuals and to show them all a good time.

Perhaps related to her extraversion, another predominant theme concerns her "hypomania." Madeline is clearly a highly active person who can work tirelessly and play tirelessly, often doing both within the same 24-hour period. She has a propensity for overextending herself, committing to too many disparate activities, but she also appears to cope reasonably well with (and seems to prefer) doing so, forgoing sleep and other mundane activities as necessary. There is no question that Madeline lives life fully, and her energy and engagement in all that life has to offer can be wonderfully contagious.

It is perhaps in part this hypomanic quality that has allowed Madeline to achieve so much, despite her relative youth and her sorely lacking early educational experiences. There is little question that Madeline is "driven." Her desire not only to succeed, but to be the best at everything she does, is well known. However, it appears that what may have begun as an attempt to prove something to herself and the wider social world has become an intrinsic passion for protecting the rights of those who have fallen prey to the same disadvantaged circumstances that colored her early life—and, for both selfish and other-oriented reasons, her goal is always to win!

It should be noted, however, that Madeline is not overly warm or empathic in the usual senses—but neither is she cold and uncaring. Madeline clearly cares deeply for her friends and would probably be the first person a friend would call if he or she required instrumental assistance of some kind. Nevertheless, Madeline can also be quick to pass judgment, and can be rather intolerant of neurotic "self-reflection"; hence friends may be less likely to seek her out as a source of emotional support, at least in the sense of having an ear to listen and a shoulder to cry on. Nonetheless, Madeline is a champion for the causes of her friends and is most willing to take on active tasks to promote, protect, or defend them.

Another of Madeline's salient qualities may be loosely termed "superficiality." Madeline is most certainly not shallow, although she is highly concerned with creating an impression. In its most pathological manifestation, this impression management takes the form of *pseudologia fantastica*—"the tendency to tell outrageous untruths while seeming, at least during the telling, to believe them" (McWilliams, 1994, p. 307). Usually these tales take the form of associating herself with famous people in order to impress upon others her own importance or social salience, but they also occasionally take the form of tales told to elicit sympathy from others. It is worth noting, however, that these tales are usually fantastical elaborations of true experiences. For example, Madeline is well acquainted with a number of musicians, some of whom are quite famous; however, she decidedly did not play the saxophone in any of their recordings (under an assumed name), despite her occasional claims of having done so. Nor has she ever been terminally ill with bone cancer, although she did undergo surgery for a joint problem.

Clearly related to this tendency toward impression management, Madeline is known for being boastful and self-aggrandizing, and there is little doubt that she does so with relish and abandon. Madeline is proud of who she is (or, more importantly, who she has become), but these tendencies also belie an underlying insecurity reflected in the fear that she does not or cannot measure up to expectations, particularly in her newer and more high-powered environments. It is likely that the more insecure she feels, the more grandiose she becomes. And in that vein, those who have known Madeline for quite some time have noted that her tendency toward embellishment has decreased as her own status and power have increased.

It is also clear that Madeline is a master of manipulation who is capable of engaging in any of a number of cunning and crafty tactics to bring about the outcomes she desires. Nevertheless, despite her obvious interests in power and control, to those who know her well she also displays an endearing vulnerability. One may need to catch her in a weak or highly comfortable moment to bring conversations back to a form of true relatedness, but with some guidance from a trusted peer she is capable of heartfelt and truthful conversation—albeit with a few divergences into the fantastical, which can generally be redirected. That said, there is little doubt that Madeline is narcissistic (perhaps even diagnostically so), but she is also intrinsically motivated by a desire to seek out and be close to others. Will she put her own needs above those of another (even a loved one)? Almost certainly, and sometimes dramatically. On the other hand, is she capable of tenderness, caring, and compassion? Yes, that too, but under the proper circumstances, with the love and acceptance of a trusted peer. Perhaps unsurprisingly, Madeline is not eager to share widely her more insecure and vulnerable side; still, she is capable of doing so in a most endearing way, with those she has come to love and trust.

It should be noted, however, that although Madeline is occasionally capable of expressing vulnerability, she is seldom susceptible to feelings of anxiety or depression. It appears that in Madeline's adult life, the only period of prolonged negative affect that she has experienced occurred following the breakup of a relationship with a man with whom she was (perhaps for the first time in her life) truly in love. There are no indications to suggest that she was clinically depressed during this time, but she was dysphoric—an emotional experience that was relatively foreign to one who is so prone to hypomania and positive emotions. Madeline reportedly "bounced back" from this episode relatively quickly, and she generally seems to be a nonanxious and "upbeat" person. Nonetheless, one must always hold out the possibility that if circumstances converged in such a way as to seriously undermine her interpersonal relationships or her career achievement, she might be prone to a depressive episode—but so, likely, would many people. However, it also seems that her "defensive armor" has served her well through a variety of potentially debilitating experiences, and we have no reason to expect it to do otherwise in the future.

With respect to Madeline's propensity for substance abuse, it would appear that although she does use substances (i.e., alcohol and marijuana), she does so in relative moderation. Within the circles in which Madeline travels, alcohol and drug use are not uncommon; in this context, Madeline does not abuse substances. Her peers (in all of their vast and varied guises) have not reported problems related to Madeline's behavior "under the influence," nor does it appear that her job performance has ever suffered from substance use. And it seems likely that Madeline's needs for control and achievement would override any desires she might have to abuse substances.

All who have spoken about Madeline in this volume have done so with enthusiasm and concern, and both impressions are warranted. Given her "rags-to-riches" story and the highly upbeat nature of the subject herself, it is perhaps easier to focus on the positive attributes that she exhibits than on the negative attributes that may also be present, although the negative attributes also warrant considerable attention.

Madeline is undoubtedly a highly dominant individual who is, first and foremost, self-protective and self-aggrandizing. She creates impressions for her own gain and is quite willing to manipulate others in order to achieve her own aims. She is deceptive in her self-presentation and is unlikely to sacrifice her desires to placate another, regardless of her relationship with the person(s) involved. And it seems that she is able to justify, on the basis of self-need rather than higher moral purposes, virtually any behavior toward which she feels inclined.

Such a combination of characteristics may seem, on the face of it, rather toxic, but consideration of her positive attributes is also in order. It seems clear that among those who are not wholly intimidated or offended by Madeline (and a vast array of high-status people may be included in this group), she presents as a very interesting and fun-loving person. She is clearly unconventional, and this characteristic appears to allow for her engagement in a wide array of activities that would appeal to different "audiences." And those who feel that they are "in her court" appear to feel privileged to be there—not in the sense of being in a "one-down" position, but in knowing that they have an active force on their side, should they ever need one. None seem to question her loyalty, although all seem to understand that her first loyalty will always be to herself. Nevertheless, all who love her seem to bask in her energy, enthusiasm, love of life, and great propensity for fun and amusement. These qualities—coupled with her ability to undertake a host of tasks at any given time, and her real concern for her friends—appear to make her a great friend to others, despite the necessary caveats and contingencies.

In sum, it is clear that Madeline has a very dominant social presence and is not easily forgotten or dismissed. She is most assuredly disinhibited and dramatic in her self-presentation, and she relishes the effect this has on others. She is grandiose and somewhat deceitful, although it appears that her goals in this regard are twofold—not only establishing dominance, but also providing an interesting social stimulus for the purpose of endearing herself to others. She also appears to care about others, although she chooses to do so in her own highly assertive and instrumental ways. It is possible that she cares most about herself and is highly aggrandizing and self-protective toward these ends. However, it is noteworthy that many of those who are closest to her acknowledge this tendency and yet continue to feel that Madeline would be readily available to them (albeit perhaps in some ways more than others) if they ever needed help. She is also highly active and hard-striving, and likely to undertake a wide range of activities within a short time period—from nude bungee jumping one day to winning a major criminal case the next. And she is a self-loving, minimally neurotic individual who enjoys a wide array of activities and pursuits. She has not only overcome considerable obstacles, but has also been willing to take them on, with the confidence of knowing that she will once again succeed in overcoming them.

The bottom line? The best we can do is to say that anyone who chooses to associate intimately with Madeline is forewarned that she is prone to selfish behavior and is capable of justifying any such actions, in her own mind at least. Coworkers are similarly forewarned, in that Madeline may be aggressive and self-promoting in her desires to achieve status and recognition. It should be noted, however, that these actions are self-focused and are not cruel or vengeful in intent or tone; rather, she may be more motivated than most to protect herself and her well-being (which probably won't be all that surprising to those who know of her upbringing). Friends, however, may benefit from her strong need to be connected with others, to entertain others, and the (instrumental) supportiveness that is engendered—not to mention the high social stimulus value that can be obtained through association with such an extraverted and well-connected individual. And intimates may perhaps enjoy brief forays into the inner workings of a highly complex and highly intelligent individual, who loves and lives life more fully than most, and who is capable of vulnerable, emotionally charged interchange.

MADELINE SINCE THE ASSESSMENTS

Another means of providing validity information involves a consideration of Madeline's current status and the events that have occurred in her life over the 3 years since she was assessed, as they relate to the various concerns and predictions made by the assessors. The predominant themes that have emerged in considerations of what might be in store for Madeline understandably fall within the categories of work and love (or agency and communion)—arguably common themes across various paradigms of personality assessment (see Chapter 6).

Madeline and the New Law Firm

Although they were not specifically asked to do so, assessors from all of the paradigms have ventured some informal "predictions" concerning how Madeline would fare in the "prestigious" law firm that she was about to join when she participated in the Life Story Interview. As it turned out, she did not fare well: After a few weeks, Madeline and her boss apparently agreed that Madeline wasn't capable of being an employee. Madeline therefore left that firm to go into private practice in criminal law, primarily defending aboriginals. Madeline describes herself as "much happier being my own boss." The views of the assessors from different paradigms on this issue follow.

• *Personological paradigm* (Chapter 7). " . . . Madeline worries that she may not fit in with the other lawyers at the new firm. Given her brash and earthy presentation, it makes sense to worry about this."
• *Psychodynamic paradigm* (Chapter 8). In line with the request of Behrends and Blatt, the psychodynamic assessment was conducted "blindly," in the absence of information from the Life Story Interview. They nevertheless were able to detect vocational concerns: " . . . her profound vulnerability to intense dysphoric feelings of helplessness and hopelessness around

issues of professional disappointment and especially around issues of interpersonal loss and loneliness."

• *Interpersonal paradigm* (Chapter 9). "We predict occupational success for Madeline. . . . However, there may also be pitfalls ahead. Indeed, she may not make the hoped-for positive interpersonal impacts on others at the law firm."

• *Multivariate paradigm* (Chapter 10). The assessors in the multivariate paradigm have not commented directly on prospects for success in the prestigious law firm, although they have provided a more general statement: "What better career for a person with this antagonistic profile to channel her aggressive tendencies into socially directed ways, than as a lawyer securing the civil rights of underdogs?"

• *Empirical paradigm* (Chapter 11). The various validity scales of the MMPI-2 have been especially effective in identifying Madeline's tendency to exaggerate, embellish, and dramatize her self-presentation. With respect to the issue of success in the new law firm, "Will Madeline be able to fit in at her new law firm? . . . In light of her history, Madeline's concerns about these issues appear more realistic than the picture of bluster and assurance she projects."

In a recent interview with Madeline, more information about her current career status was obtained. It has been nearly 3 years since Madeline began her private-practice firm, and she has continued to be highly successful, with an ever-growing practice. Madeline's law firm, "G and Company," has grown to include a staff of five, including one other attorney (also of Native American origins), a paralegal, and an accountant. Her firm continues to handle mostly criminal cases (with brief forays into protecting the other rights of her existing clients in civil cases), with far more than half of her clients being Native Americans. With respect to how Madeline feels about her work, her first response was "I keep winning, and that keeps me happy." She also went on to say that she—being originally an outsider to the mainstream, particularly where power and politics were concerned— loves the fact that she can "play by *their* rules and win." Madeline also noted that whatever her embellishment and self-promoting tendencies may be in other areas, when it comes to her legal career she works "entirely by the book" and is completely honest and above board in all of her dealings. Finally, she noted that in her first year of private practice, her firm grossed over $400,000. Madeline, however, chooses to continue to draw a salary of $1,500 every 2 weeks, and to reinvest the remainder in the firm.

Madeline and her Partner

Some comments have also been made by the assessors regarding Madeline's relationship with her partner.

- *Personological paradigm* (Chapter 7). McAdams remarks that "Her partner provides a secure base for her; his love helps to give her the confidence she needs to fight the good fight," and raises the possibility that "Should [he] fail her, she may become much more vulnerable."

- *Psychodynamic paradigm* (Chapter 8). Behrends and Blatt state: "It does appear that in Madeline's long-time relationship with her male partner, she has found in her adult life someone she can truly love and be loved by in return," and "For Madeline, their relationship appears to have been redemptive." Concern is also raised for Madeline's future well-being, in part should anything happen to her relationship: " . . . one should not underestimate her profound vulnerability to intense feelings of helplessness and hopelessness, especially around issues of interpersonal loss, professional disappointment, and loneliness."

- *Interpersonal paradigm* (Chapter 9). Pincus and Gurtman, having access to both Madeline's self-ratings and her partner's ratings of her, note significant discrepancies in their views of Madeline: "Interestingly, he shares her view that she is dominant, but contrasts in his assessment of her along the hostile–friendly dimension." Furthermore, "With regard to global interpersonal adjustment, Madeline views herself as below average in interpersonal difficulty (elevation = 37.1), whereas her partner sees her as above average (elevation = 61.7)." It is indicated that neither Madeline's own view nor the views of her partner can be seen as more or less veridical; both may be subject to biases, including that "her partner's ratings of her may also be influenced by relationship issues at the time of the assessment." Pincus and Gurtman further note: "Madeline's partner clearly holds a view of her that is divergent from the view she holds of herself. This divergence may become problematic in the future if it is not addressed," and "Madeline and her partner are likely to butt heads about this at some point, and its resolution will be critical to the stability of their relationship."

- *Multivariate paradigm* (Chapter 10). Discrepancies between Madeline's self-view and the view that her partner has of her are also apparent within the multivariate paradigm. Although much of the disagreement occurs with respect to the less "interpersonal" domains of Neuroticism and Conscientiousness, it is nonetheless apparent that her partner is negatively affected by her characteristics: " . . . Madeline has a strong, assertive personality that can easily imagine possibilities and move toward them in ways that may seem calculating and brusque, especially to her common-law husband." We also come to know that (as in the interpersonal paradigm) Madeline "sees herself more positively than her significant other sees her," and that she may experience particular difficulties in contexts "involving intimacy, nurturance, acceptance, tolerance, and forgiveness."

- *Empirical paradigm* (Chapter 11). Discussion of Madeline's relationship within the empirical assessment is rather more indirect. It can be surmised that some of her characteristics may run counter to the development of a stable intimate relationship, but the only reference made to the relationship comes in the form of Ben-Porath's agreeing with McAdams's concerns and stating: "These concerns are consistent with MMPI-2 indications that Madeline's outward presentation of confidence and poise may mask some underlying insecurity. In light of her history, Madeline's concerns about these issues appear more realistic than the picture of bluster and assurance she projects."

So what is the status of Madeline's relationship? Approximately a year and a half after the assessments were conducted, Madeline's long-term partner left her. He apparently did so somewhat surreptitiously, having bought and taken possession of a new home prior to informing her. He did, however, inform her in person, waiting for her at their shared home when she returned from a business trip. Among the myriad of things that were probably said by him at the time, Madeline remembers most clearly his saying something to the effect of "It has to be about *me* now." Madeline was both baffled and devastated.

Thinking that the book would be imminently ready for press (which wasn't yet to be), we spoke with Madeline a few months after her partner left, and we drew a few primary conclusions about Madeline's views and status at that time. Madeline was depressed, with some suicidal ideation but no plan, and she clearly stated that she had no intention of forming such a plan. She was, in part, confused and depressed about *being depressed*—a very foreign emotion for one who is usually hypomanic. At the time, however, she was not seeing herself and her behavior as having in any way contributed to her partner's leaving, and she was adamant that he would return. She was also adamant that she would welcome him back with open arms, "no questions asked."

Madeline was interviewed again within a few days of the 3-year anniversary of her assessments (and when the book *was* to be imminently ready for press). Some significant changes had occurred in her thinking in the year and a half since her partner had left, and in the year or so since she was last interviewed. Madeline began by saying that she would "never understand" why her partner left, but as the conversation proceeded it became apparent that she did understand, perhaps on levels that she would rather not think about too much. Early in the conversation (i.e., when Madeline's defenses were probably still "up"), Madeline indicated that she felt her partner had left her largely because he felt the need to appease his aging parents (who never approved of Madeline; with whom she never had a relationship; and with whom she discouraged, if not prevented, her partner's relationship). Madeline also recalled the early months of her reaction to her partner's leaving, indicating that she lost weight and couldn't sleep (sleeplessness has always been a problem for her but was now dramatically intensified), and that she obtained a prescription for sleeping pills. She poignantly told of having spent one entire night sitting at the table and looking at the bottle of pills, contemplating taking all of them, and at dawn's early light deciding that she had better get ready for work.

Madeline noted that the year after her partner left was her "hardest year ever." She added that a couple of months before our last interview (when her partner had been gone for more than a year), she and her partner spoke (they have remained friends and have seen each other regularly since he left), and he made it clear that he would not be coming back. Madeline indicated that she had held on to the belief that this was a glitch in their relationship and that he would come back; she noted that hearing him tell her that he wouldn't be returning brought back much of the earlier pain of losing him. Madeline indicated though that although she is no longer pining ("I can't; there are too many people counting on me"), she will always love him and has no interest in forming a new relationship.

As the conversation progressed, and Madeline became less characteristically "well defended," Madeline indicated that her partner was the best thing that ever happened in her life. She then spoke honestly and insightfully about how her own actions might have been problematic. Madeline recalled how her partner had said, upon leaving, that it all needed to be about *him* now. She stated that "If I'd done that 9 years ago, he never would have left." She also indicated that her partner was apparently disappointed by how busy she was and by the fact that she spent the vast majority of time away from home, but that she never knew he had felt this way. In those senses, she blamed him too, because he apparently rarely stated any grievances that she could then potentially correct. When asked if she still felt that he would come back, she said, with childlike vulnerability, "No, because he says he won't."

Madeline's Goals

When asked about her plans for the future, Madeline, perhaps unsurprisingly, noted only agentic agendas. She will continue to run (and perhaps expand) her highly successful legal practice. She indicated that she always works under a "5-year plan" and that her current plan is to save money. Madeline has never been the least bit materialistic, and none of her actions that have been designed to impress others have ever involved claiming or flaunting wealth. Madeline noted with pride, though, that she has almost completed paying off all of her debts (e.g., she recently paid off the loan on her modest car), with only a small portion of student loan debt remaining. She now has in her 5-year plan the goals of buying a house and otherwise securing her financial future.

Madeline's Reactions to Having Been Assessed

At the time when Madeline first agreed to be assessed, she was basically just beginning her legal career and was still largely caught between what she was "way back when" (i.e., an outsider from a very dysfunctional and disadvantaged background), what she had been in the interim (i.e., a student with promise but still no status), and what she was becoming (i.e., a highly successful lawyer). We believe that two of Madeline's most endearing characterics—her great sense of adventure and her desire to live life fully—were her primary motivations in agreeing to being assessed so systematically and intrusively by five assessment teams. Her narcissistic tendencies also ensured that she would enjoy telling others (especially a group of "experts") about herself. But all indications suggest that Madeline has never been particularly self-reflective, and there can be little doubt that the vast majority of individuals (even adventure-seeking ones) would *not* have agreed to partake in something so intrusive and so potentially disconcerting. That Madeline agreed to do so probably speaks largely to her Openness to Experience (and the aforementioned quality of living life fully), coupled with the fact that she had reached a point of significant accomplishment and acceptance in life. Beginning to delve into her character (for better or for worse) was now less frightening than it probably would have been at any point in the past, and although Madeline has tended to explore her tremendous curiosities in all ways *except* those related to understanding herself, she was apparently ready now; she was in the safest place she'd ever known.

Madeline has also changed (in adaptations rather than in characteristics) over the years, from the time she was approached about being assessed until the present day. In the earlier days of her anticipating being assessed, she would mention how great it would be to have part of a book written about her, and to be famous and talked about. We spoke with her about the anonymity that would be in place for her assessments, and she would joke that she couldn't wait to "go on *Oprah*" to tell the world that *she* is Madeline G! Madeline was notably less exhibitionistic about her assessments by the time that she was assessed—probably in large part because she began to worry about what they might reveal, but also in part because her career status was advancing, and even unabashedly positive reports about her would potentially relay more information to colleagues and competitors than she was now willing to share.

Although it had been our original intention to spend a significant amount of time with Madeline, to go through each and every assessment report with her, and to help her through any potential reactions, earlier attempts to coordinate schedules failed, and in the final stages Madeline indicated that she felt no need or desire for such extended contact. In a nutshell, her response was something to the effect of "I'm the expert at what I do, you're the expert at what you do—just do it!" This is not to suggest, however, that Madeline had become entirely complacent about the results of the assessments. Rather, she was satisfied that they would not reveal her true identity, and was now more truly comfortable (rather than blusteringly confident) within "her own skin"; therefore, she didn't feel the need to hear, and react to, anyone's impressions (even the experts'!).

When Madeline was interviewed for the last time, she was asked whether she had any curiosities about the assessments. She asked only one initial question: "What did my responses to the inkblots say about me?" This would be a reasonable question on any grounds, but Madeline then volunteered that she was somewhat concerned about that portion of the testing. When the assessor (Rebecca Behrends) kept asking her what Madeline remembers as something like "Where do you see that?," Madeline interpreted this as "Where do you see *that*?," and feared that her responses were bizarre and were constantly puzzling the assessor. Madeline was told that this line of inquiry would be inevitable, no matter what she had reported seeing, and Madeline was obviously relieved. Nonetheless, portions of the psychodynamic assessment were read to Madeline, and her reaction was basically "Wow!, Did everyone get me like that?" She also indicated that she was rather uncomfortable that her vulnerable side would come through so obviously, because she does everything she can to hide it so that she can keep the upper hand.

When Madeline was told that, yes, everyone "got her" (in different ways), and that all assessors had scored "hits," she enthusiastically remarked: "I love that. I love the idea of this. That's it! What a great idea this was!" She also indicated that although she recalls her earlier reaction of loving the idea of broadcasting that part of a book had been written about her, she now wants to protect her identity and ensure that no one knows that this is about her. The bulk of the "Peer Review" section about Madeline was also read to her, and she acted like a cheerleader through parts of it (e.g., "Ya!," "That's me!," "Of course!" "Who wouldn't?"). There is no question that Madeline is understandably proud of what she has overcome, pleased with who she has become, and characteristically excited and optimistic about the future. She has gone through the worst of what the assessors feared might occur (i.e., not working out at the law firm, losing her partner). She was not unscathed, but could not be undone. We place our bets alongside McAdams's, stated at the end of Chapter 7:

> The future surely looks bright. But even if things darken significantly, it is hard to imagine that life could ever return to the bleak depths Madeline ex-

perienced as a child and adolescent. The protagonist in this narrative is simply too strong now. The movement of the plot is strongly upward and progressive. The enemies have been irrevocably weakened. Even if the forces of evil manage to launch an aggressive attack as she moves into midlife, I would still put my money on Madeline.

Coda

KRISTA K. TROBST

On September 27, 2002, prior to this book being entirely ready for press, Jerry S. Wiggins, PhD, suffered a massive stroke from which he is not expected to recover in any truly meaningful sense. The book was 99% written, and it was mostly just the tedious details that were needed to send it off for publication. The last portion of that "going to press" task has been done by me (with a lot of help from our friends!). For better or worse, the present situation seems to call for something not usually provided when fully functioning authors publish—namely, a "why and how" of the author's last work. As Jerry has indicated in his Acknowledgments to this book, I am his wife and principal collaborator, and it is within those roles that I share his "hows" and "whys."

WHY *THIS* BOOK?

Jerry began writing this book in the fall of 1996. He had retired (due to mandatory retirement at the age of 65) from the University of British Columbia (where he became Professor Emeritus) at the end of June that year. We were married in May 1996, on the weekend of his retirement party; Paul Costa gave Jerry's retirement address and was then best man at our wedding, within a 3-day span. Two weeks later, Jerry and I left for New Haven, Connecticut—for me to begin my internship at Yale University School of Medicine, and for Jerry to take on a visiting fellowship at Yale. We sent the majority of our belongings via a moving company, but we drove to New Haven along the "scenic route" through Canada, and had many hours to talk during that time. Being newly retired, Jerry was in a position of feeling both loss and freedom, and was contemplating how he most wanted to spend his newfound time. He decided that he was going to write a book about agency and communion, and in the last few months before his retirement, he had some contact with David Bakan in order to stimulate his thoughts in this regard.

Jerry's vision and passion changed after we arrived at Yale. I was interning with more than a dozen others, and as happens when people are uprooted and thrown together, many of us became fast friends. As Jerry came to know many of the other interns over beers at various New Haven pubs, he delighted in "talking shop" with such a bright and enthusiastic group. In doing so, though, he came to think of how their training, expertise, and preferences seemed so largely predictable on the basis of where they had gone to school and who their research and clinical mentors were. He applauded that and them; he understood the reasons for their focused commitment; but he also wondered whether a group like this might be interested in some exposure to the other possible approaches to personality assessment, so that they could broaden their perspectives and make freer choices.

Jerry's own personality assessment training was remarkably broad, but it had probably been several decades since he had thought about the potential for breadth in clinical training and what he would come to think of as different "paradigms." Jerry had no problem at all with individuals becoming experts in the methods of any particular assessment paradigm over all others—in fact, he admired expertise in any paradigm. What he was striving for with this book was not to demand that individuals have a detailed knowledge of all of the paradigms, but rather to encourage free and informed choice among them (given that one can never become an expert in them all). Because Jerry appreciated all of the paradigms so very much, he wanted others to share his enthusiasm for them, and then to select the ones they would work with and develop expertise in—that is, not to have their choice determined entirely by where they went to graduate school and who their clinical mentors were.

WHY NOT THE *OTHER* BOOK?

Many of those who "cut their teeth" on Jerry's first book, *Personality and Prediction* (Wiggins, 1973b), often ask why Jerry never revised it—particularly after retirement, when he might have had the perfect opportunity to do so. For those who don't know about *Personality and Prediction*, it is a classic in personality assessment; it has never been updated or replaced, and is still a "must read" for anyone who is serious about developing expertise in personality assessment. The text is still often used and cited today.

Many may not know what an extraordinary effort was required to write *Personality and Prediction*; Jerry spent almost 10 years writing and perfecting it. He actually dictated the book (in the days before word processing), working in a crawl space in his tiny home (winner of a small-home award!) in Champaign–Urbana, Illinois (now Urbana–Champaign), between 5:00 and 9:00 A.M. each day. He loved the book, and was proud of the regard in which it was always held, but he had vowed that he would never do *that* again. He was asked frequently to update it, and toyed for a while with the idea of doing so, with a trusted colleague as first author. But Jerry wasn't truly enthused by the thought, and the project never took off.

Jerry also had become increasingly interested in history and theory, and felt that if he had another book or two in him, he would rather be writing in those areas. Of course, *Personality and Prediction* is strong in historical content about the *practice* (and methods) of personality assessment, but Jerry had become more interested in the history of the *theories* of personality assessment. Still, a perusal of the table of contents of *Personality and Prediction* might lead one to see the current book as, to some degree, an elaboration and extension of Part 3 of that earlier book.

One might also ask why he wrote *Paradigms of Personality Assessment* rather than the *Agency and Communion* book he had intended to write when he first retired. I think the answer to that question lies in Jerry's tremendous generativity. *Agency and Communion*, had it been written, would have been a book primarily for theorists and not so much for students. Jerry's exposure to a group of eager (albeit advanced) students at Yale ignited his generative passions to write another book for students, just as *Personality and Prediction* had been written for students.

THE *HOWS* OF THIS BOOK

As Jerry has noted in the Introduction to this book, he had a good deal of both planned and fortuitous exposure to the various personality assessment paradigms in his graduate and clinical training, and in his readings and research endeavors. Jerry was always a seeker and a voracious reader, as well as a very skilled and broad-minded researcher. There is no question that the majority of what he wrote in this book he simply pulled from his memory banks, and surprisingly little new reading was required. However, Jerry wanted to be sure that his writings were accurate—and, as he notes in the Acknowledgments, he had the tremendous benefit of dear friends who were principal representatives of each of the paradigms, and whom he could ask to review the chapters. Of course, Jerry would still take primary responsibility for any errors that might have remained in any of the paradigm chapters.

One of Jerry's primary concerns in writing this book, however, was ensuring that his complete respect and enthusiasm for *all* of the paradigms be clear. Jerry and I cotaught half of the two-semester graduate assessment course here at York University (where I am on the faculty and Jerry is an adjunct professor) for a couple of years, and we used drafts of this book's chapters as the text. The clinical students here at York take this course during their first year of graduate training, and, as such, are likely to begin the course with relatively few preconceived notions regarding the benefits and drawbacks of the various paradigms of personality assessment. Jerry's main question to our graduate students, after their reading of the chapter drafts, was "What's your favorite paradigm?" He was always delighted that no particular paradigm was favored by a majority of students. This information suggested that Jerry seemed to have achieved what he had set out to do—to write an even-handed and respectful account of *all* the paradigms. For proponents of one paradigm or another, who wish Jerry had taken a stronger stance in pointing out the flaws of an "opposing" paradigm, all I can say is that this wasn't the purpose of this book. And perhaps the greatest beauty of the book is that no one will ever know for sure which paradigm Jerry might have chosen to favor, or denigrate, if he had been forced to do so. That is also perhaps among the greatest beauties of Jerry, because I couldn't tell you which ones he would choose either—his choice was *always* to appreciate all.

AGENCY AND COMMUNION
IN THE FINAL STAGES OF THIS BOOK

Without a lot of help from our friends, this book would not have been completed as well and as quickly. As I have indicated, some finishing touches were required, following Jerry's incapacitation, in order to get the book ready for press. "Getting the book out" had become a very common phrase in our home, and therefore it seemed that the most fitting way to pay tribute to Jerry (and to the field we both love) in the aftermath of his stroke was to send the book to press as quickly as possible. Jerry and I have been very fortunate, as Jerry notes in his Acknowledgments, to have developed wonderful friendships with some of the scholars who are among the "best in the business" of personality assessment. It is unlikely that I would have had the strength, courage, and wisdom to finalize Jerry's last project as quickly and as well without significant encouragement, support, and advice from some of our comrades.

Tom Widiger continued in the role he had established with Jerry of critically appraising all chapters, and I, like Jerry, am tremendously grateful for all of Tom's substantial efforts and insights. One of the most substantive decisions required in finalizing the manuscript for this book involved deciding between various versions Jerry had written for one of the chapters, and I am indebted to Tom Widiger and Dan Ozer for assisting with that decision. Lew Goldberg read and copyedited all chapters of the book within a very short time frame—and, most importantly, he used his substantial love and guidance to make sure that I kept going through this process. Lew was also the impetus for my writing this Coda to the book. Given the unusual nature of such a thing, I was unsure about its contents and tone, and relied upon Sidney Blatt, Lew Goldberg, Dan Ozer, and Aaron Pincus to provide emotional and critical responses to that material.

The final chapter (Chapter 12) also remained incomplete, having been only partly written prior to Jerry's stroke. Although under better circumstances I probably would have handled this task alone, I called upon Dan Ozer, David Nichols, Paul Costa, Sidney Blatt, and especially Aaron Pincus for feedback regarding drafts of this last chapter. It is much better as a result of their input. One of my graduate students, Lindsay Ayearst, also read all of the chapters for Jerry at a much earlier stage and provided comments to him from a student's perspective. She also took on multiple tasks (including teaching one of my courses!) in the aftermath of Jerry's stroke, in order to free me up to nurture Jerry and complete his book. All of my students clearly came through and handled many matters that should not have been theirs to handle, but one of my undergraduate students also deserves special mention: Anthony Ruocco arranged for having photos made of the figures, found and updated references, and almost single-handedly obtained permissions for all reproduced and adapted material in this book. My undying love and gratitude go to Geoffrey Slater Wiggins (my stepson), whose commitment to and love for both his father and me led him to give up a Christmas in order to help finalize this book.

The greatest thanks are due to Madeline G (and her partner at the time), without whom Part II of this book could not have been written. Madeline volunteered to undergo an arduous and intrusive assessment process, and to embark on a process of self-discovery through those experiences. That the results of her assessments would be shared with the readers of this book would probably have led most would-be case study participants to shy away (regardless of assurances of anonymity). Perhaps equally daunting, however, is the fact that her testing results are also available to *her* within this book. As appealing as it might sound on the face of it, many of us probably don't want to know quite that much about ourselves, particularly if it comes in the form of "expert opinion." I am of the firm belief that Madeline's willingness to participate in this process is the result of her extraordinary desire to live life fully, and by whatever means we each might choose to do so, Madeline should surely serve as an inspiration toward those ends.

APPENDIX A.
THEMATIC APPERCEPTION TEST (TAT) PROTOCOL

Appendix A gives the complete transcript of Madeline G's Thematic Apperception Test (TAT) protocol. As Behrends and Blatt describe in Chapter 8, Madeline's TAT assessment was somewhat shortened because Madeline was late for the testing session. Only the following cards were presented: Cards 1, 2, 3 GF, 14, 13 MF, 5, 10, 18 GF, and 17 BM. In the transcript, each card is described first, in **boldface** with brackets (these descriptions are based on those of Murstein, 1963, pp. 16–17). Madeline's responses then follow in roman type. Questions and prompts by the assessor are given in italics with parentheses; descriptions of Madeline, and other reactions on the assessor's part, are given in roman with brackets.

Card 1. [A young boy contemplates a violin, which rests on the table in front of him.] Violin, he borrowed this from somebody. Played it, he knows he's in deep shit. "How am I going to make this right again?" But he's okay about it—not upset. (*Borrowed?*) Without permission. So intrigued by everything, he has to try it all. Knows he can get out of trouble. Not deceptive, inquisitive. But "How do I fix it?" Smart, resourceful kid. But if his mother or father comes in, he's in shit! I could do this all day. Fun, right? Gonna find somebody who knows somebody to fix it. First he thinks, "Can I fix this?" Knows somebody who fixes things. Not broken bad; a string or something. He has no money. He's complicated but not bad. Just having a look at the problem. Talks out loud.

Card 2. [Country scene: In the foreground is a young woman with books in her hand; in the background a man is working in the fields and an older woman is looking on.] She is the only daughter of this hard-working couple. Contemplating her role in family. Mother having a second child. She's not all that happy. Mother is. Wanting another child for quite some time, hoping for a son—hand around farm. He loves his daughter. She's not that strong. He works all his land. She's pretty

331

hard-working. They provide well for their daughter. Nice sweater, hair done in bow, pretty braid. Simple people. Unsure about going away to school or be like her mom. Not a bad thing. Proud of her family. Mom's happy, content. (*How does it end?*) Madeline has to say she goes away to school, becomes a whore and heroin addict!! These two characters more interesting than her. Been together since young. She is looking for more, doesn't realize depth of her own family. She's kind of boring and bland. Dad real comfortable where he's at. Salt of the earth.

Card 3 GF. [A young woman is standing with downcast head, her face covered with her right hand. Her left arm is stretched forward against a wooden door.] Oh, no! Just had fight with her boyfriend. He came over and yelled at her. She's in despair. She didn't tell him because she's pregnant. In doing that, she sealed her fate. He said some pretty nasty shit. (*Argue?*) Accused her of sleeping around. Little trollop! (*End?*) Single mother, poor, guilt-ridden, resentful, very lonely. Sad story.

Card 14. [The silhouette of a man (or woman) against a bright window. The rest of the picture is totally black.] Oh, wow, a dreamer. He can't sleep. He is up in middle of night. Throws open windows on gorgeous summer night. Enjoying the smells and the sights, pondering the meaning of life. Great sense of peace, alone but not alone. He is good by himself 'cause he is part of all of his environment. Comfortable in own skin. [Madeline stretches, rather like a cat, and pops her neck; very sensuous.]

Card 13 MF. [A young man is standing with his downcast head buried in his arm. Behind him is the figure of a woman lying in bed.] Oh, he's going home to his wife. "Thank you very much, mistress. That was great." He's happy and she's happy. She's smart, too. She loves the good sex—not the trappings of a relationship. And he likes sex with her. If his wife ever found out, his ass would be killed. Not a major age difference there. They're about the same that way. Age-old story. Nothing too complex there.

Card 5. [A middle-aged woman is standing on the threshold of a half-opened door, looking into a room.] She's his wife! She suspects something! She wasn't supposed to be home! She hears him! He's got that look on his face—"I've been caught!" She wants to know, but doesn't. If he did it, out he goes! The only one who has nothing to lose is the beautiful mistress. He should have had a shower before he went home! She's gonna be able to smell that!

Card 10. [A young man's head against a man's shoulder.] They're lovers. Very tender moment in a gay relationship, both seem very content. Nice picture. Embracing, having a little nap. Very warm, relaxed, nice because they usually fight like cats and dogs. Too tired now, take a nap. Have a friend, Martin and Matt—high drama! They can be as catty. . . !

Card 18 GF. [A woman has her hands squeezed around the throat of another woman, whom she appears to be pushing backward across the banister of a stairway.] They're having a scrap! This one's older, but this one's stronger in a way, emotionally. That one's frail, weak. This one's physically stronger and really quite mean. As she deteriorates, the woman's frustration results in hitting her—beating her a lot. It's her house. She is a bad niece. Not immediate relatives of some kind. Nasty, nasty! This poor woman's life is hellish. [Madeline seems very involved in this story.] (*End?*) It doesn't for a long time. She ends up dying in madness and mental hell. This one is a bitter old witch. With any luck, she'll get hit by a bus. Okay. This one will die falling off a ladder—she will break her neck. So *I* go in and *kick* it. This poor woman dies all dirty . . . awful. Let's make a *happy* picture!

Card 17 BM. [A naked man is clinging to a rope. He is in the act of climbing up or down.] Well, well, ain't we a little naked trapeze artist! An inmate over the wall, getting away. He gets away successfully, too! Name's Herb. For days Herb is wearing women's pants, for 2 days! Gets a pretty bad rash on his scrotum [outburst of laughter]! He'll tell his gynecologist about it later. He's got that *Cool Hand Luke* thing. He got pissed off one night. Got into some trouble. Landed in jail. Couldn't stand it! I like Herb! He does good for himself! Never goes back in again! [Madeline tells this story very dramatically, with much laughter and a kind of delicious enjoyment—total relish.]

APPENDIX B.1. RORSCHACH PROTOCOL

Appendix B.1 presents the complete transcript of Madeline's Rorschach protocol. In the double-column format employed here, Madeline's initial response to each card appears on the left, and her responses to the assessor's questions and prompts appear on the right. As recommended by Rapaport and colleagues (1946), inquiry into the responses were conducted after Madeline finished responding to each card. This inquiry was also conducted with the card out of sight. As in Appendix A, the assessor's questions and prompts are given in italics with parentheses, and the assessor's descriptions of Madeline and other reactions are given in roman with brackets. Following this transcript, the scoring of Madeline's Rorschach protocol is presented in Appendix B.2, and a summary of the scoring is presented in Appendix B.3.

I. Oh, the Rorschach! Never saw! [5"] Looks like a woman holding her hands up. Great big wings. Like she's professing. Very powerful. I like that!

(*Woman?*) The way she was standing. She's got, how her hands were held. (*Wings?*) The wings were attached, the shape. (*Professing?*) Like her back is to you. She's facing a crowd. She'd have to be giving them information. (*Powerful?*) The picture and her. Someone important in front of all these people. Like she'd have something important to say.

II. [1"] Oh! This is great! Like two panda bears dancing. Clapping, very happy, that's cute. You see the first thing and after that how it continues to define itself.

(*Panda bears?*) The shape. Standing up on their hind legs, dancing, touching hands—no paws. Looks like they're having fun. First I thought clowns, but too fat for clowns. The black and white looked like pandas. (*What else is there?*) Head was weird, not a panda head. Looks like more of a duck head. Just ignore what isn't right. You see what you want to see [emphatically].

334

III. [2"] (1) Women doing laundry. They are folding a sheet together. Very communal. They have big boobs [Madeline bursts out laughing]. Don't know if I'm supposed to say that.

(2) These look like bleeding monkeys hanging from umbilical cords. I don't like these at all! [Madeline is quite upset.] But I have to tell you. Just blot them out, then it's a nice picture. [Blocks them out with her hands over them.] They're African women.

(1) (*Laundry?*) Basket in front, awfully close. People don't get that close together unless they have to, and you would have to be close to fold a sheet.

(2) (*Monkeys?*) The shape and size relate to the women. Monkey heads. Hanging is something monkeys do! Monkey! African women! See, they're related! It's all connected. (*Bleeding?*) 'Cause of the color, the way they are hanging. Upside down by these umbilical cords—shape.

IV. Ooh! Scary monster! Great big scary monster, getting sick. Huge feet. Small head, claws. Oh, it's like fire, burning this little person. Poor bugger. Very imposing figure! Tiny head. Not very smart, dangerous! [Madeline is very involved—disturbed about the little person's being purposely burned.]

(*Sick?*) The top is his head, looking down. Spraying from his mouth. First looks like he's getting sick. Then looks like fire, very dark. (*Monster?*) The size the feet are. Closest to you. Look way up to see the head. Imposing! Not friendly at all. (*Burning?*) Fire from guy's mouth. He was burning him on purpose! Little bugger didn't stand a chance! (*Person?*) Positioning. Like it wasn't accidental. Back is to us. He's inside of the fire. Little arms hanging down there. (*Poor little guy?*) Don't you see that? God, I hope so! It's so obvious! I need to put some dancing pandas in that picture!

V. (1) Looks like a butterfly in flight. Quite majestic, out for an afternoon flight.
(2) Also looks like a kid with his back to us, wearing a flying costume. Good for Halloween.
(3) Antelope leg, small, out to each side.
(4) Looks like a cow's leg here.
(5) Maple leaf seeds. As a kid you would break them. The outside part twirls. As a kid we would throw with little propellers, quite neat. [She is now enjoying herself, with more distance.]

(1) (*Butterfly?*) Shape, so obvious! (*Flight?*) 'Cause wings were spread out. Sit with wings folded.
(2) (*Kid?*) Back of his head, a little kid with a hood on. His stature. Way he was standing. "Look at my costume."
(3) (*Legs?*) Antelope, really thin.
(4) To be honest, cows are stupid. It had a tail, so it looks like a back leg.

VI. What is that?! Hmm . . . hmm.
[30"]
(1) This top part looks like a cat splat against the wall.

(2) Bottom looks like hide that's been skinned.

(3) This part here doesn't fit—snowplow coming down road. Big snow banks on either side, all kind of snow-covered.

(4) That part doesn't fit [she covers it with her hand]. If you cover the sides it would look like shark, big shark's teeth [at bottom]. Need to trim it down. Don't know if that's allowed.

VII. Like TV, really interesting.
(1) Looks like rabbits running away from something. Side view, bushy tail. This one's weird. Shape of rabbits is so obvious.

(2) But the rest—I don't know, looks like an angry mask with a pig nose. Eyes menacing, like piercing out at you. Pig-like, but a people mask.

(2) Mask—there's no back. Not complete. Not finished. Gotta be a mask. Don't want to think it's just a scary face.

(3) Looks like [on bottom] big apple fritter shape of it, big piece of dough.

(4) Facing forward, two Indian girls or Indian boys. Indian boy and Indian girl are gonna kiss. Wearing feathers. They're young, not kids but young, Once you see something, that's what you'll see. Left eye ball more detailed, looks really mean. Frightening. This one looks more like a mask [right]. This kind of looks real [left].

(4) Look in the eye is scary. The left one is frightening. [Madeline shows assessor the card—seems disturbed.] See?

VIII. Pretty!
(1) Georgia O'Keeffe is an artist. Usually have double meanings. Orange and pink part reminds me of her work.

(1) (*Flower—double meanings?*) Like vaginas. Georgia O'Keefe. Birds stuck out [Madeline is looking at it straight on, seems a little embarassed].

(2) Four-legged animal.

(3) Top—mountains, water wilderness.

(*Mountains and water?*). The grays and greens, very earthy tones. Like panoramic view. Gray mountains. The green has a forestry-type motion to it. Also goes together

(4) These four-legged animals come from this wooded mountains area. They've done something, and not supposed to go back. Banished, can tell they want to go back. They're somehow being transformed. That flower is like a good power. Once they change back to their natural color and not the flowers' color, then go back. Feet on each side, attached in three of the four places. [Madeline enjoys weaving her story.]

(4) (*Banished?*) Where they were in relation to rest of picture. Not part of whole system, made to be outside of it. Looking towards it like they want to be part of it again. Still very much attached. Only one leg is not attached.

[Additional response] Cover this here and looks like a dinosaur leapfrogging over something [laugh], it's splitting at the top. I have to see what time the plane leaves so I won't be nervous.

IX. Oh, this is interesting. (1) Looks like a person in the middle. Something special about this person. Can't tell if it's a man or woman. Like some protective halo-aura, don't know what you'd call it. Person part is really safe. Struggle here between good and evil. Evil part is really strong-muscled. Green part is extension of the person who's good. Evil is trying to influence the person, trying to get inside. But there's way too much good. It's not bad, because there's a little evil in all of us. Hands here are pushing the evil away. So looks like the person's very safe, well protected

(1) (*Person?*) Very little definition. Outline of head, neck, shoulders, arms. Can't tell the gender. Here's the belly. Like almost holding themselves. (*Halo or aura?*) The color is really rich, warm, comforting. Surrounds the person. Blanketing, but not suffocating, wrapping—just there. (*Evil?*) Pushing itself onto the person, imposing and pushy. Forcing itself in.

(2) This looks like a great big nose sneezing and all this splattering germs and bacteria against the glass. What a sneeze would look like, a lot of crap.

(3) These alone are big moose head. Two moose. I like the person better.

X. (1) Look at this. Looks like a party in a psychedelic aquarium. Star Wars meets Disney on acid. A party—they're having fun. Everybody's smiling [gray area]. They live in an ecosystem, all in some way attached. Fine, no one's trying to get away. All enjoying themselves at the party. All so very, very, very different, but all work well together. Having a great time. [Examiner notes feeling sad and tearful herself.]

(2) This blue crab. Guy's forlorn, defeated. There is the eye. Big ole nose. Not so much sad as hopeless. This (on the other side) is not a mirror image. Otherwise, an underwater circus! A great thing going on!

(2) (*Nose?*) Nobody's nose. This is a visual of what a sneeze would be if you could see one. Colorful and messy. Could be fun to see a sneeze in color!

APPENDIX B.2. RORSCHACH SCORING

	Location	Determinants	Content qualitative
I. 5"			
1.	W	M+	H	P, Confab tend+, Fab Comb
II. 1"			
1.	D	FMC'+	(A)	P, Fab+,Fab CombS (rejected)
III. 2"			
1.	D	MC'+	H	P
2.	D	FC+/−	A	Fetus
IV.			
1.	W	Fch+	A	P, Confab tend−
2.	D	F−/+	(H)	Bugger, Confab tend−
V.			
1.	W	F+	A	P, Confab tend+, denial of color
2.	W	M+	(H)	
3.	D	F+	Ad	Cows, stupid
4.	W	F+	Na	
VI. 30"			
1.	D	F+/−	A	Agg, (P)
2.	D	F+/−	Ad	(P)
3.	D	Fv	Na	Cold
4.	Dd	F−/+	Ad	Oral, agg
VII.			
1.	Dr	F+/−	A	
2.	D	F+/−	(Ad)	Contam tend, Mask
3.	D	F−/+	oral	P, confab tend−
4.	D	M+	H	
VIII.			
1.	D	FC+/−	Na	Painting
2.	D	F+	A	P
3.	D	FC+/−	Na	
IX.			
1.	D	F−/+	H	Color symbolism
2.	D	C	(Hd)	Transparency
3.	D	F+/−	Ad	
X.			
1.	W	CF	A, circus	Transparency
2.	D	FCarb+	A	P, confab tend−

Note. A detailed explanation of scoring procedures may be found in Allison, Blatt, and Zimet (1988, pp. 135–260).

APPENDIX B.3. RORSCHACH SCORING SUMMARY

Location	Determinants	Content	Qualitative
W = 6	F+ = 4	A = 8	P = 8 + (2)
D = 18	F+/– = 5	Ad = 4	
Dd = 1	F–/+ = 4	H = 4	Confab→ = 6 (2+,4–)
Dr = 1	Fv = 1	Hd = 1	Fabcom = 1
	M = 3 (+)	(A) = 1	FabcomS = 1 (rejected)
	FC = 3 (+/–)	(H) = 2	Oral = 2
	CF = 1	(Hd) = 1	Agg = 1
	C = 1	Food = 1	Oral Agg = 1
	FCarb+	Na = 4	Transparency = 2/3
	FCh = 1 (+)	Mask = 1	Original = 1
	FMC' = 1 (+)	Fetus = 1	
	MC' = 1 (+)	Snow = 1	
	Denial of C' = 1	Art = 1	

Summary Scores

Total F = 14	Extended F = 24	F% = 54%; Extended F% = 92%
Total F+ = 9	Extended F+ = 19	F+% = 64%; Extended F+% = 79%
R = 26	Experience balance (M: Sum C) = 4.5: 4.0	

APPENDIX C.
OBJECT RELATIONS INVENTORY (ORI) PROTOCOL

Appendix C presents the complete transcript of Madeline's Object Relations Inventory (ORI) protocol. Each question is presented in **boldface**, followed by Madeline's response in roman type. As in Appendices A and B.1, the assessor's questions and prompts are given in italics with parentheses, and the assessor's descriptions and other reactions or comments are given in roman with brackets.

1. **Describe your mother.**

First word pops into mind is witch! She's greedy. (*Describe?*) . . . short, roly-poly, two-faced, phony, don't trust her. But she's tough, hard-working. I just don't know her all that well. 'Cause she won't let you. Did I say greedy? I'll say it again—she's really greedy. (*Witch first thing?*) Not good witch or bad witch. Don't think about her very much. Don't particularly like her; tolerate her—barely. Don't trust her. Worked hard all her life. Very violent marriage. Three kids really young. As a youngster, I think she had it very hard. Won't talk about it. Very closed. (*Trust?*) She has own set of motives for what she does that are unlike most people's. I don't know what she's really about. Does things if something in it for her, greedy, money hungry, complicated. She won't let you know her, so your questions remain questions. If you ask her about her childhood, she just gets up and leaves! So I'm left with just blanks. Her marriage was brutal. Good cook, though, makes great donuts. Not healthy eater. Very rarely see her. I left very young. (*Young?*) When I was 12, in foster homes for a while. They didn't work out. So I went to work. I couldn't tell you her favorite color or ice cream, no personal details. Keeps everything to herself.

2. **Describe your father.**

He's a monster. Very mean, violent monster. Not very smart. Incredibly hard worker, alcoholic, violent towards all of us. Brother got more than his share. He's mean—right to the core. He's funny, life of the party. Don't like him at all. No time or tolerance for him. (*Smart?*) He's not, hard worker, very. Been on disability for years. Used to work construction. (*Life of party?*) Very popular. Very social . . . incredibly well respected. Everyone in family knew about violence. Both of his parents were alcoholic; they died in a fire. His family doesn't talk about it much, unless drunk. Understand he has not drank in years. If drinks, he'll die.

3. Describe yourself.

I'm a combination of both. I'm quite closed. A hard worker. Hot-tempered. Very social. I love to be the life of the party. Love attention, I do so [Madeline looks wistful]. Complex [she looks off], smart. Closed—I am. It would take a lot for someone to get to know me. I can't ever leave my partner because he knows too much about me—warts and all! I love him for that. I didn't know my parents as a teenager or adult. So young when I left. Don't know if father has hobbies or interests. Haven't seen sister in 22 years. She's a born-again Christian, eight kids. Tyrant, like father, I don't like her. There was never a baby in our family. The first time I ever kissed my mother was when she was lying in the hospital, having just slit her wrists on the kitchen table. I saw my cousin brushing her hair, and I was green with envy. My brother and I talk. I've been to visit him quite often. We were like five strangers living in the same house. I recall walking downstairs with a pillow, thinking, "I gotta kill my father." Then bawling, thinking, "He'll always be stronger."

4. Describe a significant other.

Tall, dark, and handsome, fair—kind, not weak. I used to mistake kindness for weakness, but he as said to me that they are not the same thing! Very loving, funny, good teacher, good man. A lot of my friends are men. He's very jealous. Talented. Great piano player, very low-keyed, but wears being center of attention with great deal of grace. Plays beautiful background music that complements the conversation. Good cook. Holy shit. It's not fair—he doesn't do [clean] the toilet. I don't vacuum. We got housekeeping, so that solved that! [Madeline said at an earlier point (during the administration of the WAIS-III) that he is her partner, not her husband. She would never get married. She doesn't like the legalization of the partnership. He is her partner—long-standing, for over a decade.]

References

Abraham, K. (1911). Giovanni Segantini: A psychoanalytic study. In K. Abraham, *Clinical papers and essays* (pp. 210–261). New York: Basic Books, 1955.

Abraham, K. (1921). *Papers on psychoanalysis*. New York: Basic Books, 1957.

Acklin, M. W. (1999). Behavioral science foundations of the Rorschach test: Research and clinical applications. *Assessment, 6,* 319–326.

Acklin, M. W., & Oliveira-Berry, J. (1996). Return to the source: Rorschach's *Psychodiagnostics. Journal of Personality Assessment, 67,* 427–433.

Adams, H. B. (1964). "Mental illness" or interpersonal behavior? *American Psychologist, 19,* 191–197.

Aiken, L. R. (1997). *Assessment of adult personality*. New York: Springer.

Alden, L. E., & Capreol, M. J. (1993). Avoidant personality disorder: Interpersonal problems as predictors of treatment response. *Behavior Therapy, 24,* 357–376.

Alden, L. E., Wiggins, J. S., & Pincus, A. L. (1990). Construction of circumplex scales for the Inventory of Interpersonal Problems. *Journal of Personality Assessment, 55,* 521–536.

Alexander, I. E. (1990). *Personology: Method and content in personality assessment and psychobiography*. Durham, NC: Duke University Press.

Allen, J. (1998). Personality assessment with American Indians and Alaska Natives: Instrument considerations and service delivery style. *Journal of Personality Assessment, 70,* 17–42.

Allerhand, M. E., Gough, H. G., & Grais, M. L. (1950). Personality factors in neurodermatitis. *Psychosomatic Medicine, 12,* 386–390.

Allison, J., Blatt, S. J., & Zimet, C. N. (1988). *The interpretation of psychological tests*. Washington, DC: Hemisphere.

Allport, G. W. (1937). *Personality: A psychological interpretation*. New York: Holt, Rinehart & Winston.

Allport, G. W. (1942). *The use of personal documents in psychological science*. New York: Social Science Research Council.

Allport, G. W. (1965). *Letters from Jenny*. New York: Harcourt, Brace & World.

Allport, G. W. (1967). Autobiography. In E. G. Boring & G. Lindzey (Eds.), *A history of psychology in autobiography* (Vol. 5, pp. 1–25). New York: Appleton-Century-Crofts.

Allport, G. W., Bruner, J. S., & Jandorf, E. M. (1941). Personality under social catastrophe: Ninety life-histories of the Nazi revolution. *Character and Personality, 10,* 1–21.

Allport, G. W., & Odbert, H. S. (1936). Trait names: A psycho-lexical study. *Psychological Monographs, 47*(Whole No. 211).

American Psychiatric Association (APA). (1980). *Diagnostic and statistical manual of mental disorders* (3rd ed.). Washington, DC: Author.

American Psychiatric Association (APA). (1987). *Diagnostic and statistical manual of mental disorders* (3rd ed., rev.). Washington, DC: Author.

American Psychiatric Association (APA). (1994). *Diagnostic and statistical manual of mental disorders* (4th ed.). Washington, DC: Author.

American Psychological Association, Board of Professional Affairs. (1998). John E. Exner, Jr. *American Psychologist, 53,* 391–392.

Anastasi, A. (1976). *Psychological testing* (4th ed.). New York: Macmillan.

Anchin, J. C., & Kiesler, D. J. (Eds.). (1982). *Handbook of interpersonal psychotherapy*. New York: Pergamon Press.

Anderson, J. W. (1981). Psychobiographical methodology: The case of William James. In L. Wheeler (Ed.), *Review of personality and social psychology* (Vol. 2, pp. 245–272). Beverly Hills, CA: Sage.

Anderson, J. W. (1988). Henry A. Murray's early career: A psychobiographical exploration. In D. P. McAdams & R. L. Ochberg (Eds.), *Psychobiography and life narratives* (pp. 139–171). Durham, NC: Duke University Press.

Archer, R. P. (1989). Foreword. In A. F. Friedman, J. T. Webb, & R. Lewak, *Psychological assessment with the MMPI* (pp. xi–xx). Hillsdale, NJ: Erlbaum.

Archer, R. P. (1996). MMPI–Rorschach interrelationships: Proposed criteria for evaluating explanatory models. *Journal of Personality Assessment, 67,* 504–515.

Archer, R. P. (1999). Some observations on the debate currently surrounding the Rorschach. *Assessment, 6,* 309–311.

Archer, R. P., Aiduk, R., Griffin, R., & Elkins, D. E. (1996). Incremental validity of the MMPI content scales in a psychiatric sample. *Assessment, 3,* 79–90.

Archer, R. P., & Krishnamurthy, R. (1993a). Combining the Rorschach and the MMPI in the assessment of adolescents. *Journal of Personality Assessment, 61,* 132–140.

Archer, R. P., & Krishnamurthy, R. (1993b). A review of MMPI and Rorschach interrelationships in adult samples. *Journal of Personality Assessment, 61,* 277–293.

Aronow, E., Reznikoff, M., & Moreland, K. (1994). *The Rorschach technique*. Boston: Allyn & Bacon.

Aronow, E., Reznikoff, M., & Moreland, K. (1995). The Rorschach: Projective technique or psychometric test? *Journal of Personality Assessment, 64,* 213–228.

Ashton, M. C., Jackson, D. N., Paunonen, S. V., Helmes, E., & Rothstein, M. G. (1995). The criterion validity of broad factor scales versus specific facet scales. *Journal of Research in Personality, 29,* 432–442.

Atkinson, J. W. (Ed.). (1958). *Motives in fantasy, action, and society*. Princeton, NJ: Van Nostrand.

Atkinson, L. (1986). The comparative validities of the Rorschach and the MMPI: A meta-analysis. *Canadian Psychology, 27,* 238–347.

Auerbach, J. S. (1999). Psychoanalysis and projective testing: A review of *The interpretation of psychological tests*. *Journal of Personality Assessment, 72,* 147–163.

Austin, J. L. (1970). *Philosophical papers* (J. O. Urmson & G. J. Warnock, Eds.). Oxford: Oxford University Press.

Babcock, H. (1933). *A short form of the Babcock examination for the measurement of mental deterioration*. Chicago: Stoelting.

Baer, R. A., Wetter, M. W., & Berry, D. T. R. (1992). Detection of underreporting of psychopathology on the MMPI: A meta-analysis. *Clinical Psychology Review, 12,* 509–525.

Bakan, D. (1966). *The duality of human existence: Isolation and communion in Western man*. Boston: Beacon Press.

Baltes, P. B., Reese, H. W., & Lipsitt, L. P. (1980). Life-span developmental psychology. *Annual Review of Psychology, 31,* 65–110.

Barrick, M. R., & Mount, M. K. (1991). The Big Five personality dimensions and job performance: A meta-analysis. *Personnel Psychology, 44,* 1–26.

Barron, F. (1953a). An ego-strength scale which predicts response to psychotherapy. *Journal of Consulting Psychology, 17,* 327–333.

Barron, F. (1953b). Some test correlates of response to psychotherapy. *Journal of Consulting Psychology, 17,* 235–241.

Barthlow, D. L., Graham, J. R., Ben-Porath, Y. S., & McNulty, J. L. (1999). Incremental validity of the MMPI-2 content scales in an outpatient mental health setting. *Psychological Assessment, 11*, 39–47.

Bartholomew, K., & Horowitz, L. (1991). Attachment styles among young adults: A test of a four category model. *Journal of Personality and Social Psychology, 61*, 226–244.

Baumeister, R. F. (1990). Anxiety and deconstruction: On escaping the self. In J. M. Olson & M. P. Zanna (Eds.), *The Ontario Symposium: Vol. 6. Self-inference processes* (pp. 259–291). Hillsdale, NJ: Erlbaum.

Baumgarten, F. (1933). Die Charaktereigenschaften. [The character traits]. In *Beitraege zur Charakter und Persoenlichkeitsforschung* (Whole No. 1). Bern: A. Francke.

Beaver, A. P. (1953). Personality factors in choice of nursing. *Journal of Applied Psychology, 37*, 374–379.

Beck, S. J. (1936). Autism in Rorschach scoring. *American Journal of Orthopsychiatry, 6*, 83–85.

Beck, S. J. (1937). Introduction to the Rorschach method: A manual of personality study. *American Orthopsychiatric Association Monograph* (No. 1).

Beck, S. J. (1944). *Rorschach's test: Vol. 1. Basic processes.* New York: Grune & Stratton.

Beck, S. J. (1945). *Rorschach's test: Vol. 2. A variety of personality pictures.* New York: Grune & Stratton.

Beck, S. J. (1949). *Rorschach's test: Vol 1. Basic processes* (2nd ed., rev.). New York: Grune & Stratton.

Beck, S. J. (1952). *Rorschach's test: Vol. 3. Advances in interpretation.* New York: Grune & Stratton.

Beck, S. J. (1959). Rorschach. In O. K. Buros (Ed.), *The fifth mental measurements yearbook* (pp. 273–276). Highland Park, NJ: Gryphon Press.

Beck, S. J. (1960). *The Rorschach experiment: Ventures in blind diagnosis.* New York: Grune & Stratton.

Behrends, R. S., & Blatt, S. J. (1985). Internalization and psychological development through the life cycle. *Psychoanalytic Study of the Child, 40*, 11–39.

Bellack, A. S., & Hersen, M. (Series Eds.). (1998). *Comprehensive clinical psychology* (11 vols.). New York: Pergamon Press.

Benedict, R. (1934). *Patterns of culture.* Boston: Houghton Mifflin.

Benjamin, L. S. (1974). Structural analysis of social behavior. *Psychological Review, 81*, 392–425.

Benjamin, L. S. (1993). *Interpersonal diagnosis and treatment of personality disorders.* New York: Guilford Press.

Benjamin, L. S. (1996). *Interpersonal diagnosis and treatment of personality disorders* (2nd ed.) New York: Guilford Press.

Ben-Porath, Y. S. (1994). The MMPI and MMPI-2: Fifty years of differentiating normal and abnormal personality. In S. Strack & M. Lorr (Eds.), *Differentiating normal and abnormal personality* (pp. 361–401). New York: Springer.

Ben-Porath, Y. S., Butcher, J. N., & Graham, J. R. (1991). Contribution of the MMPI-2 content scales to the differential diagnosis of psychopathology. *Psychological Assessment, 3*, 634–640.

Ben-Porath, Y. S., & Graham, J. R. (1995). Scientific bases of forensic applications of the MMPI-2. In Y. S. Ben-Porath & J. R. Graham (Eds.), *Forensic applications of the MMPI-2* (Vol. 2, pp. 1–17). Thousand Oaks, CA: Sage.

Ben-Porath, Y. S., & Sherwood, N. E. (1993). *The MMPI-2 content component scales: Development, psychometric characteristics, and applications.* Minneapolis: University of Minnesota Press.

Benton, A. L. (1949). Review of Minnesota Multiphasic Personality Inventory. In O. K. Buros (Ed.), *The third mental measurements yearbook* (pp. 104–107). Highland Park, NJ: Gryphon Press.

Bergeman, C. S., Chipuer, H. M., Plomin, R., Pederse, N. L., McClearn, G. E., Nesselroade, J. R., Costa, P. T., Jr., & McCrae, R. R. (1993). Genetic and environmental effects on Openness to Experience, Agreeableness, and Conscientiousness: An adoption/twin study. *Journal of Personality, 61,* 159–179.

Berlin, I. (1958). *Two concepts of liberty.* Oxford: Clarendon Press.

Berry, D. T. R., Baer, R. A., Rinaldo, J. C., & Wetter, M. W. (2002). Assessment of malingering. In J. N. Butcher (Ed.), *Clinical personality assessment: Practical approaches* (2nd ed., pp. 269–302). New York: Oxford University Press.

Binet, A., & Henri, V. (1895–1896). La psychologie individuelle. *Anée de Psychologie, 2,* 411–465.

Bishop, D. V. M. (1977). The P scale and psychosis. *Journal of Abnormal Psychology, 86,* 127–134.

Blashfield, R. K. (1998). Diagnostic models and systems. In A. Bellack & M. Hersen (Series Eds.) & C. Reynolds (Vol. Ed.), *Comprehensive clinical psychology* (Vol. 4, pp. 57–80). New York: Pergamon Press.

Blashfield, R., Sprock, J., Pinkston, K., & Hodgin, J. (1985). Exemplar prototypes of personality disorder diagnoses. *Comprehensive Psychiatry, 26,* 11–21.

Blatt, S. J. (1974). Levels of object representation in anaclitic and introjective depression. *Psychoanalytic Study of the Child, 24,* 107–157.

Blatt, S. J. (1990). Interpersonal relatedness and self-definition: Two personality configurations and their implication for psychopathology and psychotherapy. In J. Singer (Ed.), *Repression and dissociation: Implications for personality theory, psychopathology and health* (pp. 299–335). Chicago: University of Chicago Press.

Blatt, S. J. (1992). Interpersonal relatedness and self-definition: Two personality configurations and their implications for psychopathology and psychotherapy. In J. W. Barron, M. N. Eagle, & D. L. Wolitzky (Eds.), *Interface of psychoanalysis and psychology* (pp. 299–335). Washington, DC: American Psychological Association.

Blatt, S. J., Allison, J., & Baker, B. L. (1965). The Wechsler Object Assembly subtest and bodily concerns. *Journal of Consulting Psychology, 29,* 223–230.

Blatt, S. J., & Auerbach, J. S. (1988). Differential cognitive disturbances in three types of "borderline" patients. *Journal of Personality Disorders, 2,* 198–211.

Blatt, S. J., & Blass, R. B. (1990). Attachment and separateness: A dialectic model of the products and processes of psychological development. *Psychoanalytic Study of the Child, 45,* 107–127.

Blatt, S. J., & Blass, R. B. (1992). Relatedness and self-definition: Two personality configurations and their implication for psychopathology and psychotherapy. In J. J. Barron, M. N. Eagle, & D. L. Wolitsky (Eds.), *Interface of psychoanalysis and psychology* (pp. 399–428). Washington, DC: American Psychological Association.

Blatt, S. J., & Blass, R. B. (1996). Relatedness and self-definition: A dialectical model of personality development. In G. G. Noam & K. Fischer (Eds.), *Development and vulnerabilities in close relationships* (pp. 309–338). Hillsdale, NJ: Erlbaum.

Blatt, S. J., with Blatt, E. S. (1984). *Continuity and change in art: The development of modes of representation.* Hillsdale, NJ: Erlbaum.

Blatt, S. J., Brenneis, C. B., Schimek, J. G., & Glick, M. (1976). The normal development and psychopathological impairment of the concept of the object on Rorschach. *Journal of Abnormal Psychology, 85,* 364–373.

Blatt, S. J., & Ford, R. (1994). *Therapeutic change: An object relations perspective.* New York: Plenum Press.

Blatt, S. J., & Lerner, H. (1983a). Investigations in the psychoanalytic theory of object relations and object representation. In J. Masling (Ed.), *Empirical studies of psychoanalytic theories* (pp. 189–249). Hillsdale, NJ: Erlbaum.

Blatt, S. J., & Lerner, H. (1983b). Psychodynamic perspectives on personality theory. In M. Hersen, A. Kazdin, & A. S. Bellak (Eds.), *The clinical psychology handbook* (pp. 87–106). New York: Pergamon Press.

Blatt, S. J., Quinlan, D. M., Chevron, E. S., McDonald, C., & Zuroff, D. (1982). Dependency and self-criticism: Psychological dimensions of depression. *Journal of Consulting and Clinical Psychology, 50,* 113–124.

Blatt, S. J., & Ritzler, B. A. (1974). Suicide and the representation of transparency and cross sections on the Rorschach. *Journal of Consulting and Clinical Psychology, 42,* 280–287.

Blatt, S. J., Stayner, D., Auerbach, J., & Behrends, R. S. (1996). Change in object and self representations in long-term, intensive, inpatient treatment of seriously disturbed adolescents and young adults. *Psychiatry: Interpersonal and Biological Processes, 59,* 82–107.

Blatt, S. J., & Wild, C. M. (1976). *Schizophrenia: A developmental analysis.* New York: Academic Press.

Blatt, S. J., & Zuroff, D. (1992). Interpersonal relatedness and self-definition: Two prototypes for depression. *Clinical Psychology Review, 12,* 527–562.

Block, J. (1962). *Unconfounding meaning, acquiescence and social desirability in the MMPI.* Unpublished manuscript, Institute of Human Development, University of California–Berkeley.

Block, J. (1965). *The challenge of response sets: Unconfounding meaning, acquiescence, and social desirability in the MMPI.* New York: Appleton-Century-Crofts.

Block, J. (1971). *Lives through time.* Berkeley, CA: Bancroft Books.

Block, J. (1977a). The Eysencks and psychoticism. *Journal of Abnormal Psychology, 86,* 653–654.

Block, J. (1977b). P Scale and psychosis: Continued concerns. *Journal of Abnormal Psychology, 86,* 431–434.

Block, J. (1980). The challenge of response sets: Social desirability. In W. G. Dahlstrom & L. Dahlstrom (Eds.), *Basic readings on the MMPI: A new selection on personality measurement* (pp. 188–213). Minneapolis: University of Minnesota Press.

Block, J. (1993). Studying personality the long way. In D. C. Funder, R. D. Parke, C. Tomlinson-Keasey, & K. Widaman (Eds.), *Studying lives through time: Personality and development* (pp. 9–41). Washington, DC: American Psychological Association.

Block, J. (1995). A contrarian view of the five-factor approach to personality description. *Psychological Bulletin, 117,* 187–215.

Block, J. H., & Block, J. (1979). The role of ego-control and ego-resilience in the organization of behavior. In W. A. Collins (Ed.), *Minnesota Symposia on Child Psychology* (Vol. 13, pp. 39–101). Hillsdale, NJ: Erlbaum.

Bloom, H. (1973). *The anxiety of influence: A theory of poetry.* New York: Oxford University Press.

Bloom, H. (1994). *The Western canon: The books and school of the ages.* New York: Harcourt, Brace.

Bloom, H. (1998). *Shakespeare: The invention of the human.* New York: Riverhead Books.

Blum, G. S. (1968). Assessment of psychodynamic variables by Blacky pictures. In P. McReynolds (Ed.), *Advances in psychological assessment* (Vol. 1, pp. 150–168). Palo Alto, CA: Science & Behavior Books.

Bonanno, G. A., Siddique, H. I., Keltner, D., & Horowitz, M. J. (1997). *Correlates and consequences of dispositional repression and self-deception following the loss of a spouse.* Unpublished manuscript, Catholic University of America.

Borgatta, E. F. (1964). The structure of personality characteristics. *Behavioral Science, 9,* 8–17.

Boring, E. G. (1950a). Great men and scientific progress. *Proceedings of the American Philosophical Society, 94,* 339–351.

Boring, E. G. (1950b). *A history of experimental psychology* (2nd ed.). New York: Appleton-Century-Crofts.

Bouveresse, J. (1995). *Wittgenstein reads Freud: The myth of the unconscious* (C. Cosman, Trans.). Princeton, NJ: Princeton University Press.

Bowlby, J. (1973). *Attachment and loss: Vol. 2. Separation.* New York: Basic Books.

Breuer, J., & Freud, S. (1893–1895). Studies on hysteria. *Standard Edition, 2,* 1–305.

Brissett, D., & Edgley, C. (Eds.). (1975). *Life as theater: A dramaturgical sourcebook.* Chicago: Aldine.

Broughton, R. (1990). The prototype concept in personality assessment. *Canadian Psychology, 31,* 26–37.

Browne, M. W. (1992). Circumplex models for correlation matrices. *Psychometrika, 57*, 469–497.

Browne, M. W., & Cudeck, R. (1992). Alternative ways of assessing model fit. *Sociological Methods and Research, 21*, 230–258.

Bruner, J. S. (1986). *Actual minds, possible worlds.* Cambridge, MA: Harvard University Press.

Buchwald, A. M. (1961). Verbal utterances as data. In H. Feigl & G. Maxwell (Eds.), *Current issues in the philosophy of science* (pp. 461–468). New York: Holt.

Burns, B., & Viglione, D. J. (1996). The Rorschach Human Experience variable, interpersonal relatedness, and object representation in nonpatients. *Psychological Assessment, 8*, 92–99.

Buss, D. M. (1991). Evolutionary personality psychology. *Annual Review of Psychology, 41*, 459–491.

Buss, D. M. (1996). Social adaptation and the five major factors of personality. In J. S. Wiggins (Ed.), *The five-factor model of personality: Theoretical perspectives* (pp. 180–207). New York: Guilford Press.

Buss, D. M., & Craik, K. H. (1987). Act criteria for the diagnosis of personality disorders. *Journal of Personality Disorders, 1*, 73–81.

Buss, D. M., Gomes, M., Higgins, D. S., & Lauterbach, K. (1987). Tactics of manipulation. *Journal of Personality and Social Psychology, 52*, 1219–1229.

Butcher, J. N. (Ed.). (1972). *Objective personality assessment: Changing perspectives.* New York: Academic Press.

Butcher, J. N. (1993). *User's guide for the MMPI-2 Minnesota Report: Adult clinical system.* Minneapolis, MN: National Computer Systems.

Butcher, J. N. (1996). *International adaptations of the MMPI-2: Research and clinical applications.* Minneapolis: University of Minnesota Press.

Butcher, J. N. (1999). *A beginner's guide to the MMPI-2.* Washington, DC: American Psychological Association.

Butcher, J. N., Berah, E., Ellertsen, B., Miach, P., Lim, J., Nezami, E., Pancheri, P., Derksen, J., & Almagor, M. (1998). Objective personality assessment: Computer-based Minnesota Multiphasic Personality Inventory—2 interpretation in clinical settings. In A. S. Bellack & M. Hersen (Series Eds.) & C. D. Belar (Vol. Ed), *Comprehensive clinical psychology* (Vol. 10, pp. 277–312). New York: Pergamon Press.

Butcher, J. N., Dahlstrom, W. G., Graham, J. R., Tellegen, A., & Kaemmer, B. (1989). *The Minnesota Multiphasic Personality Inventory—2 (MMPI-2): Manual for administration and scoring.* Minneapolis: University of Minnesota Press.

Butcher, J. N., Graham, J. R., Ben-Porath, Y. S., Tellegen, A., Dahlstrom, W. G., & Kaemmer, B. (2001). *The Minnesota Multiphasic Personality Inventory—2 (MMPI-2): Manual for administration, scoring, and interpretation* (rev. ed.). Minneapolis: University of Minnesota Press.

Butcher, J. N., Graham, J. R., Williams, C. L., & Ben-Porath, Y. S. (1990). *Development and use of the MMPI-2 content scales.* Minneapolis: University of Minnesota Press.

Butcher, J. N., & Han, K. (1995). Development of an MMPI-2 scale to assess the presentation of self in superlative manner: The S scale. In J. N. Butcher & C. D. Spielberger (Eds.), *Advances in personality assessment* (Vol. 10, pp. 25–50). Hillsdale, NJ: Erlbaum.

Butcher, J. N., & Tellegen, A. (1980). Objections to MMPI items. In W. G. Dahlstrom & L. Dahlstrom (Eds.), *Basic readings on the MMPI: A new selection on personality measurement* (pp. 367–379). Minneapolis: University of Minnesota Press.

Butcher, J. N., & Williams, C. L. (2000). *Essentials of MMPI-2 and MMPI-A Interpretation* (2nd ed.). Minneapolis: University of Minnesota Press.

Butcher, J. N., Williams, C. L., Graham, J. R., Archer, R. P., Tellegen, A., Ben-Porath, Y. S., & Kaemmer, B. (1992). *Minnesota Multiphasic Personality Inventory—Adolescent (MMPI-A): Manual for administration, scoring, and interpretation.* Minneapolis: University of Minnesota Press.

Caldwell, A. B. (1997). Whither goest our redoubtable mentor, the MMPI/MMPI-2? In J. A. Schinka & R. L. Greene (Eds.), *Emerging issues and methods in personality assessment* (pp. 47–67). Mahwah, NJ: Erlbaum.

Campbell, D. T., & Fiske, D. W. (1959). Convergent and discriminant validation by the multitrait–multimethod matrix. *Psychological Bulletin, 56*, 81–105.

Campbell, D. T., & Stanley, J. C. (1966). *Experimental and quasi-experimental designs for research.* Chicago: Rand McNally.

Campbell, J. (1949). *The hero with a thousand faces.* New York: Bollingen Foundation.

Campbell, M. M. (1959). *The primary dimensions of item ratings on scales designed to measure 24 of Murray's needs.* Unpublished doctoral dissertation, University of Washington.

Capwell, D. F. (1945). Personality patterns of adolescent girls: II. Delinquents and non-delinquents. *Journal of Applied Psychology, 29*, 289–297.

Carlson, R. (1998, August). Scripting lives creatively. In T. Schultz (Chair), *Psychobiography of creativity and the creativity of psychobiography.* Symposium conducted at the annual meeting of the American Psychological Association, San Francisco.

Carson, R. C. (1969a). *Interaction concepts of personality.* Chicago: Aldine.

Carson, R. C. (1969b). Interpretive manual to the MMPI. In J. N. Butcher (Ed.), *MMPI: Research developments and clinical applications* (pp. 41–53). New York: McGraw-Hill.

Carson, R. C. (1979). Personality and exchange in developing relationships. In R. I. Burgess & T. L. Huston (Eds.), *Social exchange in developing relationships* (pp. 247–269). New York: Adademic Press.

Carson, R. C. (1982). Self-fulfilling prophecy, maladaptive behavior, and psychotherapy. In J. C. Anchin & D. J. Kiesler (Eds.), *Handbook of interpersonal psychotherapy* (pp. 64–77). New York: Pergamon Press.

Carson, R. C. (1991). Dilemmas in the pathway of DSM-IV. *Journal of Abnormal Psychology, 100*, 302–307.

Carson, R. C. (1996). Seamlessness in personality and its derangements. *Journal of Personality Assessment, 66*, 240–247.

Cattell, H. E. P. (1994). Development of the 16 PF fifth edition. In S. R. Conn & M. L. Rieke (Eds.), *The 16 PF fifth edition technical manual* (pp. 3–20). Champaign, IL: Institute of Personality and Ability Testing.

Cattell, H. E. P. (1996). The original Big-Five: A historical perspective. *European Review of Applied Psychology, 46*, 5–14.

Cattell, R. B. (1933). Temperament tests. II: Tests. *British Journal of Psychology, 23*, 308–329.

Cattell, R. B. (1943). The description of personality: Basic traits resolved into clusters. *Journal of Abnormal and Social Psychology, 38*, 476–506.

Cattell, R. B. (1944). Interpretation of the twelve primary factors. *Character and Personality, 13*, 55–91.

Cattell, R. B. (1945). The diagnosis and classification of neurotic states: A re-interpretation of Eysenck's factors. *Journal of Nervous and Mental Disease, 102*, 576–589.

Cattell, R. B. (1946). *The description and measurement of personality.* Yonkers-on-Hudson, N Y: World Book.

Cattell, R. B. (1949). *The Sixteen Personality Factor Questionnaire.* Champaign, IL: Institute for Personality and Ability Testing.

Cattell, R. B. (1953). Research designs in psychological genetics with special reference to the multiple variance analysis method. *American Journal of Human Genetics, 5*, 76–93.

Cattell, R. B. (1957). *Personality and motivation structure and measurement.* Yonkers-on-Hudson, NY: World Book.

Cattell, R. B. (1966). Guest editorial: Multivariate behavioral research and the integrative challenge. *Multivariate Behavioral Research, 1*, 4–23.

Cattell, R. B. (1973). *Personality and mood by questionnaire.* San Francisco: Jossey-Bass.

Cattell, R. B. (1979). *Personality and learning theory: Vol. 1. The structure of personality in its environment.* New York: Springer

Cattell, R. B. (1984). The voyage of a laboratory, 1928–1984. *Multivariate Behavioral Research, 19*, 121–174.

Cattell, R. B. (1994). Constancy of global, second-order personality factors over a twenty-year-plus period. *Psychological Reports, 75*, 3–9.

Cattell, R. B., Cattell, A. K., & Cattell, H. E. P. (1993). *Sixteen Personality Factor Questionnaire* (5th ed.). Champaign, IL: Institute of Personality and Ability Testing.

Cattell, R. B., Eber, H. W., & Tatsuoka, M. M. (1970). *Handbook for the Sixteen Personality Factor Questionnaire (16PF)*. Champaign, IL: Institute for Personality and Ability Testing.

Challman, R. C. (1947). The clinical psychology program at Winter V. A. Hospital, the Menninger Foundation, and the University of Kansas. *Journal of Clinical Psychology, 3*, 21–28.

Chapman, A. H. (1976). *Harry Stack Sullivan: His life and work*. New York: Putnam.

Chatelaine, K. (1981). *Harry Stack Sullivan: The formative years*. Washington, DC: University Press of America.

Chayatte, C. (1949). Psychological traits of professional actors. *Occupations, 27*, 245–250.

Cicchetti, D., & Grove, W. M. (Eds.). (1991). *Thinking clearly about psychology: Essays in honor of Paul E. Meehl* (Vol. 1). Minneapolis: University of Minnesota Press.

Cicchetti, D., & Toth, S. L. (Eds.). (1995). *Rochester Symposium on Developmental Psychopathology: Vol. 6. Emotion, cognition, and representation*. Rochester, NY: University of Rochester Press.

Clark, L. A. (1993). Personality disorders: Limitations of the five-factor model. *Psychological Inquiry, 4*, 100–104.

Clark, L. A., & Watson, D. (1999). Personality disorder, and personality disorder: Towards a more rational conceptualization. *Journal of Personality Disorders, 13*, 142–151.

Coan, R. W. (1974). *The optimal personality*. New York: Columbia University Press.

Cofer, C. N., Chance, J., & Judson, A. J. (1949). A study of malingering on the MMPI. *Journal of Psychology, 27*, 491–499.

Coffey, H., Freedman, M. B., Leary, T. F., & Ossorio, A. G. (1950). Community service and social research: Group psychotherapy in a church setting. *Journal of Social Issues, 6*, 1–65.

Coles, R. (1989). *The call of stories: Teaching and the moral imagination*. Boston: Houghton Mifflin.

Conn, S. R., & Rieke, M. L. (1994a). Construct validation of the 16 PF fifth edition. In S. R. Conn & M. L. Rieke (Eds.), *The 16 PF fifth edition technical manual* (pp. 103–142). Champaign, IL: Institute of Personality and Ability Testing.

Conn, S. R., & Rieke, M. L. (Eds.). (1994b). *The 16 PF fifth edition technical manual*. Champaign, IL: Institute of Personality and Ability Testing.

Cook, W. W., & Medley, D. M. (1954). Proposed hostility and Pharisaic-virtue scales for the MMPI. *Journal of Applied Psychology, 38*, 414–418.

Cooley, C. H. (1930). *Sociological theory and social research*. New York: Holt.

Coolidge, F. L., Becker, L. A., Dirito, D. C. Durham, R. L., Kinlaw, M. M., & Philbrick, P. B. (1994). On the relationship of the five-factor personality model to personality disorders: Four reservations. *Psychological Reports, 75*, 11–21.

Costa, P. T., Jr., & McCrae, R. R. (1985). *The NEO Personality Inventory manual*. Odessa, FL: Psychological Assessment Resources.

Costa, P. T., Jr., & McCrae, R. R. (1988). From catalog to classification: Murray's needs and the five-factor model. *Journal of Personality and Social Psychology, 55*, 258–265.

Costa, P. T., Jr., & McCrae, R. R. (1990). Personality disorders and the five-factor model of personality. *Journal of Personality Disorders, 4*, 362–371.

Costa, P. T., Jr., & McCrae, R. R. (1992). *Revised NEO Personality Inventory (NEO PI-R) and NEO Five-Factor Inventory (NEO-FFI) professional manual*. Odessa, FL: Psychological Assessment Resources.

Costa, P. T., Jr., & McCrae, R. R. (1994). "Set like plaster"?: Evidence for the stability of adult personality. In T. Heatherton & J. Weinberger (Eds.), *Can personality change?* (pp. 21–40). Washington, DC: American Psychological Association.

Costa, P. T., Jr., & McCrae, R. R. (1998). *Manual supplement for the NEO-4*. Odessa, FL: Psychological Assessment Resources.

Costa, P. T., Jr., & McCrae, R. R. (Eds.). (2000). Innovations in assessment using the revised NEO Personality Inventory [Special issue]. *Assessment, 7*, 323–419.

Costa, P. T., Jr., McCrae, R. R., & PAR Staff. (1994). *NEO Software System*. Odessa, FL: Psychological Assessment Resources (PAR).

Costa, P. T., Jr., McCrae, R. R., & PAR Staff. (2000). *NEO PI-R interpretive report*. Lutz, FL: Psychological Assessment Resources (PAR).

Costa, P. T., Jr., & Widiger, T. A. (1994). *Personality disorders and the five-factor model of personality*. Washington, DC: American Psychological Association.

Craik, K. H. (1986). Personality research methods: An historical perspective. *Journal of Personality, 54*, 18–51.

Craik, K. H. (1988). Assessing the personalities of historical figures. In W. M. Runyan (Ed.), *Psychology and historical interpretation* (pp. 196–218). New York: Oxford University Press.

Craik, K. H. (1997). Circumnavigating the personality as a whole: The challenges of methodological pluralism. *Journal of Personality, 65*, 1087–1111.

Craik, K. H., Hogan, R., & Wolfe, R. N. (Eds.). (1993). *Fifty years of personality psychology*. New York: Plenum Press.

Cramer, P. (1996). *Storytelling, narrative, and the Thematic Apperception Test*. New York: Guilford Press.

Crews, F. C. (1980, July). Analysis terminable. *Commentary*, pp. 25–34.

Crews, F. C. (1988). Commentary on "The problem of subjectivity in history." In W. M. Runyan (Ed.), *Psychology and historical interpretation* (pp. 187–195). New York: Oxford University Press.

Crews, F. C. (1993, November 18). The unknown Freud. *The New York Review of Books*, pp. 55–66.

Crews, F. C. (1994, November 17). The revenge of the repressed. *The New York Review of Books*, pp. 54–60.

Crews, F. C. (Ed.). (1995). *The memory wars: Freud's legacy in dispute*. New York: The New York Review of Books.

Crews, F. C. (Ed.). (1998). *Unauthorized Freud: Doubters confront a legend*. New York: Viking.

Cronbach, L. J. (1960). *Essentials of psychological testing* (2nd ed.). New York: Harper & Brothers.

Cronbach, L. J., & Gleser, G. C. (1957). *Psychological tests and personnel decisions*. Urbana: University of Illinois Press.

Cronbach, L. J., & Meehl, P. E. (1955). Construct validity in psychological tests. *Psychological Bulletin, 52*, 281–302.

Crowne, D. P., & Marlowe, D. (1960). A new scale of social desirability independent of psychopathology. *Journal of Consulting Psychology, 24*, 349–354.

Dahlstrom, W. G., & Dahlstrom, L. E. (Eds.). (1980). *Basic readings on the MMPI: A new selection on personality measurement*. Minneapolis: University of Minnesota Press.

Dahlstrom, W. G., & Welsh, G. S. (1960). *An MMPI handbook: A guide to use in clinical practice and research*. Minneapolis: University of Minnesota Press.

Dahlstrom, W. G., Welsh, G. S., & Dahlstrom, L. E. (1972). *An MMPI handbook* (rev. ed.): Vol. 1. Clinical interpretation. Minneapolis: University of Minnesota Press.

Dahlstrom, W. G., Welsh, G. S., & Dahlstrom, L. E. (1975). *An MMPI handbook* (rev. ed.): Vol. 2. Research applications. Minneapolis: University of Minnesota Press.

Dana, R. H. (1993). *Multicultural assessment perspectives for professional psychology*. Boston: Allyn & Bacon.

Dana, R. H. (1994). Testing and assessment ethics for all persons: Beginnings and agenda. *Professional Psychology: Research and Practice, 25*, 349–354.

Darwin, E. (1794–1796). *Zoonomia, or the laws of organic life* (3 parts in 2 vols.). Dublin: Byrne & Jones.

Davison, M. L. (1994). Multidimensional scaling models of personality responding. In S. Strack & M. Lorr (Eds.), *Differentiating normal and abnormal personality* (pp. 196–215). New York: Springer.

Dawes, R. M. (1994). *House of cards: Psychology and psychotherapy built on myth*. New York: The Free Press.

Dawes, R. M. (1999). Two methods for studying the incremental validity of a Rorschach variable. *Psychological Assessment, 11,* 297–302.

Departments of the Army and the Air Force. (1951). *Military clinical psychology* (Technical Manual No. TM 8–242 AFM 160–45). Washington, DC: U.S. Government Printing Office.

Derman, D., French, J. W., & Harman, H. H. (1974). *Verification of self-report temperament factors* (ETS Project Report No. PR-74–21). Princeton, NJ: Educational Testing Service.

Derman, D., French, J. W., & Harman, H. H. (1978). *Guide to factor-referenced temperament scales: 1978.* Princeton, NJ: Educational Testing Service.

Dickinson, K. A., & Pincus, A. L. (2003). Interpersonal analysis of grandiose and vulnerable narcissism. *Journal of Personality Disorders, 17,* 188–207.

Dickinson, K. A., Wilson, K. R., & Pincus, A. L. (1999, June). *An interpersonal analysis of grandiose and vulnerable narcissism.* Paper presented at the annual meeting of the Society for Interpersonal Theory and Research, Madison, WI.

Diener, E., Emmons, R. A., Larson, R., & Griffin, S. (1985). The Satisfaction with Life Scale. *Journal of Personality Assessment, 49,* 71–76.

Digman, J. M. (1979). *The five major domains of personality variables: Analysis of personality questionnaire data in the light of the five robust factors emerging from studies of rated characteristics.* Paper presented at the annual meeting of the Society for Multivariate Experimental Psychology, Los Angeles.

Digman, J. M. (1994). Historical antecedents of the five-factor model. In P. T. Costa, Jr., & T. A. Widiger (Eds.), *Personality disorders and the five-factor model of personality* (pp. 13–18). Washington, DC: American Psychological Association.

Digman, J. M. (1996). The curious history of the five-factor model. In J. S. Wiggins (Ed.), *The five-factor model of personality: Theoretical perspectives* (pp. 1–20). New York: Guilford Press.

Digman, J. M. (1997). Higher order factors of the Big Five. *Journal of Personality and Social Psychology, 73,* 1246–1256.

Dollard, J. (1935). *Criteria for the life history.* New Haven, CT: Yale University Press.

Duff, F. L. (1965). Item subtlety in personality inventory scales. *Journal of Consulting Psychology, 28,* 565–570.

Duijsens, I. J., & Diekstra, R. F. W. (1996). DSM-III-R and ICD-10 personality disorders and their relationship with the Big Five dimensions of personality. *Personality and Individual Differences, 21,* 119–133.

Dyce, J. A., & O'Connor, B. P. (1998). Personality disorders and the five-factor model: A test of facet level predictions. *Journal of Personality Disorders, 12,* 31–45.

Eagle, M. (2000). A miniparadigm shift in psychoanalysis [Review of S. A. Mitchell & L. Aron (Eds.), *Relational psychoanalysis*]. *Contemporary Psychology: APA Review of Books, 45,* 673–676.

Edwards, A. L. (1953). *Edwards Personal Preference Schedule.* New York: Psychological Corporation.

Edwards, A. L. (1957). *The social desirability variable in personality assessment and research.* New York: Dryden Press.

Edwards, A. L. (1959). *Edwards Personal Preference Schedule.* New York: Psychological Corporation.

Edwards, A. L. (1980). Social desirability and performance on the MMPI. In W. G. Dahlstrom & L. Dahlstrom (Eds.), *Basic readings on the MMPI: A new selection on personality measurement* (pp. 152–158). Minneapolis: University of Minnesota Press.

Edwards, A. L., & Heathers, L. B. (1962). The first factor of the MMPI: Social desirability or ego strength? *Journal of Consulting Psychology, 26,* 99–100.

Einstein, A., & Infeld, L. (1938). *The evolution of physics.* New York: Simon & Schuster.

Eldridge, S. (1925). *The organization of life.* New York: Crowell.

Ellenberger, H. F. (1954). The life and work of Hermann Rorschach (1884–1922). *Bulletin of the Menninger Clinic, 18,* 173–213.

Elms, A. C. (1987). The personalities of Henry A. Murray. In R. Hogan & W. H. Jones (Eds.), *Perspectives in personality* (Vol. 2, pp. 1–14). Greenwich, CT: JAI Press.

Elms, A. C. (1988). Freud as Leonardo: Why the first psychobiography went wrong. *Journal of Personality, 56,* 19–40.

Elms, A. C. (1994). *Uncovering lives: The uneasy alliance of biography and psychology.* New York: Oxford University Press.

Emmons, R. A. (1986). Personal strivings: An approach to personality and subjective well-being. *Journal of Personality and Social Psychology, 51,* 1058–1068.

Endler, N. S. (1975). The case for person–situation interactions. *Canadian Psychological Review, 16,* 12–21.

Endler, N. S. (1983). Interactionism: A personality model, but not yet a theory. In M. M. Page (Ed.), *Nebraska Symposium on Motivation: Vol. 30. Personality—current theory and research* (pp. 155–200). Lincoln: University of Nebraska Press.

Erikson, E. H. (1937). Configurations in play—clinical notes. *Psychoanalytic Quarterly, 6,* 139–214.

Erikson, E. H. (1950). *Childhood and society.* New York: Norton.

Erikson, E. H. (1958). *Young man Luther: A study in psychoanalysis and history.* New York: Norton.

Erikson, E. H. (1963). *Childhood and society* (2nd ed.). New York: Norton.

Erikson, E. H. (1968). *Identity: Youth and crisis.* New York: Norton.

Erikson, E. H. (1969). *Gandhi's truth: On the origins of militant nonviolence.* New York: Norton.

Erlenmeyer-Kimling, L., Golden, R. R., & Cornblatt, B. A. (1989). A taxometric analysis of cognitive and neuromotor variables in children at risk for schizophrenia. *Journal of Abnormal Psychology, 98,* 203–208.

Erlich, H. S., & Blatt, S. J. (1985). Narcissism and object love: The metapsychology of experience. *Psychoanalytic Study of the Child, 40,* 57–79.

Eron, L. D. (1965). Rorschach. In O. K. Buros (Ed.), *The sixth mental measurements yearbook* (pp. 495–501). Highland Park, NJ: Gryphon Press.

Exner, J. E., Jr. (1969). *The Rorschach systems.* New York: Grune & Stratton.

Exner, J. E., Jr. (1974). *The Rorschach: A comprehensive system. Vol. 1.* New York: Wiley.

Exner, J. E., Jr. (1978). *The Rorschach: A comprehensive system. Vol. 2. Current research and advanced interpretation.* New York: Wiley.

Exner, J. E., Jr. (1986). *The Rorschach: A comprehensive system* (2nd ed., Vol. 1). New York: Wiley.

Exner, J. E., Jr. (1989). Searching for projection in the Rorschach. *Journal of Personality Assessment, 53,* 520–536.

Exner, J. E., Jr. (1990). *A Rorschach workbook for the comprehensive system.* Asheville, NC: Rorschach Workshops.

Exner, J. E., Jr. (1991). *The Rorschach: A comprehensive system* (2nd ed., Vol. 2). New York: Wiley.

Exner, J. E., Jr., (1993). *The Rorschach: A comprehensive system* (3rd ed., Vol. 1.). New York: Wiley.

Exner, J. E., Jr. (1994). *The Rorschach: A comprehensive system. Assessment of children and adolescents.* New York: Wiley.

Exner, J. E., Jr. (1995a). Comment on "Narcissism in the Comprehensive System for the Rorschach." *Clinical Psychology: Science and Practice, 2,* 200–206.

Exner, J. E., Jr. (Ed.). (1995b). *Issues and methods in Rorschach research.* Mahwah, NJ: Erlbaum.

Exner, J. E., Jr. (1996). A comment on "The Comprehensive System for the Rorschach: A critical examination." *Psychological Science, 7,* 11–13.

Exner, J. E., Jr. (1997). The future of Rorschach in personality assessment. In J. A. Schinka & R. L. Greene (Eds.), *Emerging issues and methods in personality assessment* (pp. 37–46). Mahwah, NJ: Erlbaum.

Exner, J. E., Jr. (2001). A comment on "The misperception of psychopathology: Problems with the norms of the Comprehensive System for the Rorschach." *Clinical Psychology: Science and Practice, 8,* 386–388.

Exner, J. E., Jr., & Exner, D. E. (1972). How clinicians use the Rorschach test. *Journal of Personality, 36,* 403–408.

Exner, J. E., Jr., & Weiner, I. B. (1982). *The Rorschach: A comprehensive system* (Vol. 3). New York: Wiley.

Exner, J. E., Jr., & Weiner, I. B. (1995). *The Rorschach: A comprehensive system* (2nd ed.): *Vol. 3. Assessment of children and adolescents.* New York: Wiley.

Eysenck, H. J. (1944). Types of personality: A factorial study of seven hundred neurotics. *Journal of Mental Science, 90,* 851–861.

Eysenck, H. J. (1947). *Dimensions of personality.* London: Routledge & Kegan Paul.

Eysenck, H. J. (1953). *The structure of human personality.* New York: Wiley.

Eysenck, H. J. (1959). Rorschach. In O. K. Buros (Ed.), *The fifth mental measurements yearbook* (pp. 276–278). Highland Park, NJ: Gryphon Press.

Eysenck, H. J. (Ed.). (1960). *Handbook of abnormal psychology: An experimental approach.* New York: Basic Books.

Eysenck, H. J. (Ed.). (1970–1971). *Readings in extraversion and introversion* (3 vols.). London: Staples Press.

Eysenck, H. J. (1990). *Rebel with a cause.* London: Allen.

Eysenck, H. J. (1992). Four ways five factors are *not* basic. *Personality and Individual Differences, 6,* 667–673.

Eysenck, H. J. (1994). Normality–abnormality and the three-factor model of personality. In S. Strack & M. Lorr (Eds.), *Differentiating normal and abnormal personality* (pp. 3–25). New York: Springer.

Eysenck, H. J., & Eysenck, S. B. G. (1993). *The Eysenck Personality Questionnaire—Revised.* London: Hodder & Stoughton.

Fabrigar, L. R., Visser, P. S., & Browne, M. W. (1997). Conceptual and methodological issues in testing the circumplex structure of data in personality and social psychology. *Personality and Social Psychology Review, 1,* 184–203.

Fairbairn, W. R. D. (1952). *Psychoanalytic studies of the personality: The object relations theory of personality.* London: Routledge & Kegan Paul.

Fenichel, O. (1941). *Problems of psychoanalytic technique.* New York: Psychoanalytic Quarterly.

Feynman, R. (1985). *Surely you're joking, Mr. Feynman!* New York: Norton.

Finney, J. C. (1965). Development of a new set of MMPI scales. *Psychological Reports, 17,* 707–713.

Fisher, R. A. (1930). *The genetical theory of natural selection.* Oxford: Oxford University Press.

Fisher, R. A. (1937). *The design of experiments.* Edinburgh: Oliver & Boyd.

Fiske, D. W. (1949). Consistency of the factorial structure of personality ratings from different sources. *Journal of Abnormal and Social Psychology, 44,* 329–344.

Fiske, D. W. (1971). *Measuring the concepts of personality.* Chicago: Aldine.

Foa, U. G. (1961). Convergences in the analysis of the structure of interpersonal behavior. *Psychological Review, 68,* 341–353.

Foa, U. G. (1965). New developments in facet design and analysis. *Psychological Review, 72,* 262–274.

Foa, U. G., & Foa, E. B. (1974). *Societal structures of the mind.* Springfield, IL: Thomas.

Foreman, M. (1988). *Psychopathy and interpersonal behavior.* Unpublished doctoral dissertation, University of British Columbia.

Forrester, J. (1998). *Dispatches from the Freud wars: Psychoanalysis and its passions.* Cambridge, MA: Harvard University Press.

Fowler, K. C., Hilsenroth, M. J., & Piers, C. (2001). An empirical study of seriously disturbed suicidal patients. *Journal of the American Psychoanalytic Association, 49,* 161–186.

Frank, L. K. (1939). Projective methods for the study of personality. *Journal of Personality, 8*, 389–413.

Freedman, M. B. (1950). *The social dimensions of personality: Concepts and quantification methods.* Unpublished doctoral dissertation, University of California–Berkeley.

Freedman, M. B. (1985). Symposium: Interpersonal circumplex models: 1948–1983. *Journal of Personality Assessment, 49*, 622–625.

Freedman, M. B., Leary, T. F., Ossorio, A. G., & Coffey, H. S. (1951). The interpersonal dimension of personality. *Journal of Personality, 20*, 143–161.

French, J. W. (1953). *The description of personality measurements in terms of rotated factors.* Princeton, NJ: Educational Testing Service.

French, J. W. (1973). *Toward the establishment of self-report temperament factors through literature search and interpretation* (ETS Project Report No. PR-73–29). Princeton, NJ: Educational Testing Service.

Freud, S. (1900). The interpretation of dreams. *Standard Edition, 4*, 1–338; *5*, 339–621.

Freud, S. (1901). The psychopathology of everyday life. *Standard Edition, 6*, 1–289.

Freud, S. (1905). Fragment of an analysis of a case of hysteria. *Standard Edition, 7*, 1–122.

Freud, S. (1908). Character and anal erotism. *Standard Edition, 9*, 169–175.

Freud, S. (1910). Leonardo da Vinci and a memory of his childhood. *Standard Edition, 11*, 59–137.

Freud, S. (1915–1917). Papers on metapsychology. *Standard Edition, 14*, 103–260.

Freud, S. (1917). A metapsychological supplement to the theory of dreams. *Standard Edition, 14*, 217–235.

Freud, S. (1923). The ego and the id. *Standard Edition, 19*, 3–66.

Freud, S. (1925a). An autobiographical study. *Standard Edition, 20*, 3–74.

Freud, S. (1925b). Negation. *Standard Edition, 19*, 235–239.

Freud, S. (1930). *Civilization and its discontents* (J. Riviere, Trans.). New York: Cape & Smith.

Freud, S. (1931). Libidinal types. *Standard Edition, 21*, 215–222.

Freud, S. (1937). Analysis terminable and interminable. *Standard Edition, 22*, 211–253.

Friedman, A. F., Webb, J. T., & Lewak, R. (1989). *Psychological assessment with the MMPI.* Hillsdale, NJ: Erlbaum.

Fromm, E. (1947). *Man for himself.* Greenwich, CT: Fawcett.

Galton, F. (1869). *Hereditary genius.* London: Macmillan.

Galton, F. (1884). Measurement of character. *Fortnightly Review, 42*, 179–185.

Galton, F. (1885). Regression towards mediocrity in hereditary stature. *Journal of the Anthropological Institute, 15*, 246–263.

Galton, F. (1888). Co-relations and their measurement, chiefly from Anthropometric data. *Proceedings of the Royal Society, 45*, 135–145.

Ganellen, R. J. (1996a). Comparing the diagnostic efficiency of the MMPI, MCMI-II, and Rorschach: A review. *Journal of Personality Assessment, 67*, 219–243.

Ganellen, R. J. (1996b). *Integrating the Rorschach and the MMPI-2 in personality assessment.* Mahwah, NJ: Erlbaum.

Garb, H. N. (1998). *Studying the clinician: Judgment research and psychological assessment.* Washington, DC: American Psychological Association.

Garb, H. N. (1999). Call for a moratorium on the use of the Rorschach inkblot test in clinical and forensic settings. *Assessment, 6*, 313–315.

Garb, H. N., Florio, C. M., & Grove, W. M. (1998). The validity of the Rorschach and the Minnesota Multiphasic Personality Inventory: Results from meta-analyses. *Psychological Science, 9*, 402–404.

Gardner, H. (1999, July 24). The enigma of Erik Erikson. *The New York Review of Books*, pp. 51–56.

Gay, P. (1988). *Freud: A life for our time.* New York: Norton.

Gay, P. (Ed.). (1989). *The Freud reader.* New York: Norton.

Gergen, K. J. (1992). *The saturated self: Dilemmas of identity in contemporary life.* New York: Basic Books.

Gifford, R. (1991). Mapping nonverbal behavior on the Interpersonal Circle. *Journal of Personality and Social Psychology, 61,* 279–288.

Gilberstadt, H., & Duker, J. (1965). *A handbook for clinical and actuarial MMPI interpretation.* Philadelphia: Saunders.

Gill, M. M. (Ed.). (1967). *The collected papers of David Rapaport.* New York: Basic Books.

Gill, M. M., & Klein, G. S. (1967). The structuring of drive and reality: David Rapaport's contributions to psychoanalysis and psychology. In M. M. Gill (Ed.), *The collected papers of David Rapaport* (pp. 8–34). New York: Basic Books.

Goffman, E. (1959). *The presentation of self in everyday life.* Garden City, NY: Doubleday/Anchor.

Goffman, E. (1961). *Asylums.* Garden City: Doubleday/Anchor.

Goldberg, L. R. (1971). A historical survey of personality scales and inventories. In P. McReynolds (Ed.), *Advances in psychological assessment* (Vol. 2, pp. 293–382). Palo Alto, CA: Science & Behavior Books.

Goldberg, L. R. (1977, August). *Language and personality: Developing a taxonomy of trait descriptive terms.* Invited address to the Division of Evaluation and Measurement at the annual meeting of the American Psychological Association, San Francisco.

Goldberg, L. R. (1980, May). *Some ruminations about the structure of individual differences: Developing a common lexicon for the major characteristics of human personality.* Paper presented at the annual meeting of the Western Psychological Association, Honolulu, HI.

Goldberg, L. R. (1981). Language and individual differences: The search for universals in personality lexicons. In L. Wheeler (Ed.), *Review of personality and social psychology* (Vol. 2, pp. 141–165). Beverly Hills, CA: Sage.

Goldberg, L.R. (1990). An alternative "description of personality": The Big-Five factor structure. *Journal of Personality and Social Psychology, 59,* 1216–1229.

Goldberg, L. R. (1992). The development of markers for the Big-Five factor structure. *Psychological Assessment, 1,* 26–42.

Goldberg, L. R. (1993). The structure of personality traits: Vertical and horizontal aspects. In D. C. Funder, R. D. Parke, C. Tomlinson-Keasey, & K. Widman (Eds.), *Studying lives through time: Personality and development* (pp. 169–188). Washington, DC: American Psychological Association.

Goldberg, L. R. (1995). What the hell took so long?: Donald Fiske and the Big Five factor structure. In P. E. Shrout & S. T. Fiske (Eds.), *Personality research, methods, and theory: A festschrift honoring Donald W. Fiske* (pp. 29–43), Hillsdale, NJ: Erlbaum.

Goldberg, L. R. (1999). A broad-bandwidth, public domain, personality inventory measuring the lower-level facets of several five-factor models. In I. Mervielde, I. J. Deary, F. De Fruyt, & F. Ostendorf (Eds.), *Personality psychology in Europe* (Vol. 7, pp. 7–28). Tilburg, The Netherlands: Tilburg University Press.

Goldberg, L. R. (in press). The comparative validity of adult personality inventories: Applications of a consumer-testing framework. In S. R. Briggs, J. M. Cheek, & E. M. Donahue (Eds.), *Handbook of adult personality inventories.*

Goldberg, L. R., & Digman, J. M. (1994). Revealing structure in the data: Principles of exploratory factor analysis. In S. Strack & M. Lorr (Eds.), *Differentiating normal and abnormal personality* (pp. 216–242). New York: Springer.

Goldberg, L. R., & Rosolack, T. K. (1994). The Big Five factor structure as an integrative framework: An empirical comparison with Eysenck's P-E-N model. In C. F. Halverson, Jr., G. A. Kohnstamm, & R. P. Martin (Eds.), *The developing structure of temperament and personality from infancy to adulthood* (pp. 7–35). New York: Erlbaum.

Golden, R. R., & Meehl, P. E. (1979). Detection of the schizoid taxon with MMPI indicators. *Journal of Abnormal Psychology, 88,* 217–233.

Goldstein, K., & Scheerer, M. (1941). Abstract and concrete behavior: An experimental study with special tests. *Psychological Monographs, 53,* 1–53.

Gottesman, I. I., & Prescott, A. A. (1989). Abuses of the MacAndrew MMPI Alcoholism scale: A critical review. *Clinical Psychology Review, 9,* 223–242.

Gough, H. G. (1946). Diagnostic patterns on the MMPI. *Journal of Clinical Psychology, 2*, 23–37.

Gough, H. G. (1948). A new dimension of status: I. Development of a personality scale. *American Sociological Review, 13*, 401–409.

Gough, H. G. (1952). Predicting social participation. *Journal of Social Psychology, 35*, 227–233.

Gough, H. G. (1956). Some common misconceptions about neuroticism. In G. S. Welsh & W. G. Dahlstrom (Eds.), *Basic readings on the MMPI in psychology and medicine* (pp. 51–57). Minneapolis: University of Minnesota Press.

Gough, H. G. (1957). Imagination—undeveloped resource. In *Proceedings of the first conference on research development*. Los Angeles: Institute of Industrial Relations, University of California.

Gough, H. G. (1987). *California Psychological Inventory*. Palo Alto, CA: Consulting Psychologists Press.

Gough, H. G., & Heilbrun, A. B., Jr. (1965). *The Adjective Check List manual*. Palo Alto, CA: Consulting Psychologists Press.

Gough, H. G., & Heilbrun, A. B., Jr. (1980). *The Adjective Check List manual* (rev. ed.). Palo Alto, CA: Consulting Psychologists Press.

Gough, H. G., McClosky, H., & Meehl, P. E. (1951). A personality scale for dominance. *Journal of Abnormal and Social Psychology, 46*, 360–366.

Gough, H. G., McClosky, H., & Meehl, P. E. (1952). A personality scale for social responsibility. *Journal of Abnormal and Social Psychology, 47*, 73–80.

Gough, H. G., McKee, M. G., & Yandell, R. J. (1953). *Adjective Check List analysis of a number of selected psychometric and assessment variables*. Berkeley: Institute of Personality Assessment and Research, University of California.

Graham, J. R. (2000). *The MMPI-2: Assessing personality and psychopathology* (3rd ed.). New York: Oxford University Press.

Graham, J. R., Tinbrook, R. E., Ben-Porath, Y. S., & Butcher, J. N. (1991). Code-type congruence between MMPI and MMPI-2: Separating fact from artifact. *Journal of Personality Assessment, 57*, 197–205.

Gray, P. (1993, November 29). The assault on Freud. *Time.*

Greenberg, J. R. (1998). A clinical moment. *Psychoanalytic Dialogues, 8*, 217–224.

Greenberg, J. R., & Mitchell, S. A. (1983). *Object relations in psychoanalytic theory*. Cambridge, MA: Harvard University Press.

Greene, R. L. (1980). *The MMPI: An interpretive manual*. New York: Grune & Stratton.

Grossman, W. I., & Simon, B. (1969). Anthropomorphism: Motive, meaning, and causality in psychoanalytic theory. *Psychoanalytic Study of the Child, 24*, 78–114.

Grove, W. M., & Cicchetti, D. (Eds.). (1991). *Thinking clearly about psychology: Essays in honor of Paul E. Meehl* (Vol. 2). Minneapolis: University of Minnesota Press.

Grove, W. M., & Meehl, P. E. (1996). Comparative efficiency of informal (subjective, impressionistic) and formal (mechanical, algorithmic) prediction procedures: The clinical–statistical controversy. *Psychology, Public Policy, and Law, 2*, 293–323.

Grunbaum, A. (1993). *Validation in the clinical theory of psychoanalysis: A study in the philosophy of psychoanalysis*. Madison, CT: International Universities Press.

Guilford, J. P. (1959). *Personality*. New York: McGraw-Hill.

Guilford, J. P., Christensen, P. R., & Bond, N. A. (1954). *The DF opinion survey: Manual of instructions and interpretations*. Beverly Hills, CA: Sheridan Supply.

Guilford, J. P., & Guilford, R. B. (1936). Personality factors S, E, and M, and their measurement. *Journal of Psychology, 2*, 109–127.

Guilford, J. P., & Guilford, R. B. (1939). Personality factors D, R, T, and A. *Journal of Abnormal and Social Psychology, 34*, 21–36.

Guntrip, H. (1961). *Personality structure and human interaction: The developing synthesis of psychodynamic theory*. New York: International Universities Press.

Guntrip, H. (1967). The concept of psychodynamic science. *International Journal of Psycho-Analysis, 48*, 32–43.

Gurtman, M. B. (1991). Evaluating the interpersonalness of personality scales. *Personality and Social Psychology Bulletin, 17*, 670–677.

Gurtman, M. B. (1992). Construct validity of interpersonal personality measures: The interpersonal circumplex as a nomological net. *Journal of Personality and Social Psychology, 63*, 105–118.

Gurtman, M. B. (1994). The circumplex as a tool for studying normal and abnormal personality: A methodological primer. In S. Strack & M. Lorr (Eds.), *Differentiating normal and abnormal personality* (pp. 243–263). New York: Springer.

Gurtman, M. B. (1995). Personality structure and interpersonal problems: A theoretically-guided item analysis of the Inventory of Interpersonal Problems. *Assessment, 3*, 343–361.

Gurtman, M. B. (1996). Interpersonal problems in the psychotherapy context: The construct validity of the Inventory of Interpersonal Problems. *Psychological Assessment, 8*, 241–255.

Gurtman, M. B. (1999). Social competence: An interpersonal reformulation. *European Journal of Psychological Assessment, 15*, 233–245.

Gurtman, M. B., & Balakrishnan, J. D. (1998). Circular measurement redux: The analysis and interpretation of interpersonal circle profiles. *Clinical Psychology: Science and Practice, 5*, 344–360.

Gurtman, M. B., & Pincus, A. L. (2000). Interpersonal Adjective Scales: Confirmation of circumplex structure from multiple perspectives. *Personality and Social Psychology Bulletin, 26*, 374–384.

Gurtman, M. B., & Pincus, A. L. (2003). The circumplex model: Methods and research applications. In J. A. Schinka & W. F. Velicer (Eds.), *Comprehensive handbook of psychology. Volume 2: Research methods in psychology* (pp. 407–428). New York: Wiley.

Guttman, L. (1954). A new approach to factor analysis: The radex. In P. R. Lazarsfeld (Ed.), *Mathematical thinking in the social sciences* (pp. 258–348). Glencoe, IL: Free Press.

Halbower, C. C. (1955). *A comparison of actuarial versus clinical prediction to classes discriminated by MMPI.* Unpublished doctoral dissertation, University of Minnesota.

Hall, C. S., & Lindzey, G. (1978). *Theories of personality* (3rd ed.). New York: Wiley.

Hampshire, S. (1959). *Thought and action.* New York: Viking Press.

Hampson, S. E., John, O. J., & Goldberg, L. R. (1986). Category breadth and hierarchical structure in personality: Studies of asymmetries in judgments of trait implications. *Journal of Personality and Social Psychology, 51*, 37–54.

Han, K., Weed, N., Calhoun, R. F., & Butcher, J. N. (1995). Psychometric characteristics of the MMPI-2 Cook–Medley Hostility Scale. *Journal of Personality Assessment, 65*, 567–585.

Handler, L. (1994). Bruno Klopfer, a measure of the man and his work: A review of *Developments in the Rorschach technique: Volumes I, II, and III. Journal of Personality Assessment, 62*, 562–577.

Handler, L. (1996). John Exner and the book that started it all: A review of *The Rorschach systems. Journal of Personality Assessment, 66*, 650–658.

Hanfmann, E., & Kasanin, J. (1937). A method for the study of concept formation. *Journal of Psychology, 3*, 521–540.

Hansell, A. G., Lerner, H. D., Milden, R. S., & Ludolph, P. S. (1988). Single-sign Rorschach suicide indicators: A validity study using a depressed inpatient population. *Journal of Personality Assessment, 52*, 658–669.

Harris, G. T., Rice, M. E., & Quinsey, V. L. (1994). Psychopathy as a taxon: Evidence that psychopaths are a discrete class. *Journal of Consulting and Clinical Psychology, 62*, 387–397.

Harris, R., & Lingoes, J. (1955). *Subscales for the Minnesota Multiphasic Personality Inventory.* Unpublished mimeograph, Langley Porter Clinic, San Francisco.

Hartmann, H. (1939). *Ego psychology and the problem of adaptation* (D. Rapaport, Trans.). New York: International Universities Press, 1958.

Hartshorne, H., & May, M. A. (1928). *Studies in the nature of character: Vol. 1. Studies in deceit.* New York: Macmillan.

Hathaway, S. R. (1960). Foreword. In W. G. Dahlstrom & G. S. Welsh, *An MMPI handbook: A guide to use in clinical practice and research* (pp. vii–xi). Minneapolis: University of Minnesota Press.

Hathaway, S. R. (1972). Where have we gone wrong? The mystery of the missing progress. In J. N. Butcher (Ed.), *Objective personality assessment: Changing perspectives* (pp. 21–43). New York: Academic Press.

Hathaway, S. R., & McKinley, J. C. (1940). A multiphasic personality schedule (Minnesota): I. Construction of the schedule. *Journal of Psychology, 10*, 249–254.

Hathaway, S. R., & McKinley, J. C. (1943). *The Minnesota Multiphasic Personality Inventory manual*. Minneapolis: University of Minnesota Press.

Hathaway, S. R., & Meehl, P. E. (1951a). *An atlas for the clinical use of the MMPI*. Minneapolis: University of Minnesota Press.

Hathaway, S. R., & Meehl, P. E. (1951b). The MMPI. In *Departments of the Army and Air Force, Military clinical psychology* (Technical Manual No. TM 8-242 AFM 160-45, pp. 71–111). Washington, DC: U.S. Government Printing Office.

Hathaway, S. R., & Monachesi, E. E. (Eds.). (1953). *Analyzing and predicting juvenile delinquency with the MMPI*. Minneapolis: University of Minnesota Press.

Havens, L. L. (1965). Emil Kraepelin. *Journal of Nervous and Mental Disease, 141*, 16–28.

Heath, A. C., Neale, M. C., Kessler, R. C., Eaves, L. J., & Kendler, K. S. (1992). Evidence for genetic influences on personality from self-reports and informant ratings. *Journal of Personality and Social Psychology, 63*, 85–96.

Heck, S. A., & Pincus, A. L. (2001). Agency and communion in the structure of parental representations. *Journal of Personality Assessment, 76*, 180–184.

Hendriks, A. A. J. (1997). *The construction of the Five-Factor Personality Inventory (FFPI)*. Groningen, The Netherlands: Rijksuniversiteit Groningen.

Henry, W. P. (1996). Structural Analysis of Social Behavior as a common metric for programmatic psychopathology and psychotherapy research. *Journal of Consulting and Clinical Psychology, 64*, 1263–1275.

Hertz, M. (1970). Bruno Klopfer: An appreciation. In B. Klopfer, M. Meyer, F. Brawer, & W. Klopfer (Eds.), *Developments in the Rorschach technique: Vol. 3. Aspects of personality structure* (pp. ix–xiv). Yonkers-on-Hudson, NY: World Book.

Hiller, J. B., Rosenthal, R., Bornstein, R. F., Berry, D. T. R., & Brunell-Neuleib, S. (1999). A comparative meta-analysis of Rorschach and MMPI validity. *Psychological Assessment, 11*, 278–296.

Hilsenroth, M., & Handler, L. (1995). A survey of graduate students' experiences, interests, and attitudes about learning the Rorschach. *Journal of Personality Assessment, 64*, 243–257.

Hjemboe, S., Almagor, M., & Butcher, J. N. (1992). Empirical assessment of marital distress: The Marital Distress Scale (MDS) for the MMPI-2. In C. D. Spielberger & J. N. Butcher (Eds.), *Advances in personality assessment* (Vol. 9, pp. 141–152). Hillsdale, NJ: Erlbaum.

Hjemboe, S., & Butcher, J. N. (1991). Couples in marital distress: A study of demographic and personality factors as measured by the MMPI-2. *Journal of Personality Assessment, 57*, 216–237.

Hofstee, W. K. B., De Raad, B., & Goldberg, L. R. (1992). Integration of the Big Five and circumplex approaches to trait structure. *Journal of Personality and Social Psychology, 63*, 146–163.

Hofstee, W. K. B., Kiers, H. A. L., De Raad, B., Goldberg, L. R., & Ostendorf, F. (1997). A comparison of Big-Five structures of personality traits in Dutch, English, and German. *European Journal of Personality, 11*, 15–31.

Hogan, R. (1983). A socioanalytic theory of personality. In M. M. Page (Ed.), *Nebraska Symposium on Motivation 1982: Personality—current theory and research* (pp. 55–89). Lincoln: University of Nebraska Press.

Hogan, R. (1986). *Hogan Personality Inventory manual*. Minneapolis, MN: National Computer Systems.

Hogan, R. (1994). Reinventing ourselves [Review of D. P. McAdams, *The stories we live by*]. *Contemporary Psychology, 39*, 355–356.

Hogan, R. (1996). A socioanalytic perspective on the five-factor model. In J. S. Wiggins (Ed.), *The five-factor model of personality: Theoretical perspectives* (pp. 163–179). New York: Guilford Press.

Hogan, R., & Hogan, J. (1992). *Hogan Personality Inventory manual.* Tulsa, OK: Hogan Assessment Systems.

Hogan, R., & Johnson, J. A. (1981, August). *The structure of personality.* Paper presented at the annual meeting of the American Psychological Association, Los Angeles.

Holt, R. R. (1951). The Thematic Apperception Test. In H. A. Anderson & G. L. Anderson (Eds.), *An introduction to projective techniques* (pp. 181–229). New York: Prentice-Hall.

Holt, R. R. (1958). Clinical *and* statistical prediction: A reformulation and some new data. *Journal of Abnormal and Social Psychology, 56,* 1–12.

Holt, R. R. (1965). A review of some of Freud's biological assumptions and their influence on his theories. In N. S. Greenfield & W. C. Lewis (Eds.), *Psychoanalysis and current biological thought* (pp. 93–124). Madison: University of Wisconsin Press.

Holt, R. R. (1966). Measuring libidinal aggressive motives and their control by means of the Rorschach Test. In *Nebraska Symposium on Motivation* (Vol. 14, pp. 1–47). Lincoln: University of Nebraska Press.

Holt, R. R., & Havel, J. (1960). A method for assessing primary and secondary process in Rorschach responses. In M. A. Rickers-Ovsiankina (Ed.), *Rorschach psychology* (pp. 263–315). New York: Wiley.

Home, H. J. (1966). The concept of mind. *International Journal of Psycho-Analysis, 47,* 42–49.

Hoorens, V. (1995). Self-favoring biases, self-presentation, and the self–other asymmetry in social comparison. *Journal of Personality, 63,* 180–191.

Horowitz, L. M. (1979). On the cognitive structure of interpersonal problems treated in psychotherapy. *Journal of Consulting and Clinical Psychology, 47,* 5–15.

Horowitz, L. M., Alden, L. E., Wiggins, J. S., & Pincus, A. L. (2000). *IIP Inventory of Interpersonal Problems: Manual.* San Antonio, TX: Psychological Corporation.

Horowitz, L, M., Rosenberg, S. E., & Bartholomew, K. (1993). Interpersonal problems, attachment styles, and outcome in brief, dynamic psychotherapy. *Journal of Consulting and Clinical Psychology, 61,* 549–560.

Horowitz, L. M., Rosenberg, S. E., Baer, B. A., Ureno, G., & Villasenor, V. S. (1988). The Inventory of Interpersonal Problems: Psychometric properties and clinical applications. *Journal of Consulting and Clinical Psychology, 56,* 885–892.

Hough, L. (1992). The "Big Five" personality variables—construct confusion: Description versus prediction. *Human Performance, 5,* 139–155.

Hovey, H. B. (1964). Brain lesions and five MMPI items. *Journal of Consulting Psychology, 28,* 78–79.

Howard, G. S. (1991). Culture tales: A narrative approach to thinking, cross-cultural psychology and psychotherapy. *American Psychologist, 46,* 187–197.

Humm, D. G., & Humm, K. A. (1944). Validity of the Humm–Wadsworth Temperament Scale: With consideration of the effects of subjects' response bias. *Journal of Psychology, 18,* 55–64.

Humm, D. G., & Wadsworth, G. W. (1935). The Humm–Wadsworth Temperament Scale. *Journal of Applied Psychology, 92,* 163–200.

Hurley, J. R., & Cattell, R. B. (1962). The Procrustes program: Producing direct rotation to test a hypothesized factor structure. *Behavioral Science, 7,* 258–262.

Huxley, J. (1942). *Evolution: The modern synthesis.* London: Allen & Unwin.

Jackson, D. N. (1967). *Personality Research Form: Manual.* Goshen, NY: Research Psychologists Press.

Jackson, D. N. (1970). A sequential system for personality scale development. In C. D. Spielberger (Ed.), *Current topics in clinical and community psychology* (Vol. 2, pp. 61–96). New York: Academic Press.

Jackson, D. N. (1971). The dynamics of structured personality tests: 1971. *Psychological Review, 78,* 229–248.

Jackson, D. N. (1984). *Personality Research Form manual* (3rd ed.). Port Huron, MI: Sigma Assessment Systems.

Jackson, D. N. (1987). *Personality Research Form manual* (3rd ed.). Port Huron, MI: Research Psychologists Press.

Jackson, D. N., & Messick, S. J. (1958). Content and style in personality assessment. *Psychological Bulletin, 55,* 243–252.

Jackson, D. N., & Messick, S. J. (1961). Acquiescence and desirability as response determinants on the MMPI. *Educational and Psychological Measurement, 21,* 771–792.

Jackson, D. N., & Messick, S. (1980). Response styles and the assessment of psychopathology. In W. G. Dahlstrom & L. Dahlstrom (Eds.), *Basic readings on the MMPI: A new selection on personality measurement* (pp. 159–167). Minneapolis: University of Minnesota Press.

Jackson, D. N., Paunonen, S. V., Fraboni, M., & Goffin, R. D. (1996). A five-factor versus six-factor model of personality structure. *Personality and Individual Differences, 20,* 33–45.

Jacobson, E. (1954). *The self and the object world.* New York: International Universities Press.

Jang, K. L., Livesley, W. J., & Vernon, P. A. (1996). Heritability of the Big Five personality dimensions and their facets: A twin study. *Journal of Personality, 64,* 577–591.

Jensen, A. R. (1965). Rorschach. In O. K. Buros (Ed.), *The sixth mental measurements yearbook* (pp. 501–509). Highland Park, NJ: Gryphon Press.

John, O. P. (1990). The "Big Five" factor taxonomy: Dimensions of personality in the natural language and in questionnaires. In L. A. Pervin (Ed.), *Handbook of personality: Theory and research* (pp. 66–100). New York: Guilford Press.

John, O. P., Hampson, S. E., Goldberg, L. R. (1991). The basic level in personality trait hierarchies: Studies of trait use and accessibility in different contexts. *Journal of Personality and Social Psychology, 60,* 348–361.

John, O. P., & Srivastava, S. (1999). The Big Five factor model. In L. A. Pervin & O. P. John (Eds.), *Handbook of personality: Theory and research* (2nd ed., pp. 102–138). New York: Guilford Press.

Johnson, J. A. (2000). Predicting observers' ratings of the Big Five from the CPI, HPI, and NEO-PI-R: A comparative validity study. *European Journal of Personality, 14,* 1–19.

Johnson, J. H., Butcher, J. N., Null, C., & Johnson, K. N. (1984). Replicated item level factor analysis of the full MMPI. *Journal of Personality and Social Psychology, 47,* 105–114.

Jones, E. (1910). The Oedipus complex as an explanation of Hamlet's mystery: A study in motive. *American Journal of Psychology, 21,* 72–113.

Jones, E. (1953–1957). *The life and work of Sigmund Freud* (3 vols.). New York: Basic Books.

Jourard, S. M. (1964). *The transparent self.* Princeton, NJ: Van Nostrand.

Jung, C. G. (1923). *Psychological types* (H. G. Baynes, Trans.; revised by R. F. C. Hull, Ed.). Princeton, NJ: Princeton University Press, 1971.

Kaiser, H. J. (1958). The varimax criterion for analytic rotation in factor analysis. *Psychometrika, 23,* 187–200.

Kantor, J. R. (1924–1926). *Principles of psychology* (2 vols.). Bloomington, IN: Principia Press.

Kantor, J. R. (1953). *The logic of modern science.* Bloomington, IN: Principia Press.

Kazdin, A. E. (1992). Foreword. In C. L. Williams, J. N. Butcher, Y. S. Ben-Porath, & J. R. Graham, *MMPI-A content scales: Assessing psychopathology in adolescents.* Minneapolis: University of Minnesota Press.

Kelly, E. L., & Fiske, D. W. (1951). *The prediction of performance in clinical psychology.* Ann Arbor: University of Michigan Press.

Kelly, G. A. (1955). *The psychology of personal constructs* (2 vols.). New York: Norton.

Keniston, K. (1965). *The uncommitted: Alienated youth in American society.* New York: Harcourt Brace Jovanovich.

Kernberg, O. F. (1984). *Severe personality disorders: Psychotherapeutic strategies.* New Haven, CT: Yale University Press.

Kernberg, O. F. (1992). *Aggression in the personality disorders and perversions.* New Haven, CT: Yale University Press.

Kernberg, O. F. (1996). A psychoanalytic theory of personality disorders. In J. Clarkin & M. Lenzenweger (Eds.), *Major theories of personality disorder* (pp. 106–140). New York: Guilford Press.

Kiesler, D. J. (1979). An interpersonal communication analysis of relationship in psychotherapy. *Psychiatry, 42,* 299–311.

Kiesler, D. J. (1983). The 1982 interpersonal circle: A taxonomy for complementarity in human transactions. *Psychological Review, 90,* 185–214.

Kiesler, D. J. (1986). The 1982 interpersonal circle: An analysis of DSM-III personality disorders. In T. Millon & G. L. Klerman (Eds.), *Contemporary directions in psychopathology* (pp. 57–59). New York: Guilford Press.

Kiesler, D. J. (1987). *Research manual for the Impact Message Inventory.* Palo Alto, CA: Consulting Psychologists Press.

Kiesler, D. J. (1988). *Therapeutic metacommunication: Therapist impact disclosure as feedback in psychotherapy.* Palo Alto, CA: Consulting Psychologists Press.

Kiesler, D. J. (1992). Interpersonal Circle inventories: Pantheoretical applications to psychotherapy research and practice. *Journal of Psychotherapy Integration, 2,* 77–79.

Kiesler, D. J. (1996). *Contemporary interpersonal theory and research: Personality, psychopathology, and psychotherapy.* New York: Wiley.

Kiesler, D. J. (2001). *Empirical studies that used the Impact Message Inventory: An annotated bibliography (original or octant scale versions).* Richmond: Virginia Commonwealth University.

Kiesler, D. J., Goldston, C. S., & Schmidt, J. A. (1991). *Manual for the Check List of Interpersonal Transactions—Revised (CLOIT-R) and the Check List of Psychotherapy Transactions—Revised (CLOPT-R).* Richmond: Virginia Commonwealth University.

Kiesler, D. J., & Schmidt, J. A. (1993). *The Impact Message Inventory: Form IIA Octant Scale Version.* Palo Alto, CA: Mind Garden.

Kiesler, D. J., Schmidt, J. A., & Wagner, C. C. (1997). A circumplex inventory of impact messages: An operational bridge between emotion and interpersonal behavior. In R. Plutchik & H. R. Conte (Eds.), *Circumplex models of personality and emotions* (pp. 221–244). Washington, DC: American Psychological Association.

Klages, L. (1926). *The science of character* (W. H. Johnston, Trans.). London: Allen & Unwin, 1929.

Kleiger, J. H. (1993). The enduring contributions of David Rapaport. *Journal of Personality Assessment, 61,* 198–205.

Klein, G. S. (1967). Premptory ideation: Structure and force in motivated ideas. In R. R. Holt (Ed.), Motives and thought: Psychoanalytic essays in honor of David Rapaport. *Psychological Issues, 5*(2–3, Monograph No. 18–19), 78–128.

Klerman, G. L. (1978). The evolution of a scientific nosology. In J. C. Shershow (Ed.), *Schizophrenia: Science and practice* (pp. 99–121). Cambridge, MA: Harvard University Press.

Klopfer, B. (1936). Foreword. *Rorschach Research Exchange, 1,* 2.

Klopfer, B., Ainsworth, M. D., Klopfer, W. G., & Holt, R. R. (1954). *Developments in the Rorschach technique: Vol. 1. Theory and technique.* Yonkers-on-Hudson, NY: World Book.

Klopfer, B., et al. (1956). *Developments in the Rorschach technique: Vol. 2. Fields of application.* Yonkers-on-Hudson, NY: World Book.

Klopfer, B., & Davidson, H. (1962). *The Rorschach technique: An introductory manual.* New York: Harcourt, Brace & World.

Klopfer, B., & Kelley, D. (1942). *The Rorschach technique.* Yonkers-on-Hudson, NY: World Book.

Klopfer, B., Meyer, M., Brawer, F., & Klopfer, W. (Eds.). (1970). *Developments in the Rorschach technique: Vol. 3. Aspects of personality structure.* Yonkers-on-Hudson, NY: World Book.

Klopfer, B., & Sender, S. (1936). A system of refined scoring symbols. *Rorschach Research Exchange, 2,* 19–22.

Kluckhohn, C., & Murray, H. A. (1953). Personality formation: The determinants. In C.

Kluckhohn, H. A. Murray, & D. M. Schneider (Eds.), *Personality in nature, society, and culture* (pp. 53–67). New York: Knopf.

Koffka, K. (1935). *Principles of Gestalt psychology*. New York: Harcourt, Brace.

Kohler, K. (1929). *Gestalt psychology*. New York: Liveright.

Kohut, H. (1971). *The analysis of the self: A systematic psychoanalytic approach to the treatment of narcissistic personality disorders*. New York: International Universities Press.

Kohut, H. (1977). *The restoration of the self*. New York: International Universities Press.

Korfine, L., & Lenzenweger, M. F. (1995). The taxonicity of schizotypy: A replication. *Journal of Abnormal Psychology, 104*, 26–31.

Kraepelin, E. (1896). *Clinical psychiatry: A text-book for students and physicians* (6th ed., A. R. Diefendorf, Trans.). London: Macmillan, 1902.

Kramer, R. L. (1991). The Rorschach M response: A return to its roots. *Journal of Personality Assessment, 57*, 30–36.

Krug, S. E. (1994). Personality: A Cattellian perspective. In S. Strack & M. Lorr (Eds.), *Differentiating normal and abnormal personality* (pp. 65–78). New York: Springer.

Kuhn, T. S. (1996). *The structure of scientific revolutions* (3rd ed.). Chicago: University of Chicago Press.

Kuhn, T. S. (2000). *The road since structure: Philosophical essays, 1970–93* (J. Conant & J. Haugeland, Eds.). Chicago: University of Chicago Press.

La Place, J. P. (1954). An exploratory study of personality and its relationship to success in professional baseball. *Research Quarterly, 25*, 313–319.

Lacan, J. (1977). *Écrits: A selection*. New York: Norton.

LaForge, R. (1952). *The conceptualization of personality phenomena*. Unpublished doctoral dissertation, University of California–Berkeley.

LaForge, R. (1977). *Using the ICL: 1976*. Unpublished manuscript, Mill Valley, CA.

LaForge, R. (1985). The early development of the Freedman–Leary–Coffey Interpersonal System. *Journal of Personality Assessment, 49*, 613–621.

LaForge, R., Leary, T., Naboisek, H., Coffey, H. S., & Freedman, M. B. (1954). The interpersonal dimension of personality: II. An objective study of repression. *Journal of Personality, 23*, 129–153.

LaForge, R., & Suczek, R. F. (1955). The interpersonal dimension of personality: III. An interpersonal check list. *Journal of Personality, 24*, 94–112.

Lakoff, R. T., & Coyne, J. C. (1993). *Father knows best: The use and abuse of power in Freud's case of Dora*. New York: Teachers College Press.

Landis, C., & Katz, S. E. (1934). The validity of certain questions which purport to measure neurotic tendencies. *Journal of Applied Psychology, 18*, 343–356.

Landis, C., Zubin, J., & Katz, S. E. (1935). Empirical validation of three personality adjustment inventories. *Journal of Educational Psychology, 26*, 321–330.

Lanyon, R. I., & Goodstein, L. D. (1997). *Personality assessment* (3rd ed.). New York: Wiley.

Lapsley, H. (1999). *Margaret Mead and Ruth Benedict: The kinship of women*. Amherst: University of Massachusetts Press.

Leary, T. F. (1950). *The social dimensions of personality: Group structure and process*. Unpublished doctoral dissertation, University of California–Berkeley.

Leary, T. F. (1957). *Interpersonal diagnosis of personality: A functional theory and methodology for personality evaluation*. New York: Ronald Press.

Leary, T. F. (1983). *Flashbacks: An autobiography*. Los Angeles: J. P. Tarcher.

Leary, T. F. (1996). Commentary. *Journal of Personality Assessment, 66*, 301–307.

Lehman, B. (1986, October 20). Around the world in a study of solitude. *The Boston Globe*, pp. 55–57.

Lenzenweger, M. F., & Korfine, L. (1992). Confirming the latent structure and base rate of schizotypy: A taxometric analysis. *Journal of Abnormal Psychology, 101*, 567–571.

Leonard, R. (1997). Theorizing the relationship between agency and communion. *Theory and Psychology, 7*, 823–835.

Levinson, D. J. (1978). *The seasons of a man's life*. New York: Knopf.

Lewin, K. (1935). *A dynamic theory of personality*. New York: McGraw-Hill.

Lewin, K. (1939). Field theory and experiment in social psychology. In D. Cartwright (Ed.), *Field theory in social science: Selected theoretical papers* (pp. 262–278). Washington, DC: American Psychological Association, 1997.

Lewin, K. (1946). Behavior and development a function of the total situation. In D. Cartwright (Ed.), *Field theory in social science: Selected theoretical papers* (pp. 337–381). Washington, DC: American Psychological Association, 1997.

Liff, Z. A. (1998). Freud and psychoanalysis bashed again: This time paranoid accusations [Review of J. Farrell, *Freud's paranoid quest: Psychoanalysis and modern suspicion*]. *Contemporary Psychology*, 43, 785–786.

Linton, R. (1945). *The cultural background of personality*. New York: Appleton-Century.

Livesley, W. J., Schroeder, M. L., Jackson, D. N., & Jang, K. L. (1994). Categorical distinctions in the study of personality disorder: Implications for classification. *Journal of Abnormal Psychology*, 103, 6–17.

Loehlin, J. C. (1992). *Genes and environment in personality development*. Newbury Park, CA: Sage.

Loehlin, J. C., & Nichols, R. C. (1976). *Heredity, environment, and personality: A study of 850 sets of twins*. Austin: University of Texas Press.

Loevinger, J. (1957). Objective tests as instruments of psychological theory. *Psychological Reports*, 3 (Monograph No. 9), 635–694.

Loewenstein, R. M., Newman, L. M., Schur, M., & Solnit, A. J. (Eds.). (1966). *Psychoanalysis—A general psychology: Essays in honor of Heinz Hartmann*. New York: International Universities Press.

Lorr, M., & McNair, D. M. (1963). An interpersonal behavior circle. *Journal of Abnormal and Social Psychology*, 2, 823–830.

MacAndrew, C. (1965). The differentiation of male alcoholic outpatients from nonalcoholic psychiatric outpatients by means of the MMPI. *Quarterly Journal on Studies of Alcohol*, 26, 238–246.

MacKinnon, D. W. (1944). The structure of personality. In J. M. Hunt (Ed.), *Personality and the behavior disorders* (Vol. 1, pp. 3–48). New York: Ronald Press.

MacKinnon, D. W. (1975). IPAR's contribution to the conceptualization and study of creativity. In I. A. Taylor & J. W. Getzels (Eds.), *Perspectives in creativity* (pp. 60–89). Chicago: Aldine.

Main, M., Kaplan, N., & Cassidy, J. (1985). Security in infancy, childhood, and adulthood: A move to the level of representation. In I. Bretherton & E. Waters (Eds.), Growing points of attachment theory and research. *Monographs of the Society for Research in Child Development*, 50(1–2, Serial No. 209), 66–104.

Marks, P. A., & Seeman, W. (1963). *The actuarial description of abnormal personality: An atlas for use with the MMPI*. Baltimore: Williams & Wilkins.

Marks, P. A., Seeman, W., & Haller, D. L. (1974). *The actuarial use of the MMPI with adolescents and adults*. Baltimore: Williams & Wilkins.

Maruna, S. (1997). Going straight: Desistance from crime and life narratives of reform. In A. Lieblich & R. Josselson (Eds.), *The narrative study of lives* (Vol. 5, pp. 59–93). Thousand Oaks, CA: Sage.

Marx, K. (1845). Theses on Feuerbach. In L. Feuer (Ed.), *Basic writings on poilitics and philosophy: Karl Marx and Friedrich Engels* (pp. 243–245). Garden City, NY: Doubleday/Anchor, 1959.

Masson, J. (Ed.). (1985). *The complete letters of Sigmund Freud to Wilhelm Fliess*. Cambridge, MA: Harvard University Press.

Mayman, M. (1967). Object representations and object relationships in Rorschach responses. *Journal of Projective Techniques*, 31, 17–25.

Mayman, M., Schafer, R., & Rapaport, D. (1951). Interpretation of the Wechsler-Bellevue intelligence test and personality appraisal. In H. H. Anderson & G. L. Anderson (Eds.), *An introduction to projective techniques* (pp. 541–580). New York: Prentice-Hall.

McAdams, D. P. (1980). A thematic coding system for the intimacy motive. *Journal of Research in Personality, 14*, 413–432.

McAdams, D. P. (1985a). Motivation and friendship. In S. Duck & D. Perlman (Eds.), *Understanding personal relationships: An interdisciplinary approach* (pp. 85–105). Beverly Hills, CA: Sage

McAdams, D. P. (1985b). *Power, intimacy, and the life story: Personological inquiries into identity.* Homewood, IL: Dorsey.

McAdams, D. P. (1988). Biography, narrative, and lives: An introduction. *Journal of Personality, 56*, 1–18.

McAdams, D. P. (1989). *Intimacy: The need to be close.* New York: Doubleday.

McAdams, D. P. (1990). *The person: An introduction to personality psychology.* New York: Harcourt Brace Jovanovich.

McAdams, D. P. (1992). The five-factor model of personality: A critical appraisal. *Journal of Personality, 60*, 329–361.

McAdams, D. P. (1993). *The stories we live by: Personal myths and the making of the self.* New York: Morrow.

McAdams, D. P. (1994). *The person: An introduction to personality psychology* (2nd ed.). Fort Worth, TX: Harcourt, Brace.

McAdams, D. P. (1995). What do we know when we know a person? *Journal of Personality, 63*, 365–396.

McAdams, D. P. (1996). Personality, modernity, and the storied self: A contemporary framework for studying persons [Target article]. *Psychological Inquiry, 7*, 295–321.

McAdams, D. P. (2001). *The person: An integrated introduction to personality psychology* (3rd ed.). Fort Worth, TX: Harcourt Brace College.

McAdams, D. P., & Bowman, P. J. (2001). Narrating life's turning points: Redemption and contamination. In D. P. McAdams, R. Josselson, & A. Lieblich (Eds.), *Turns in the road: Narrative studies of lives in transition* (pp. 3–34). Washington, DC: American Psychological Association.

McAdams, D. P., & de St. Aubin, E. (1992). A theory of generativity and its assessment through self-report, behavioral acts, and narrative themes in autobiography. *Journal of Personality and Social Psychology, 62*, 1003–1015.

McAdams, D. P., de St. Aubin, E. & Logan, R. L. (1993). Generativity among young, middle, and older adults. *Psychology and Aging, 8*, 221–230.

McAdams, D. P., Diamond, A., de St. Aubin, E., & Mansfield, E. (1997). Stories of commitment: The psychosocial construction of generative lives. *Journal of Personality and Social Psychology, 72*, 678–694.

McAdams, D. P., Hoffman, B. J., Mansfield, E. D., & Day, R. (1996). Themes of agency and communion in significant autobiographical scenes. *Journal of Personality, 64*, 339–377.

McAdams, D. P., & Ochberg, R. L. (Eds.). (1988). *Psychobiography and life narratives.* Durham, NC: Duke University Press.

McAdams, D. P., & West, S. G. (1997). Introduction: Personality and the case study. *Journal of Personality, 65*, 757–783.

McClelland, D. C. (1951). *Personality.* New York: Dryden Press.

McClelland, D. C. (1961). *The achieving society.* Princeton, NJ: Van Nostrand.

McClelland, D. C. (1996). Does the field of personality have a future? [Commentary]. *Journal of Research in Personality, 30*, 429–434.

McClelland, D. C., Atkinson, J. W., Clark, R. A., & Lowell, E. L. (1953). *The achievement motive.* Princeton, NJ: Van Nostrand.

McCrae, R. R. (1993). Agreement of personality profiles across observers. *Multivariate Behavioral Research, 28*, 25–40.

McCrae, R. R. (1994a). Psychopathology from the perspective of the five-factor model. In S.

Strack & M. Lorr (Eds.), *Differentiating normal and abnormal personality* (pp. 26–39). New York: Springer.

McCrae, R. R. (1994b). A reformulation of Axis II: Personality and personality-related problems. In P. T. Costa, Jr., & T. A. Widiger (Eds.), *Personality disorders and the five-factor model of personality* (pp. 303–309). Washington, DC: American Psychological Association.

McCrae, R. R., & Costa, P. T., Jr. (1985). Comparison of EPI and psychoticism scales with measures of the five-factor model of personality. *Personality and Individual Differences, 6,* 587–597.

McCrae, R. R., & Costa, P. T., Jr. (1987). Validation of the five-factor model across instruments and observers. *Journal of Personality and Social Psychology, 52,* 81–90.

McCrae, R. R., & Costa, P. T., Jr. (1989). The structure of interpersonal traits: Wiggins' circumplex and the five-factor model. *Journal of Personality and Social Psychology, 56,* 586–595.

McCrae, R. R., & Costa, P. T., Jr. (1990). *Personality in adulthood.* New York: Guilford Press.

McCrae, R. R., & Costa, P. T., Jr. (1996). Toward a new generation of personality theories: Theoretical contexts for the five-factor model. In J. S. Wiggins (Ed.), *The five-factor model of personality: Theoretical perspectives* (pp. 51–87). New York: Guilford Press.

McCrae, R. R., Costa, P. T., Jr., Lima, M. P., Simoes, A., Ostendorf, F., Angleitner, A., Marusic, I., Bratko, D., Caprara, G. V., Barbaranelli C., Chae, J. H., & Piedmont, R. L. (1999). Age differences in personality across the adult lifespan: Parallels in five cultures. *Developmental Psychology, 35,* 466–477.

McCrae, R. R., Costa, P. T., Jr., Ostendorf, F., Angleitner, A., Hrebrikova, M., Avia, M. D., Sanz, J., Sanchez-Bernardos, M. L., Kusdil, M. E., Woodfield, R., Saunders, P. T., & Smith, P. B. (2000). Nature over nurture: Temperament, personality, and lifespan development. *Journal of Personality and Social Psychology, 78,* 173–186.

McCrae, R. R., & John, O. P. (1992). An introduction to the five-factor model and its applications. *Journal of Personality, 60,* 175–215.

McCrae, R. R., Stone, S. V., Fagan, P. J., & Costa, P. T., Jr. (1998). Identifying causes of disagreement between self-reports and spouse ratings of personality. *Journal of Personality, 66,* 285–313.

McGuire, W. (Ed.). (1974). *The Freud/Jung letters: The correspondence between Sigmund Freud and C. G. Jung* (R. Manheim & R. F. C. Hull, Trans.). Princeton, NJ: Princeton University Press.

McKinley, J. C., & Hathaway, S. R. (1940). A Multiphasic Personality Schedule (Minnesota): II. A differential study of hypochondriasis. *Journal of Psychology, 10,* 255–268.

McLemore, C. W., & Benjamin, L. S. (1979). Whatever happened to interpersonal diagnosis?: A psychosocial alternative to DSM-III. *American Psychologist, 34,* 17–34.

McWilliams, N. (1994). *Psychoanalytic diagnosis: Understanding personality structure in the clinical process.* New York: Guilford Press.

Mead, G. H. (1934). *Mind, self, and society.* Chicago: University of Chicago Press.

Meehl, P. E. (1945). The dynamics of "structured" personality tests. *Journal of Clinical Psychology, 1,* 296–303.

Meehl, P. E. (1950). Configural scoring. *Journal of Consulting Psychology, 14,* 165–171.

Meehl, P. E. (1954). *Clinical versus statistical prediction: A theoretical analysis and review of the evidence.* Northvale, NJ: Aronson, 1996.

Meehl, P. E. (1956). Wanted—A good cookbook. *American Psychologist, 11,* 263–272.

Meehl, P. E. (1962). Schizotaxia, schizotypy, schizophrenia. *American Psychologist, 17,* 827–838.

Meehl, P. E. (1973). *Psychodiagnosis: Selected papers.* Minneapolis: University of Minnesota Press.

Meehl, P. E. (1989). Autobiography. In G. Lindzey (Ed.), *A history of psychology in autobiography* (Vol. 3, pp. 337–389). Stanford, CA: Stanford University Press.

Meehl, P. E. (1995). Bootstrap taxometrics: Solving the classification problem in psychopathology. *American Psychologist, 50*, 266–275.

Meehl, P. E., & Hathaway, S. R. (1946). The *K* factor as a suppressor variable in the MMPI. *Journal of Applied Psychology, 30*, 524–564.

Meehl, P. E., & Yonce, L. J. (1994). Taxometric analysis: I. Detecting taxonicity with two quantitative indicators using means above and below a sliding cut (MAMBAC procedure). *Psychological Reports, 74*, 1059–1274.

Meehl, P. E., & Yonce, L. J. (1996). Taxometric analysis: II. Detecting taxonicity with two quantitative indicators in successive intervals of a third indicator (MAXCOV procedure). *Psychological Reports, 78*, 1091–1227.

Mershon, B., & Gorsuch, R. L. (1988). Number of factors in the personality sphere: Does increase in factors increase predictability of real-life criteria? *Journal of Personality and Social Psychology, 55*, 675–680.

Meston, C. M., Heiman, J. R., Trapnell, P. D., & Paulhus, D. L. (1998). Socially desirable responding in self-reports of sexual behavior. *Journal of Sex Research, 35*, 148–157.

Meyer, A. (1907). Fundamental conceptions of dementia praecox. *Journal of Nervous and Mental Disease, 34*, 331–336.

Meyer, G. J. (1997a). Assessing reliability: Critical corrections for a critical examination of the Rorschach Comprehensive System. *Psychological Assessment, 9*, 480–489.

Meyer, G. J. (1997b). Thinking clearly about reliability: More critical corrections regarding the Rorschach Comprehensive System. *Psychological Assessment, 9*, 495–498.

Meyer, G. J. (Ed.). (1999). I. The utility of the Rorschach in clinical assessment [Special section]. *Psychological Assessment, 11*, 235–302.

Meyer, G. J. (2000). On the science of Rorschach research. *Journal of Personality Assessment, 75*, 46–81.

Meyer, G. J. (2001). Evidence to correct misperceptions about Rorschach norms. *Clinical Psychology: Science and Practice, 8*, 389–396.

Meyer, G. J., Finn, S. E., Eyde, L. D., Kay, G. G., Moreland, K. L., Dies, R. R., Eisman, E. J., Kubiszyn, T. W., & Reed, G. M. (2001). Psychological testing and psychological assessment: A review of evidence and issues. *American Psychologist, 56*, 128–165.

Miller, T. R. (1991). The psychotherapeutic utility of the five-factor model of personality: A clinician's experience. *Journal of Personality Assessment, 57*, 415–433.

Millon, T. (1969). *Modern psychopathology.* Philadelphia: Saunders.

Millon, T. (1981). *Disorders of personality.* New York: Wiley.

Millon, T. (1987). *Manual for the MCMI-II* (2nd ed.). Minneapolis, MN: National Computer Systems.

Millon, T. (1994). *Manual for the MCMI-III.* Minneapolis, MN: National Computer Systems.

Minnesota Casualty Study. (1954). St. Paul, MN: Jacob Schmidt Brewing.

Mischel, W. (1968). *Personality and assessment.* New York: Wiley.

Mitchell, S. A., & Aron, L. (Eds.). (1999). *Relational psychoanalysis: The emergence of a tradition.* Hillsdale, NJ: Analytic Press.

Mohr, D. C., Beutler, L. E., Engle, D., Shoham-Salomon, V., Bergen, J., Kaszniak, A. W., & Yost, E. B. (1990). Identification of patients at risk for nonresponse and negative outcome in psychotherapy. *Journal of Consulting and Clinical Psychology, 58*, 622–628.

Monte, C. F. (1999). *Beneath the mask: An introduction to theories of personality* (6th ed.). Forth Worth, TX: Harcourt Brace College.

Morey, L. C., Gunderson, J., Quigley, B. D., & Lyons, M. (2000). Dimensions and categories: The "Big Five" factors and the DSM personality disorders. *Assessment, 7*, 203–216.

Morey, L. C., Waugh, M. H., & Blashfield, R. K. (1985). MMPI scales for DSM-III personality disorders: Their derivation and correlates. *Journal of Personality Assessment, 49*, 245–251.

Morgan, C. D., & Murray, H. A. (1935). A method for investigating fantasies: The Thematic Apperception Test. *Archives of Neurology and Psychiatry, 34*, 289–306.

Morgan, W. G. (1995). Origin and history of the Thematic Apperception Test. *Journal of Personality Assessment, 65*, 237–254.

Morris, W. M. (1947). A preliminary evaluation of the Minnesota Multiphasic Personality Inventory. *Journal of Clinical Psychology, 3*, 370–374.

Mosher, D. (1972). Alternative viewpoints. *Contemporary Psychology, 17*, 522–523.

Moskowitz, D. S. (1994). Cross-situational generality and the interpersonal circumplex. *Journal of Personality and Social Psychology, 66*, 921–933.

Mullahy, P. (1948). *Oedipus myth and complex: A review of psychoanalytic theory*. New York: Hermitage Press.

Muran, J. C., Segal, Z. V., Samstag, L. W., & Crawford, C. E. (1994). Patient pretreatment interpersonal problems and therapeutic alliance in short-term cognitive therapy. *Journal of Consulting and Clinical Psychology, 62*, 185–190.

Muraven, M., & Baumeister, R. F. (2000). Self-regulation and depletion of limited resources: Does self-control resemble a muscle? *Psychological Bulletin, 126*, 247–259.

Murphy, L., Stone, L. J., Hutt, M., Deri, S., & Frank, L. K. (1947). Editorial comments. *Rorschach Research Exchange and Journal of Projective Techniques, 11*, 3–8.

Murray, H. A. (1938). *Explorations in personality*. New York: Oxford University Press.

Murray, H. A. (1943). *The Thematic Apperception Test: Manual*. Cambridge, MA: Harvard University Press.

Murray, H. A. (1959). Preparations for the scaffold of a comprehensive system. In S. Koch (Ed.), *Psychology: A study of a science* (Vol. 3, pp. 7–54). New York: McGraw-Hill.

Murray, H. A. (1967a). The case of Murr. In E. G. Boring & G. Lindzey (Eds.), *A history of psychology in autobiography* (Vol. 5, pp. 285–310). New York: Appleton-Century-Crofts.

Murray, H. A. (1967b). Dead to the world: On the passions of Herman Melville. In E. J. Schneidman (Ed.), *Essays in self-destruction* (pp. 7–29). New York: Science House.

Murstein, B. I. (1963). *Theory and research in projective techniques, emphasizing the TAT*. New York: Wiley.

Nasby, W., & Read, N. W. (1997a). The life voyage of a solo circumnavigator: Integrating theoretical and methodological perspectives. *Journal of Personality, 65*, 785–1068.

Nasby, W., & Read, N. W. (Eds.). (1997b). Patterns of consistency and change: The five-factor and life-history models in the life of Dodge Morgan [Special issue]. *Journal of Personality. 65*(4), 757–1111.

Nichols, D. S. (1987). Interpreting the Wiggins MMPI content scales. In K. L. Moreland & J. N. Butcher (Eds.), *Clinical notes on the MMPI* (No. 10). Minneapolis, MN: National Computer Systems.

Nichols, D. S. (1992). Minnesota Multiphasic Personality Inventory—2. In J. J. Kramer & J. C. Conley (Eds.), *Eleventh mental measurements yearbook* (pp. 562–565). Lincoln, NE: Buros Institute of Mental Measurements.

Nichols, D. S., & Greene, R. L. (1988, March). *Adaptive or defensive: An evaluation of Paulhus' two-factor model of social desirability responding in the MMPI with non-college samples*. Paper presented at the 23rd annual symposium on Recent Developments in the Use of the MMPI, St. Petersburg Beach, FL.

Nichols, D. S., & Greene, R. L. (1995). *MMPI-2 Structural Summary: Interpretive manual*. Odessa, FL: Psychological Assessment Resources.

Norman, W. T. (1963). Toward an adequate taxonomy of personality attributes: Replicated factor structure in peer nomination personality ratings. *Journal of Abnormal and Social Psychology, 66*, 574–583.

Norman, W. T. (1967). *2800 personality trait descriptors: Normative operating characteristics in a university population*. Ann Arbor: University of Michigan, Department of Psychology.

Norman, W. T. (1972). Psychometric considerations for a revision of the MMPI. In J. N. Butcher (Ed.), *Objective personality assessment: Changing perspectives* (pp. 59–83). New York: Adademic Press.

Oettel, A. (1953). *Leadership: A psychological study*. Unpublished doctoral dissertation, University of California–Berkeley.

Office of Strategic Service (OSS) Assessment Staff. (1948). *Assessment of men*. New York: Rinehart.

Ossorio, A. (1950). *The social dimensions of personality: Individual process and structure*. Unpublished doctoral dissertation, University of California–Berkeley.

Overstreet, H. A. (1949). *The mature mind*. New York: Norton.

Ozer, D. J., & Reise, S. P. (1994). Personality assessment. *Annual Review of Psychology, 45*, 357–388.

Panton, J. H. (1960). A new MMPI scale for the indentification of homosexuality. *Journal of Clinical Psychology, 16*, 17–21.

Parker, K. C. H. (1983). A meta-analysis of the reliability and validity of the Rorschach. *Journal of Personality Assessment, 47*, 227–231.

Parker, K. C. H., Hanson, R., & Hunsley, J. (1988). MMPI, Rorschach, and WAIS: A meta-analytic comparison of reliability, stability, and validity. *Psychological Bulletin, 103*, 367–373.

Parsons, R., & Bales, R. F. (1955). *Family, socialization and interaction process*. Glencoe, IL: Free Press.

Paulhus, D. L. (1984). Two-component models of social desirability. *Journal of Personality and Social Psychology, 46*, 598–609.

Paulhus, D. L. (1988). *Manual for the Balanced Inventory of Desirability Responding (BIDR-7)*. Unpublished manual, University of British Columbia.

Paulhus, D. L. (1998a). Interpersonal and intrapsychic adaptiveness of trait self-enhancement: A mixed blessing? *Journal of Personality and Social Psychology, 74*, 1197–1208.

Paulhus, D. L. (1998b). *Paulhus Deception Scales: Manual for The Balanced Inventory of Desirable Responding, Version 7*. Toronto: Multi-Health Systems.

Paulhus, D. L. (2002). Socially desirable responding: Evolution of a construct. In H. Braun, D. N. Jackson, & D. Wiley (Eds.), *The role of constructs in psychological and educational measurement* (pp. 49–69). Mahwah, NJ: Erlbaum.

Paulhus, D. L., & John, O. P. (1998). Egoistic and moralistic biases in self-perception: The interplay of self-deceptive styles with basic traits and motives. *Journal of Personality, 66*, 1025–1060.

Payne, F. D., & Wiggins, J. S. (1972). MMPI profile types and the self-report of psychiatric patients. *Journal of Abnormal Psychology, 79*, 1–8.

Pearson, J. S., Swenson, W. M., & Rome, H. P. (1965). Age and sex differences related to MMPI frequency response in 25,000 medical patients. *American Journal of Psychiatry, 121*, 988–995.

Pearson, K. (1896). Mathematical contributions to the theory of evolution: Regression, heredity, and panmixia. *Philosophical Transactions of the Royal Society of London, Series A, 187*, 235–318.

Pennebaker, J. W. (1992, August). *Putting stress into words: Health, linguistics, and therapeutic implications*. Paper presented at the annual meeting of the American Psychological Association, Washington, DC.

Pepper, S. (1942). *World hypotheses*. Berkeley: University of California Press.

Perry, H. S. (1982). *Psychiatrist of America: The life of Harry Stack Sullivan*. Cambridge, MA: Harvard University Press.

Pervin, L. A. (1994). A critical analysis of current trait theory. *Psychological Inquiry, 5*, 103–113.

Peterson, R. A. (1978). Rorschach. In O. K. Buros (Ed.), *The eighth mental measurements yearbook* (Vol. 1, pp. 1042–1045). Highland Park, NJ: Gryphon Press.

Phillips, L., & Smith, J. G. (1953). *Rorschach interpretation: Advanced technique*. New York: Grune & Stratton.

Phillips, W. (1983). *A partisan view: Five decades of the literary life*. New York: Stein & Day.

Piedmont, R. L. (1998). *The Revised NEO Personality Inventory: Clinical and research applications*. New York: Plenum Press.

Pincus, A. L. (1994). The interpersonal circumplex and the interpersonal theory: Perspectives on personality and its pathology. In S. Strack & M. Lorr (Eds.), *Differentiating normal and abnormal personality* (pp. 114–136). New York: Springer.

Pincus, A. L. (1997, August). Beyond complementarity: An object-relations perspective. In M. B. Gurtman (Chair), *Interpersonal complementarity: Critical issues and future directions*. Symposium conducted at the annual meeting of the American Psychological Association, Chicago.

Pincus, A. L. (1999, June). *Reciprocal interpersonal processes in personality development*. Paper presented at the annual meeting of the Society for Interpersonal Theory and Research, Madison, WI.

Pincus, A. L., & Ansell, E. B. (2003). Interpersonal theory of personality. In T. Millon & M. J. Lerner (Eds.), *Comprehensive handbook of psychology. Volume 5: Personality and social psychology* (pp. 209–229). New York: Wiley.

Pincus, A. L., Boekman, L. F., & Laurenceau, J. P. (1994, August). The interpersonal problems circumplex: Descriptive, theoretical, and applied marital research. In M. B. Gurtman (Chair), *Inventory of Interpersonal Problems: Clinical and research applications*. Symposium conducted at the annual meeting of the American Psychological Association, Los Angeles.

Pincus, A. L., Dickinson, K. A., Schut, A. J., Castonguay, L. G., & Bedics, J. (1999). Integrating interpersonal assessment and adult attachment using SASB. *European Journal of Psychological Assessment, 15*, 206–220.

Pincus, A. L., & Wiggins, J. S. (1990). Interpersonal problems and conceptions of personality disorders. *Journal of Personality Disorders, 4*, 342–352.

Piotrowski, C., & Zalewski, C. (1993). Training in psychodiagnostic testing in APA-approved PsyD and PhD clinical psychology programs. *Journal of Personality Assessment, 6*, 394–405.

Piotrowski, Z. A. (1957). *Perceptanalysis*. New York: Macmillan.

Plutchik, R. (1997). The circumplex as a general model of the structure of emotions and personality. In R. Plutchik & H. R. Conte (Eds.), *Circumplex models of personality and emotions* (pp. 17–45). Washington, DC: American Psychological Association.

Plutchik, R., & Conte, H. R. (1986). Quantitative assessment of personality disorders. In R. Michels & J. O. Cavenar, Jr. (Eds.), *Psychiatry* (Vol. 1, pp. 1–13). Philadelphia: Lippincott.

Plutchik, R., & Conte, H.R. (Eds.). (1997). *Circumplex models of personality and emotions*. Washington, DC: American Psychological Association.

Plutchik, R., & Platman, S. R. (1977). Personality connotations of psychiatric diagnosis. *Journal of Nervous and Mental Disease, 165*, 418–422.

Polanyi, M. (1966). *The tacit dimension*. Garden City, NY: Doubleday.

Potter, S. (1950). *Gamesmanship*. New York: Holt, Rinehart & Winston.

Prelinger, E., & Zimet, C. N. (1964). *An ego-psychological approach to character assessment*. Glencoe, IL: Free Press.

Pressey, S. L. (1921). A group scale for investigating the emotions. *Journal of Abnormal and Social Psychology, 16*, 55–64.

Rapaport, D. (1942). Principles underlying projective techniques. In M. M. Gill (Ed.), *The collected papers of David Rapaport* (pp. 91–97). New York: Basic Books, 1967.

Rapaport, D. (1944–1946). *Manual of diagnostic psychological testing* (2 vols.). New York: Josiah Macy, Jr. Foundation.

Rapaport, D. (1946). Principles underlying nonprojective tests of personality. In M. M. Gill (Ed.), *The collected papers of David Rapaport* (pp. 221–229). New York: Basic Books, 1967.

Rapaport, D. (1951). The conceptual model of psychoanalysis. In M. M. Gill (Ed.), *The collected papers of David Rapaport* (pp. 221–229). New York: Basic Books, 1967.

Rapaport, D. (1959a). Introduction: A history of psychoanalytic ego psychology. *Psychological Issues, 1*(1, Monograph No. 1).

Rapaport, D. (1959b). The structure of psychoanalytic theory: A systematizing attempt. In S. Koch (Ed.), *Psychology: A study of a science* (Vol. 3, pp. 55–183). New York: McGraw-Hill.

Rapaport, D., & Gill, M. M. (1959). The points of view and assumptions of metapsychology. In

M. M. Gill (Ed.), *The collected papers of David Rapaport* (pp. 795–811). New York: Basic Books, 1967.

Rapaport, D., Gill, M., & Schafer, R. (1946). *Diagnostic psychological testing* (2 vols.). Chicago: Year Book.

Rapaport, D., Gill, M., & Schafer, R. (1968). *Diagnostic psychological testing* (rev. ed.; R. Holt, Ed.). New York: International Universities Press.

Rapaport, D., Menninger, K. A., & Schafer, R. (1947). The new role of psychological testing in psychiatry. In M. M. Gill (Ed.), *The collected papers of David Rapaport* (pp. 245–250). New York: Basic Books, 1967.

Rapaport, D., & Schafer, R. (1946). The psychological internship training program of the Menninger Clinic. In M. M. Gill (Ed.), *The collected papers of David Rapaport* (pp. 230–236). New York: Basic Books, 1967.

Redfield, R. (1960). How society operates. In H. L. Shapiro (Ed.), *Man, culture, and society* (pp. 345–368). New York: Oxford University Press.

Reich, W. (1933). *Character analysis*. New York: Orgone Institute Press, 1949.

Reznikoff, M. (1972). Rorschach. In O. K. Buros (Ed.), *The seventh mental measurements yearbook* (Vol. 1, pp. 446–449). Highland Park, NJ: Gryphon Press.

Rickers-Ovsiankina, M. A. (Ed.). (1960). *Rorschach psychology*. New York: Wiley.

Riemann, R., Angleitner, A., & Strelau, J. (1997). Genetic and environmental influences on personality: A study of twins reared together using the self- and peer report NEO-FFI scales. *Journal of Personality, 65*, 449–475.

Rierdan, J., Lange, E., & Eddy, S. (1978). Suicide and transparency responses on the Rorschach: A replication. *Journal of Consulting and Clinical Psychology, 46*, 1162–1163.

Roazen, P. (1968). *Freud: Political and social thought*. New York: Knopf.

Robinson, F. G. (1992). *Love's story told: A life of Henry A. Murray*. Cambridge, MA: Harvard University Press.

Roessel, F. P. (1954). *MMPI results for high school drop-outs and graduates*. Unpublished doctoral dissertation, University of Minnesota.

Rogers, C. R. (1961). *On becoming a person: A therapist's view of psychotherapy*. Boston: Houghton Mifflin.

Rolland, R. (1924). *Mahatma Gandhi* (C. D. Groth, Trans.). New York: Century.

Rorschach, H. (1921). *Psychodiagnostics*. New York: Grune & Stratton, 1942.

Rorschach, H., & Oberholzer, E. (1924). The application of the interpretation of form to psychoanalysis. *Journal of Nervous and Mental Disease, 60*, 225–248, 359–379.

Rosch, E., Mervis, C. B., Gray, W. D., Johnson, D. M., & Boyes-Braem, P. (1976). Basic objects in natural categories. *Cognitive Psychology, 8*, 382–439.

Rose, R. J. (1995). Genes and human behavior. *Annual Review of Psychology, 46*, 625–654.

Rosenhan, D. L. (1973). On being sane in insane places. *Science, 179*, 250–258.

Roth, D., & Blatt, S. J. (1974). Spatial representations of transparency and the suicide potential. *International Journal of Psycho-Analysis, 55*, 287–293.

Runyan, W. M. (1982). *Life histories and psychobiography: Explorations in theory and method*. New York: Oxford University Press.

Runyan, W. M. (Ed.). (1988a). *Psychology and historical interpretation*. New York: Oxford University Press.

Runyan, W. M. (1988b). Reconceptualizing the relationships between history and psychology. In W. M. Runyan (Ed.), *Psychology and historical interpretation* (pp. 247–295). New York: Oxford University Press.

Runyan, W. M. (1994). Coming to terms with the life, loves, and work of Henry A. Murray. *Contemporary Psychology, 39*, 701–704.

Russell, J. A., Weiss, A., & Mendelsohn, G. A. (1989). Affect Grid: A single-item scale of pleasure and arousal. *Journal of Personality and Social Psychology, 57*, 493–502.

Rycroft, C. (1966). Introduction: Causes and meaning. In C. Rycroft (Ed.), *Psychoanalysis observed* (pp. 7–22). London: Constable.

Ryle, G. (1949). *The concept of mind*. New York: Barnes & Noble.

Sackeim, H. A., & Gur, R. C. (1978). Self-deception, self-confrontation and self-consciousness. In G. E. Schwartz & D. Shapiro (Eds.), *Consciousness and self-regulation: Advances in research* (Vol. 2, pp. 139–197). New York: Plenum Press.

Safran, J. D., & Segal, Z. (1990). *Interpersonal process in cognitive therapy.* New York: Basic Books.

Sandler, J. (1981). Unconscious wishes and human relationships. *Contemporary Psychoanalysis, 17,* 180–196.

Sandler, J., & Rosenblatt, B. (1962). The concept of the representational world. *Psychoanalytic Study of the Child, 17,* 128–145.

Sapir, E. (1935). Language. In *Encyclopedia of the social sciences* (Vol. 9, pp. 155–169). New York: Macmillan.

Sarbin, T. R. (Ed.). (1986). *Narrative psychology: The storied nature of human conduct.* New York: Oxford University Press.

Sarbin, T. R. (1997). On the futility of psychiatric diagnostic manuals (DSMs) and the return of personal agency. *Applied and Preventive Psychology, 6,* 233–243.

Saucier, G., & Goldberg, L. R. (1996a). Evidence for the Big Five in analyses of familiar English personality inventories. *European Journal of Personality, 10,* 61–77.

Saucier, G., & Goldberg, L. R. (1996b). The language of personality: Lexical perspectives on the five-factor model. In J. S. Wiggins (Ed.), *The five-factor model of personality: Theoretical perspectives* (pp. 21–50). New York: Guilford Press.

Schaefer, E. S. (1961). Converging conceptual models for maternal behavior and for child behavior. In J. G. Glidewell (Ed.), *Parental attitudes and child behavior* (pp. 124–146). Springfield, IL: Thomas.

Schafer, R. (1948). *The clinical application of psychological tests.* New York: International Universities Press.

Schafer, R. (1954). *Psychoanalytic interpretation in Rorschach testing: Theory and application.* New York: Grune & Stratton.

Schafer, R. (1967). *Projective testing and psychoanalysis.* New York: International Universities Press.

Schafer, R. (1968). *Aspects of internalization.* New York: International Universities Press.

Schafer, R. (1976). *A new language for psychoanalysis.* New Haven, CT: Yale University Press.

Schmidt, J. A., Wagner, C. C., & Kiesler, D. J. (1993). DSM-IV Axis II: Dimensionality ratings? "Yes"; Big five? "Perhaps later." *Psychological Inquiry, 4,* 119–121.

Schofield, W. (1952). Critique of scatter and profile analysis in psychometric data. *Journal of Clinical Psychology, 8,* 16–22.

Sechrist, L., Stickle, T. R., & Stewart, M. (1998). The role of assessment in clinical psychology. In A. Bellack & M. Hersen (Series Eds.) & C. R. Reynolds (Vol. Ed.), *Comprehensive clinical psychology* (Vol. 4, pp. 1–32). New York: Pergamon Press.

Shakespeare, W. (ca. 1599). As you like it. In G. B. Evans (Ed.), *The Riverside Shakespeare* (pp. 365–402). Boston: Houghton Mifflin, 1974.

Shannon, C., & Weaver, W. (1949). *The mathematical theory of communication.* Urbana: University of Illinois Press.

Shapiro, D. (1965). *Neurotic styles.* New York: Basic Books.

Shapiro, D. (1981). *Autonomy and rigid character.* New York: Basic Books.

Sheldon, W. H., & Stevens, S. S. (1942). *The varieties of temperament.* New York: Harper.

Shepard, R. N. (1978). The circumplex and related topological manifolds in the study of perception. In S. Shye (Ed.), *Theory construction and data analysis in the behavioral sciences* (pp. 29–80). San Francisco: Jossey-Bass.

Shontz, F., & Green, P. (1992). Trends in research on the Rorschach: Review and recommendations. *Applied and Preventive Psychology, 1,* 149–156.

Shopshire, M. S., & Craik, K. H. (1994). The five factor model of personality and the DSM-III-R personality disorders: Correspondence and differentiation. *Journal of Personality Disorders, 8,* 41–52.

Silver, B. L. (1998). *The ascent of science*. New York: Oxford University Press.

Sines, J. O. (1966). Actuarial methods in personaltity assessment. In B. Maher (Ed.), *Progress in experimental personality research* (pp. 133–193). New York: Academic Press.

Skrzypek, G. J., & Wiggins, J. S. (1966). Contrasted groups versus repeated measurement designs in the evaluation of social desirability scales. *Educational and Psychological Measurement, 26*, 131–138,

Slocum, J. (1900). Sailing alone around the world. In W. M. Teller (Ed.), *The voyages of Joshua Slocum* (pp. 225–384). New Brunswick, NJ: Rutgers University Press, 1958.

Soldz, S., Budman, S., Demby, A., & Merry, J. (1993). Representation of personality disorders in circumplex and five-factor space: Explorations with a clinical sample. *Psychological Assessment, 5*, 41–52.

Spearman, C. (1904). "General intelligence" objectively determined and measured. *American Journal of Psychology, 15*, 201–292.

Spence, D. P. (1982). *Narrative truth and historical truth: Meaning and interpretation in psychoanalysis*. New York: Norton.

Steiger, J. H. (1980). Tests for comparing elements in a correlation matrix. *Psychological Bulletin, 87*, 195–201.

Stern, G. G. (1958). *Preliminary manual: Activities Index—College Characteristics Index*. Syracuse, NY: Syracuse University Psychological Research Center.

Stern, G. G. (1970). *People in context: Measuring person–environment congruence in education and industry*. New York: Wiley.

Stern, G. G., Stein, M. I., & Bloom, B. S. (1956). *Methods in personality assessment*. Glencoe, IL: Free Press.

Stewart, A. J., Franz, C., & Layton, L. (1988). The changing self: Using personal documents to study lives. *Journal of Personality, 56*, 41–74.

Stolorow, R. D., & Atwood, G. E. (1979). *Faces in a cloud: Subjectivity in personality theory*. New York: Aronson.

Strack, S. (1987). Development and validation of an adjective checklist to assess the Millon personality types in a normal population. *Journal of Personality Assessment, 51*, 572–587.

Strack, S. (1991). *Manual for the Personality Adjective Check List (PACL)*. South Pasadena, CA: 21st Century Assessment.

Strack, S. (Ed.). (1996). Interpersonal theory and the interpersonal circumplex: Timothy Leary's legacy [Special series]. *Journal of Personality Assessment, 66*, 212–307.

Stricker, L. J. (1978). Eysenck Personality Questionnaire. In O. K. Buros (Ed.), *The eighth mental measurement yearbook* (Vol. 1, pp. 810–814). Highland Park, NJ: Gryphon Press.

Strong, D. R., Greene, R. L., & Schinka, J. A. (2000). A taxometric analysis of MMPI-2 infrequency scales [F and F(p)] in clinical settings. *Psychological Assessment, 12*, 166–173.

Strong, E. K., Jr. (1927). *Vocational Interest Blank (Form A)*. Stanford, CA: Stanford University Press.

Strong, E. K., Jr. (1943). *Vocational interests of men and women*. Stanford, CA: Stanford University Press.

Strong, E. K., Jr. (1959). *Strong Vocational Interest Blank*. Palo Alto, CA: Consulting Psychologists Press.

Sullivan, H. S. (1936). A note on the implications of psychiatry, the study of interpersonal relations, for investigations in the social sciences. *American Journal of Sociology, 42*, 848–861.

Sullivan, H. S. (1940). Conceptions of modern psychiatry: The first William Alanson White Memorial Lectures. *Psychiatry, 3*, 1–117.

Sullivan, H. S. (1948a). The meaning of anxiety in psychiatry and in life. *Psychiatry, 11*, 1–13.

Sullivan, H. S. (1948b). Ruth Fulton Benedict, Ph.D., D.Sc. 1887–1948. *Psychiatry, 11*, 5–6.

Sullivan, H. S. (1949). Multidisciplined coordination of interpersonal data. In S. S. Sargent & M. W. Smith (Eds.), *Culture and personality* (pp. 175–194). New York: Viking Fund.

Sullivan, H. S. (1950). The illusion of personal individuality. In H. S. Sullivan, *The fusion of psychiatry and social science* (pp. 198–226). New York: Norton, 1964.

Sullivan, H. S. (1953a). *Conceptions of modern psychiatry*. New York: Norton.

Sullivan, H. S. (1953b). *The interpersonal theory of psychiatry*. New York: Norton.

Sullivan, H. S. (1954). *The psychiatric interview*. New York: Norton.

Sullivan, H. S. (1956). *Clinical studies in psychiatry*. New York: Norton.

Szasz, T. (1961). *The myth of mental illness*. New York: Hoeber–Harper.

Tellegen, A., & Ben-Porath, Y. S. (1992). The new uniform T-scores for the MMPI-2: Rationale, derivation, and appraisal. *Psychological Assessment, 4*, 145–155.

Thompson, C. (1964). *Interpersonal psychoanalysis: The selected papers of Clara M. Thompson* (M. Green, Ed.). New York: Basic Books.

Thurstone, L. L. (1934). The vectors of mind. *Psychological Review, 41*, 1–32.

Tomkins, S. S. (1947). *The Thematic Apperception Test*. New York: Grune & Stratton.

Tomkins, S. S. (1979). Script theory: Differential magnification of affects. In H. E. Howe, Jr., & R. A. Dienstbier (Eds.), *Nebraska Symposium on Motivation* (Vol. 26, pp. 201–236). Lincoln: University of Nebraska Press.

Tracey, T. J. G., & Rounds, J. B. (1997). Circular structure of vocational interests. In R. Plutchik & H. R. Conte (Eds.), *Circumplex models of personality and emotions* (pp. 183–201). Washington, DC: American Psychological Association.

Trapnell, P. D., & Wiggins, J. S. (1990). The extension of the Interpersonal Adjective Scales to include the Big Five dimensions of personality. *Journal of Personality and Social Psychology, 59*, 781–790.

Triandis, H. C. (1990). Cross-cultural studies of individualism and collectivism. In J. J. Berman (Ed.), *Nebraska Symposium on Motivation: Vol. 37. Cross-cultural perspectives* (pp. 41–133). Lincoln: University of Nebraska Press.

Trilling, L. (1950). *The liberal imagination*. Garden City, NY: Doubleday & Co.

Trilling, L., & Marcus, S. (Eds.). (1961). *The life and work of Sigmund Freud*. New York: Basic Books.

Trobst, K. K. (1999). Social support as an interpersonal construct. *European Journal of Psychological Assessment, 15*, 246–255.

Trobst, K. K. (2000). An interpersonal conceptualization and quantification of social support transactions. *Personality and Social Psychology Bulletin, 26*, 971–986.

Trobst, K. K., & Hemphill, K. J. (2000). *Raising questions regarding social support processes: Provisional answers from an interpersonal analysis of chronic fatigue syndrome patients and their providers*. Unpublished manuscript, York University, Toronto.

Trull, T. J., Widiger, T. A., & Guthrie, P. (1990). Categorical versus dimensional status of borderline personality disorder. *Journal of Abnormal Psychology, 99*, 40–48.

Tupes, E. C., & Christal, R. E. (1958). *Stability of personality trait rating factors obtained under diverse conditions* (USAF WADC Technical Note No. 58–61). Lackland Air Force Base, TX: U.S. Air Force.

Tupes, E. C., & Christal, R. E. (1961). *Recurrent personality factors based on trait ratings* (USAF ASD Tech. Rep. No. 61–97). Lackland Air Force Base, TX: U.S. Air Force.

Vernon, P. E. (1950). *The structure of human abilities*. London: Methuen.

Viglione, D. J., Jr. (1993). A review of Beck's *The Rorschach experiment: Ventures in blind diagnosis. Journal of Personality Assessment, 61*, 406–413.

Walker, C. E. (1980). The effect of eliminating offensive items on the reliability and validity of the MMPI. In W. G. Dahlstrom & L. Dahlstrom (Eds.), *Basic readings on the MMPI: A new selection on personality measurement* (pp. 380–385). Minneapolis: University of Minnesota Press.

Waller, N. G., & Meehl, P. E. (1998). *Multivariate taxometric procedures: Distinguishing types from continua*. Thousand Oaks, CA: Sage.

Waller, N. G., Putnam, F. W., & Carlson, E. (1996). Types of dissociation and dissociative types: A taxometric analysis of the Dissociative Experiences Scale. *Psychological Methods, 3*, 300–321.

Webster, R. (1997, May 16). The bewildered visionary. *Times Literary Supplement*.

Wechsler, D. (1939). *The measurement of adult intelligence.* Baltimore: Williams & Wilkins.

Wechsler, D. (1941). *The measurement of adult intelligence* (2nd ed.). Baltimore: Williams & Wilkins.

Wechsler, D. (1958). *The measurement and appraisal of adult intelligence* (4th ed.). Baltimore: Williams & Wilkins.

Weed, N. C., Butcher, J. N., McKenna, T., & Ben-Porath, Y. S. (1992). New measures for assessing alcohol and drug abuse with the MMPI-2: The *APS* and *AAS. Journal of Personality Assessment, 58,* 389–404.

Weiner, I. B. (1994). The Rorschach Inkblot Method (RIM) is not a test: Implications for theory and practice. *Journal of Personality Assessment, 62,* 498–504.

Weiner, I. B. (1995). Variable selection in Rorschach research. In J. E. Exner, Jr. (Ed.), *Issues and methods in Rorschach research* (pp. 73–98). Mahwah, NJ: Erlbaum.

Weiner, I. B. (1996). Some observations on the validity of the Rorschach inkblot method. *Psychological Assessment, 8,* 206–213.

Weiner, I. B. (1997). Current status of the Rorschach inkblot method. *Journal of Personality Assessment, 68,* 5–19.

Weiner, I. B. (1999). What the Rorschach can do for you: Incremental validity in clinical applications. *Assessment, 6,* 327–338.

Weiner, I. B. (2000a). Making Rorschach interpretation as good as it can be. *Journal of Personality Assessment, 74,* 164–174.

Weiner, I. B. (2000b). Using the Rorschach properly in practice and research. *Journal of Clinical Psychology, 56,* 435–438.

Wellek, R., & Warren, A. (1963). *Theory of literature* (3rd ed.). London: Harmondsworth.

Welsh, G. S. (1948). An extension of Hathaway's MMPI profile coding system. *Journal of Consulting Psychology, 12,* 343–344.

Welsh, G. S. (1956). Factor dimensions A and R. In G. S. Welsh & W. G. Dahlstrom (Eds.), *Basic readings on the MMPI in psychology and medicine* (pp. 264–281). Minneapolis: University of Minnesota Press.

Welsh, G. S., & Dahlstrom, W. G. (Eds.). (1956). *Basic readings on the MMPI in psychology and medicine.* Minneapolis: University of Minnesota Press.

Welsh, G. S., & Dahlstrom, W. G. (Eds.)(1980). *Basic readings on the MMPI in psychology and medicine: A new selection on personality measurement.* Minneapolis: University of Minnesota Press.

Wertheimer, M. (1912). Experimentelle Studien uber das Sehen von Bewegung. *Zeitschrift für Psychologie, 61,* 161–265.

West, S. G., & Graziano, W. G. (Eds.). (1989). Long-term stability and change in personality [Special issue]. *Journal of Personality, 57,* 175–245.

Westen, D. (1990). Psychoanalytic approaches to personality. In L. Pervin (Ed.), *Handbook of personality: Theory and research* (pp. 21–65). New York: Guilford Press.

Westen, D. (1991). Clinical assessment of object relations using the TAT. *Journal of Personality Assessment, 56,* 56–74.

Westen, D. (1998). The scientific legacy of Sigmund Freud: Toward a psychodynamically informed psychological science. *Psycholological Bulletin, 124,* 333–371.

Wheeler, W. M., Little, K. B., & Lehner, G. F. J. (1951). The internal structure of the MMPI. *Journal of Consulting Psychology, 15,* 134–141.

Whipple, G. M. (1910). *Manual of mental tests and physical tests.* Baltimore: Warwick & York.

White, R. W. (1943). The personality of Joseph Kidd. *Character and Personality, 11,* 183–208.

White, R. W. (1952). *Lives in progress.* New York: Holt, Rinehart & Winston.

White, R. W. (1963a). Ego and reality in psychoanalytic theory. *Psychological Issues, 3*(3, Monograph No. 11).

White, R. W. (1963b). Sense of interpersonal competence: Two case studies and some reflections on origins. In R. W. White (Ed.), *The study of lives: Essays on personality in honor of Henry A. Murray* (pp. 73–93). New York: Atherton Press.

White, R. W. (Ed.). (1963c). *The study of lives: Essays on personality in honor of Henry A. Murray.* New York: Atherton Press.

White, R. W. (1966). *Lives in progress* (2nd ed.). New York: Holt, Rinehart & Winston.

White, R. W. (1975). *Lives in progress* (3rd ed.). New York: Holt, Rinehart & Winston.

White, R. W. (1981). Exploring personality the long way: The study of lives. In A. I. Rabin, J. Arnoff, A. M. Barclay, & R. A. Zucker (Eds.), *Further explorations in personality* (pp. 3–19). New York: Wiley.

White, W. A. (1922). *Outline of psychiatry.* New York: Nervous and Mental Disease Publishing.

Widiger, T. A. (1991). Personality disorder dimensional models proposed for DSM-IV. *Journal of Personality Disorders, 5,* 386–398.

Widiger, T. A. (2001). The best and the worst of us? *Clinical Psychology: Science and Practice, 8,* 374–377.

Widiger, T. A., & Frances, A. J. (1985). The DSM-III personality disorders: Perspectives from psychology. *Archives of General Psychiatry, 42,* 615–623.

Widiger, T. A., & Frances, A. J. (1994). Toward a dimensional model for the personality disorders. In P. T. Costa, Jr., & T. A. Widiger (Eds.), *Personality disorders and the five-factor model of personality* (pp. 19–39). Washington, DC: American Psychological Association.

Widiger, T. A., & Saylor, K. I. (1998). Personality assessment. In A. Bellack & M. Hersen (Series Eds.) & N. R. Schooler (Vol. Ed.), *Comprehensive clinical psychology* (Vol. 3, pp. 145–167). New York: Pergamon Press.

Widiger, T. A., Trull, T. J., Clarkin, J. F. , Sanderson, C. & Costa, P. T., Jr. (1994). A description of the DSM-III-R and DSM-IV personality disorders with the five-factor model of personality. In P. T. Costa, Jr. & T. A. Widiger (Eds.), *Personality disorders and the five-factor model of personality* (pp. 41–56). Washington, DC: American Psychological Association.

Widiger, T. A., Trull, T. J., Clarkin, J. F. , Sanderson, C. & Costa, P. T., Jr. (2002). A description of the DSM-III-R and DSM-IV personality disorders with the five-factor model of personality. In P. T. Costa, Jr. & T. A. Widiger (Eds.), *Personality disorders and the five-factor model of personality* (2nd ed., pp. 89–99). Washington, DC: American Psychological Association.

Wiener, D. N., & Harmon, L. R. (1946). *Subtle and obvious keys for the MMPI: Their development* (Advisement Bulletin No. 16). Minneapolis, MN: Regional Veterans Administrative Office.

Wiggins, J. S. (1959). Interrelationships among MMPI measures of dissimulation under standard and social desirability instructions. *Journal of Consulting Psychology, 23,* 419–427.

Wiggins, J. S. (1962). Strategic, method, and stylistic variance in the MMPI. *Psychological Bulletin, 59,* 224–242.

Wiggins, J. S. (1964). Convergences among stylistic response measures from objective personality tests. *Educational and Psychological Measurement, 24,* 551–562.

Wiggins, J. S. (1966). Substantive dimensions of self-report in the MMPI item pool. *Psychological Monographs, 80*(22, Whole No. 630).

Wiggins, J. S. (1968). Personality structure. *Annual Review of Psychology, 19,* 293–350.

Wiggins, J. S. (1973a). Despair and optimism in Minneapolis [Review of J. N. Butcher (Ed.), *Objective personality assessment: Changing perspectives*]. *Contemporary Psychology, 18,* 605–606.

Wiggins, J. S. (1973b). *Personality and prediction: Principles of personality assessment.* Malabar, FL: Krieger, 1988.

Wiggins, J. S. (1979). A psychological taxonomy of trait descriptive terms: The interpersonal domain. *Journal of Personality and Social Psychology, 37,* 395–412.

Wiggins, J. S. (1980a). Circumplex models of interpersonal behavior. In L. Wheeler (Ed.), *Review of personality and social psychology* (Vol. 1, pp. 265–294). Beverly Hills, CA: Sage.

Wiggins, J. S. (1980b). Content dimensions in the MMPI. In W. G. Dahlstrom & L. Dahlstrom (Eds.), *Basic readings on the MMPI: A new selection on personality measurement* (pp. 300–327). Minneapolis: University of Minnesota Press.

Wiggins, J. S. (1982). Circumplex models of interpersonal behavior in clinical psychology. In P.

C. Kendall & J. N. Butcher (Eds.), *Handbook of research methods in clinical psychology* (pp. 183–221). New York: Wiley.

Wiggins, J. S. (1985). Symposium: Interpersonal circumplex models: 1949–1983 [Commentary]. *Journal of Personality Assessment, 49,* 626–631.

Wiggins, J. S. (1989). Personality Research Form. In J.V. Mitchell (Ed.), *The tenth mental measurements yearbook* (pp. 633–634). Lincoln: University of Nebraska Press.

Wiggins, J. S. (1990). Foreword. In J. N. Butcher, J. R. Graham, C. L. Williams, & Y. Ben-Porath, *Development and use of the MMPI-2 content scales* (pp. vii–ix). Minneapolis: University of Minnesota Press.

Wiggins, J. S. (1991). Agency and communion as conceptual coordinates for the understanding and measurement of interpersonal behavior. In W. Grove & D. Cicchetti (Eds.), *Thinking clearly about psychology: Essays in honor of Paul E. Meehl* (Vol. 2, pp. 89–113). Minneapolis: University of Minnesota Press.

Wiggins, J. S. (1995). *Interpersonal Adjective Scales: Professional manual.* Odessa, FL: Psychological Assessment Resources.

Wiggins, J. S. (Ed.). (1996a). *The five-factor model of personality: Theoretical perspectives.* New York: Guilford Press.

Wiggins, J. S. (1996b). An informal history of the interpersonal circumplex tradition. *Journal of Personality Assessment, 66,* 217–233.

Wiggins, J. S. (1996c). Preface. In J. S. Wiggins (Ed.), *The five-factor model of personality: Theoretical perspectives* (pp. vii–xi). New York: Guilford Press.

Wiggins, J. S. (1997). Circumnavigating Dodge Morgan's interpersonal style. *Journal of Personality, 65,* 1069–1086.

Wiggins, J. S., & Broughton, R. (1985). The interpersonal circle: A structural model for the integration of personality research. In R. Hogan & W. H. Jones (Eds.), *Perspectives in personality* (Vol. 1, pp. 1–48). Greenwich, CT: JAI Press.

Wiggins, J. S., & Broughton, R. (1991). A geometric taxonomy of personality scales. *European Journal of Personality, 5,* 343–365.

Wiggins, J. S., Phillips, N., & Trapnell, P. (1989). Circular reasoning about interpersonal behavior: Evidence concerning some untested assumptions underlying diagnostic classification. *Journal of Personality and Social Psychology, 56,* 296–305.

Wiggins, J. S., & Pincus, A. L. (1989). Conceptions of personality disorders and dimensions of personality. *Psychological Assessment, 1,* 305–316.

Wiggins, J. S., & Pincus, A. L. (1992). Personality: Structure and assessment. *Annual Review of Psychology, 43,* 473–504.

Wiggins, J. S., & Pincus, A. L. (1994). Personality structure and the structure of personality disorders. In P. T. Costa, Jr., & T. A. Widiger (Eds.), *Personality disorders and the five-factor model of personality* (pp. 73–93). Washington DC: American Psychological Association.

Wiggins, J. S., Renner, K. E., Clore, G. L., & Rose, R. J. (1971). *The psychology of personality.* Reading, MA: Addison-Wesley.

Wiggins, J. S., Steiger, J. H., & Gaelick, L. (1981). Evaluating circumplexity in personality data. *Multivariate Behavioral Research, 16,* 263–289.

Wiggins, J. S., & Trapnell, P. D. (1996). A dyadic-interactional perspective on the five-factor model. In J. S. Wiggins (Ed.), *The five-factor model of personality: Theoretical perspectives* (pp. 88–162). New York: Guilford Press.

Wiggins, J. S., & Trapnell, P. D. (1997). Personality structure: The return of the Big Five. In R. Hogan, J. A. Johnson, & S. R. Briggs (Eds.), *Handbook of personality psychology* (pp. 737–765). San Diego, CA: Academic Press.

Wiggins, J. S., & Trobst, K. K. (1997a). Prospects for the assessment of normal and abnormal interpersonal behavior. In J. A. Schinka & R. L. Greene (Eds.), *Emerging issues and methods in personality assessment* (pp. 113–129). Mahwah, NJ: Erlbaum.

Wiggins, J. S., & Trobst, K. K. (1997b). When is a circumplex an "interpersonal circumplex"?: The case of supportive actions. In R. Plutchik & H. R. Conte (Eds.), *Circumplex models of personality and emotions* (pp. 57–80). Washington, DC: American Psychological Association.

Wiggins, J. S., & Trobst, K. K. (1999). The fields of interpersonal behavior. In L. A. Pervin & O. P. John (Eds.), *Handbook of personality: Theory and research* (2nd ed., pp. 653–670). New York: Guilford Press.

Wiggins, J. S., & Vollmar, J. (1959). The content of the MMPI. *Journal of Clinical Psychology, 15*, 45–47.

Wilde, O. (1887). The critic as artist. In *The complete works of Oscar Wilde* (pp. 948–998). Leicester, England: Blitz, 1990.

Williams, C. L., Butcher, J. N., Ben-Porath, Y. S., & Graham, J. R. (1992). *MMPI-A content scales: Assessing psychopathology in adolescents.* Minneapolis: University of Minnesota Press.

Winnicott, D. W. (1965). *The maturational process and the facilitating environment.* New York: International Universities Press.

Winter, D. G. (1973). *The power motive.* New York: Free Press.

Winter, D. G. (1993). Gordon Allport and *Letters from Jenny.* In K. H. Craik, R. Hogan, & R. N. Wolfe (Eds.), *Fifty years of personality psychology* (pp. 147–163). New York: Plenum Press.

Winter, D. G., & Barenbaum, N. B. (1999). History of modern personality theory and research. In L. A. Pervin & O. P. John (Eds.), *Handbook of personality: Theory and research* (2nd ed., pp. 3–27). New York: Guilford Press.

Wittenborn, J. R. (1949). Rorschach. In O. K. Buros (Ed.), *Personality tests and reviews* (pp. 394–395). Highland Park, NJ: Gryphon Press, 1970.

Wittgenstein, L. (1958). *The blue and brown books.* New York: Harper Torchbooks.

Wolfe, T. (1969). *The electric Kool-Aid acid test.* New York: Bantam Books.

Wood, J. M., & Lilienfeld, S. W. (1999). The Rorschach Inkblot Test: A case of overstatement? *Assessment, 6*, 341–351.

Wood, J. M., Lilienfeld, S. O., Garb, H. N., & Nezworski, M. T. (2000). The Rorschach test in clinical diagnosis: A critical review, with a backward look at Garfield (1947). *Journal of Clinical Psychology, 56*, 395–430.

Wood, J. M., Nezworski, M. T., Garb, H. N., & Lilienfeld, S. O. (2001). The misperception of psychopathology: Problems with the norms of the Comprehensive System for the Rorschach. *Clinical Psychology: Science and Practice, 8*, 397–402.

Wood, J. M., Nezworski, M. T., & Stejskal, W. J. (1997). The Comprehensive System for the Rorschach: A comment on Meyer (1997). *Psychological Assessment, 9*, 490–494.

Wood, J. M., Nezworski, M. T., Stejskal, W. J., & Garven, S. (2001). Advancing scientific discourse in the controversy surrounding the Comprehensive System for the Rorschach: A rejoinder to Meyer (2000). *Journal of Personality Assessment, 76*, 369–378.

Wood, J. M., Nezworski, M. T., Stejskal, W. J., Garven, S., & West, S. G. (1999). Methodological issues in evaluating Rorschach validity: A comment on Burns and Viglione (1996), Weiner (1996) and Ganellen (1996). *Assessment, 6*, 115–120.

Woodworth, R. S. (1917). *Personal Data Sheet.* Chicago: Stoelting.

Zubin, J. (1967). Classification of behavior disorders. *Annual Review of Psychology, 28*, 373–406.

Index

Page numbers followed by *f* indicate figure; *t*, table

379